Perfection's Therapy

Perfection's Therapy

An Essay on Albrecht Dürer's Melencolia I

Mitchell B. Merback

ZONE BOOKS · NEW YORK

2017

© 2017 Mitchell B. Merback

ZONE BOOKS
633 Vanderbilt Street
Brooklyn, NY 11218

Printed in the United States of America.

Distributed by The MIT Press,
Cambridge, Massachusetts, and London, England

Library of Congress Cataloging-in-Publication Data
Names: Merback, Mitchell B., author.
Title: Perfection's therapy : An Essay on Albrecht Dürer's
    Melencolia I / Mitchell B. Merback.
Description: New York : Zone Books, 2017. | Includes
    bibliographical references and index.
Identifiers: LCCN 2017013718 | ISBN 9781942130000 (hardcover)
Subjects: LCSH: Dürer, Albrecht, 1471–1528. Melencolia I. |
    Dürer, Albrecht, 1471–1528 — Criticism and interpretation. |
    Dürer, Albrecht, 1471–1528 — Psychology. | Personality
    and creative ability.
Classification: LCC NE654.D9 A673 2017 | DDC 759.3 — dc23
LC record available at https://lccn.loc.gov/2017013718

To my teachers

Contents

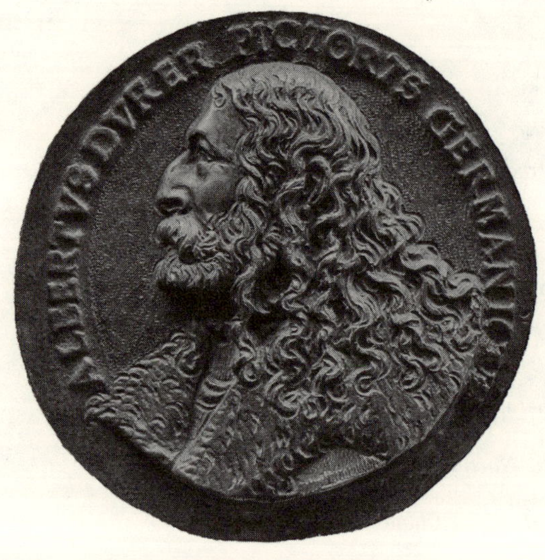

Figure I.1. Hans Schwarz, portrait medallion of Albrecht Dürer, 1519–20, bronze, 5.6 cm dia. (Hannover, Kestner-Museum).

Introduction

It may be difficult . . . for many of us, to abandon the belief that there is an instinct toward perfection at work in human beings, which has brought them to their present high level of intellectual achievement and ethical sublimation and which may be expected to watch over their development into supermen. I have no faith, however, in the existence of any such internal instinct and I cannot see how this benevolent illusion is to be preserved. . . . What appears in a minority of human individuals as an untiring impulsion towards perfection can easily be understood as a result of the instinctual repression upon which is based all that is most precious in human civilization.
—Sigmund Freud, *Beyond the Pleasure Principle*

"Just as Miserable as Ever"
Imagine an exclusive television interview with one of the luminaries of the European Renaissance—a Petrarch, a Pico della Mirandola, an Alberti, an Erasmus, or the subject of this book, Albrecht Dürer of Nuremberg (figure I.1)—and consider asking him how it felt to wake up on the threshold of modernity, to be alive amidst such a great flowering of civilization, to emerge into light after such a long dark. What was it like to participate in the revival of classical thought, literature, science, and the fine arts, you might ask, to free the project of human perfectibility from its theological burdens, to exalt human dignity, and bring it to its realization? How glorious was it to experience every day reason's brilliant ascendance, the mastery of *geometria, eruditio,* and *eloquentia,* and the arts based upon them? Now that the spell of primitive superstition had been broken, the tyrannous fear of demons and pagan gods overcome, and a rational knowledge of the world embraced, what great happiness had settled upon humanity? If you, starry-eyed as I would be to share in such great company,

were to inquire, simply, "What was it like to *experience* all this?" it's a fair bet each man would reply as the proverbial Zen monk did after the news spread that he, a relative novice, had become enlightened. "Is it true?" the other novices reportedly asked, gathering around. "It is true," he told them, radiating serenity in the eyes of witnesses. "And how does it feel to be enlightened?" they all inquired. "I'll tell you," the monk replied, "just as miserable as ever."[1]

Now this amusing little Zen kōan, so rich with paradox, conveys an unmistakably Buddhist attitude toward human perfectibility, the nature of wisdom, the cosmic necessity of suffering (*dukkha*), and the close interrelationship of the three. At the same time, it's not hard to find parallels between the tale's resigned awareness of the divided, earthbound reality we all endure and a distinctly European-Christian style of misery whose first flourishing was the Renaissance. Generalizations about collective mentalities and psychological dispositions in history are inherently fraught and risky, the interpretation of emotions and cultural "moods" all the more so, and though our leading lights of the Renaissance would have been familiar with the metaphors of rebirth and revival, darkness and light, with which we still celebrate their modernity, it would be unfair to expect them to picture their own age as a closed historical whole or to portray their own suffering in crisp contours and accurate colors.

Nevertheless, Renaissance misery does have a peculiar character we can identify, and doing so is the crucial first step, I submit, toward a fresh understanding of one of the most talked-about pictures in the European canon, a portrait of creative endeavor poised between inspired breakthrough and demoralizing breakdown: Albrecht Dürer's shimmering allegory of 1514, the engraving called *Melencolia I* (see figure 1.1). Referring to the print's technical perfection, one of its earliest commentators, the Florentine biographer and artist Giorgio Vasari (1511–74), called it a work that puts the whole world in awe—*che feciono stupire il mondo*—and more than four hundred years of ardent acclaim and zealous interpretation has only etched that judgment deeper.[2] The awesomeness of that achievement, however, stems from a certain kind of misery the work is also at pains to diagnose and symbolize—a misery itself borne of the pursuit of perfection.

Every age has its evils and miseries, its peculiar forms of fear, despair, and loss, its syndromes and psychic disturbances, its dark moods. Likewise, every age has its compensations and consolations in times of crisis—its methods for coping and its forms of escape, remedies for the ailing body and therapies for the suffering soul. Where do we look to a get a handle on *Renaissance* misery? What, if anything, makes it exceptional? Over the past several decades, social historians, literary historians, and art historians have filled in many details in our inherited picture of the extravagant misfortunes that befell Europe in the period stretching from the time of the Black Death (mid-fourteenth century) to the Wars of Religion (early sixteenth to mid-seventeenth centuries)—roughly coincident with what we call the Renaissance—and that picture is bleak indeed.[3] Warfare became more frequent and wars themselves more destructive, exposing both rural and urban populations to untold ravages and insecurities. A heightened state of conflict and public alarm settled on a Europe whose boundaries were steadily contracting after the failure of the Crusades, especially in the decades framed by the fall of Constantinople in 1453 and the siege of Vienna in 1529, when the Ottoman Turks menaced Christendom directly at Europe's eastern door. Peasant insurgents were on the move across the breadth of imperial South Germany, upending both temporal and spiritual governance and, under the sway of radical theologians, obliterating the distinctions between them. Unprecedented ecological breakdowns revealed the fragility of the human environment and the human body. Along with recurrences of pestilence and ancient diseases such as leprosy, "modern" ones such as syphilis appeared on the scene, stoking fears and challenging established medical opinion (figure I.2).[4] Most terrifying of all were the celestial portents of doom—comets and apparitions and prognostications of a "second flood," which reached a skittish public through the medium of print. Divine judgment was imminent, and total apocalyptic destruction seemed close at hand (figure I.3).[5] For what wrath was not deserved by a world so mired in sin and depravity, so overtaken by folly and ignorance, so forgetful of wisdom, so reprobate in the eyes of God? In the eyes of church reformers, the religion of the common folk had degenerated into a hysterical pursuit of the holy. Start-up pilgrimage cults appeared to authorities as false, materialistic rites that exposed God to ridicule and revealed the idolater lurking in the heart of every Christian. Everywhere the ceaseless labor of the Devil and his minions could be felt: in the insults and blasphemies hurled upon Christianity by

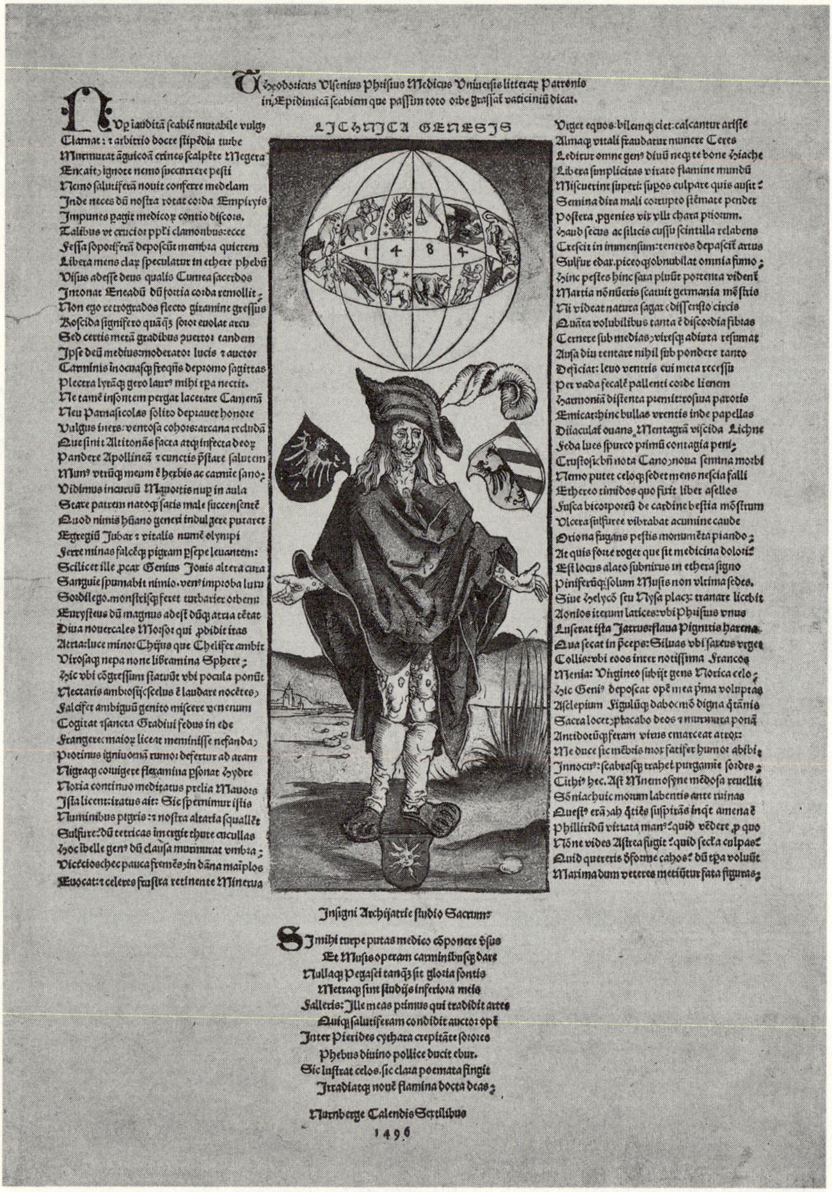

Figure I.2. Albrecht Dürer (attrib.), *Syphilitic Man*, hand-colored woodcut broadsheet, with didactic poem by Dirk van Ulsen, 1496, 2nd ed. (Ausburg: Johann Froschauer, 1496–97) (Berlin, Staatliche Museen, Kupferstichkabinett) (photo: bpk Bildagentur / Jörg P. Anders / Art Resource, NY).

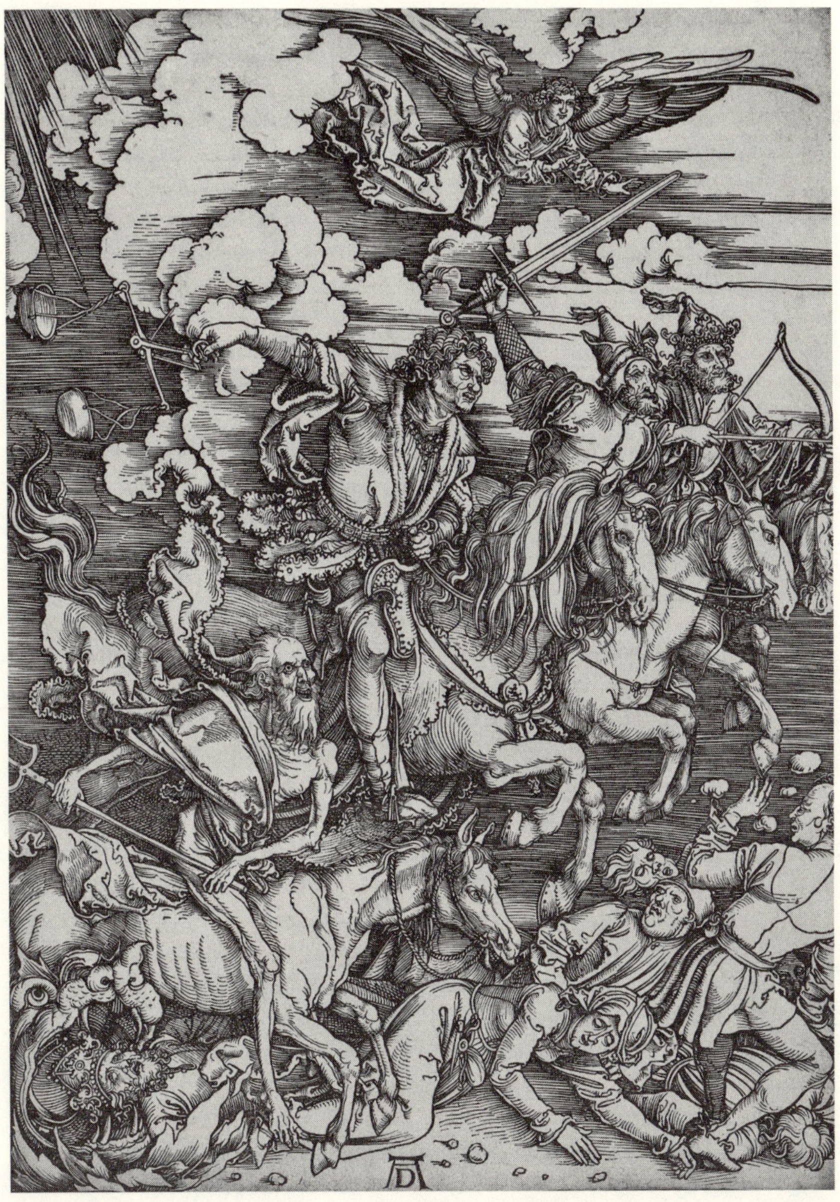

Figure I.3. Albrecht Dürer, *Four Horsemen*, woodcut from the *Apocalypse* series, ca. 1496–98, 45.7 x 31.5 cm (Washington, D.C., National Gallery of Art, Ferdinand Lammot Belin Fund and William Nelson Cromwell Fund).

heretics, by the depredation of "bloodthirsty" Jews and legions of sorcerers and witches—a pervasive domestic terrorism against which no one could defend.

To historians of the era, this is a familiar litany of woes—yet woefully comparable to the disasters and disarrays of any other preatomic age. What takes us aback in surveying the landscape of Renaissance misery, with its blending of objective plights and inner syndromes, worldly tribulations and religious sorrows, is the striking contrast it forms with the era's vigorous idealism: the dignity of man as created in the image and likeness of God; the intellectual liberation from scholasticism and—in much of Northern Europe—from the Roman Church as well; and the sustained belief in the human potential "to refashion [the] mind and will in accord with the noblest intellectual and moral values set forth in classical moral philosophy in harmony with the Christian doctrine of redemption."[6] In recognizing the radical disjunction between image and reality in the appraisal of the Renaissance, we are not unlike the very people who lived it; our own sense of contradiction has its counterpart, if not its mirror image, in the era's self-perception. Thinkers of the age truly felt the rub: aspiration toward dignity, order, eloquence, and virtue would always take place in a world overrun by perversity, indolence, error, and sin. Contemplation of this irony, the perpetual frustration of achievement, became one occasion for a uniquely European "philosophical" melancholy. The resulting complex forms an important backdrop for understanding Dürer's great engraving.

Melancholia, so closely related in the western tradition to *acedia*, or "spiritual sloth," and *tristia*, or "spiritual sadness," may be perfection's antithesis or its constant companion—centuries of philosophical, literary, medical, and psychological investigation have not provided a clear answer. For all the efforts to trace its genealogy backward from the *ennui* and *Weltschmerz* of Romanticism, or from the Kantian sublime, or from the revelatory "boredom" of the existentialists,[7] we still await a basic cultural history of frustrated exertion in the pursuit of perfection: technical perfection, moral perfection, aesthetic perfection.[8] One suspects such a history could explain a lot. Trying too hard, whether in the service of some ideal or simply as neurotic behavior, lies behind humankind's greatest achievements and its bitterest disappointments. In his *Pensées*, Blaise Pascal (1623–62) writes:

Men have a hidden instinct that prompts them to seek diversion and occupation from without, stemming from resentment at their unceasing misery. And they have another secret instinct remaining from the grandeur of the primary nature which makes them aware that happiness resides only in tranquility. And from those two contrary instincts is formed a confused plan hidden from sight at the bottom of their soul that leads them to reach for tranquility through agitation and always to imagine that the satisfaction they lack will come to them if, by surmounting certain obstacles they face, they can thus open the doors to peace and tranquility.[9]

And then there's the toll on health. Freud was probably right to doubt the instinctual basis for a compulsion toward perfection; if anything, it tends to be more trouble than it's worth for the ego, not to mention the body. Overtax the system, doctors since antiquity have been warning their patients, and disequilibrium sets in; push too hard, and you have total breakdown. For all the demands he made on his students, Dürer, himself an incurable aesthetic and technical perfectionist, was likewise at pains to alert the next generation to the pitfalls of overexertion. In his advice manual for the education of artists, *Ein Speis der Malerknaben* (Nourishment for young painters, ca. 1512–13), an unfinished treatise that survives only as a draft in the British Museum, he explains that during one's training, there is always the temptation to go beyond one's limits. But if the apprentice "exerts himself too much" (*zw fill vbte*) he might "fall under the hand of melancholy" (*do fan jm dÿ Melecoley vber hant mocht nemen*).[10]

Unless we count the letters boldly displayed upon the wings of *Melencolia*'s nocturnal messenger (see figure I.9), this passage, remarkably, is the only place in Dürer's surviving writings where he invoked the term "melancholy" (*Melecoley*). Should it surprise us that Dürer had trouble following his own advice? Whatever doubts he might have entertained about the possibility of perfection, it was the artist's obligation to strive for it. "Because we cannot altogether attain unto perfection, shall we therefore wholly cease from our learning?" Dürer the preceptor asks in his *Vier Bücher von menschlicher Proportionen* (Four books on human proportions); naturally, for him, the answer was foregone (he calls such doubts "fit for cattle").[11] Alongside the many virtues—excellence of character, physical beauty, preternatural skill with pen and brush, piety, morality—

celebrated by the painter's first biographer, Joachim Camerarius (1500–74), there was but one fault to ascribe to his famous friend. It was "his excessive industry, which often made unfair demands on him."[12]

Misery wrought by perfection was never merely a physical exhaustion, of course, and artists were hardly its most privileged victims. Those Renaissance thinkers who most vigorously advanced the cause of ethical education, spiritual self-knowledge, the dignity of humanity, and the rule of reason felt the "sickness of the soul" most acutely. It was the poet, philosopher, and humanist scholar Francesco Petrarca (1304–74) (figure I.4) who, more than any other, recast anew the problems raised by a ceaseless striving toward happiness in the face of adversity. When Petrarch's alter ego in the dialogue known as *De secreto conflictu curarum mearum* (On the Private Conflict of my Thoughts, better known as the *Secretum*) complains to his mentor, the philosopher Augustinus, about the failure of his meditations to help him overcome his sorrows or to cope with the blows delivered by Fortune, the feebleness of all his efforts are suddenly laid bare. Until the storm of the passions is calmed, Augustinus warns, until "that plague of phantasms which shatter and wreck your thoughts"[13] is dispersed, the ego will remain bound to the world, with tears and suffering its only companions. Submitting the passions to rational control is the archproject of the moral perfectibilist, according to John Passmore in his great book on the subject.[14] Afflicted by the insight that any and all successes in reaching for this mode of well-being—the "natural end" of *eudaimonia* toward which all humans strive, according to Aristotle—are destined to be provisional and immediately qualified, if not doomed to failure, Petrarch took up the project nonetheless.

In the deeply personal "inner discord" of his own mind that Petrarch tracked and examined, he also recognized humankind's historical plight. The march toward universal truth, the common project of prophets and saints, philosophers and poets, ancient and modern, had always been riddled with frustrations, setbacks, reversals, and wrong turns. Despite their brilliance and eloquence, the Roman authors Petrarch admired most—Virgil, Cicero, Seneca—had been ill-fated to live amidst pervasive error and gloom, unillumined by the advent of Christ. "But they failed to arrive at the destination they sought," the real Augustine (not Petrarch's Augustinus) once said of

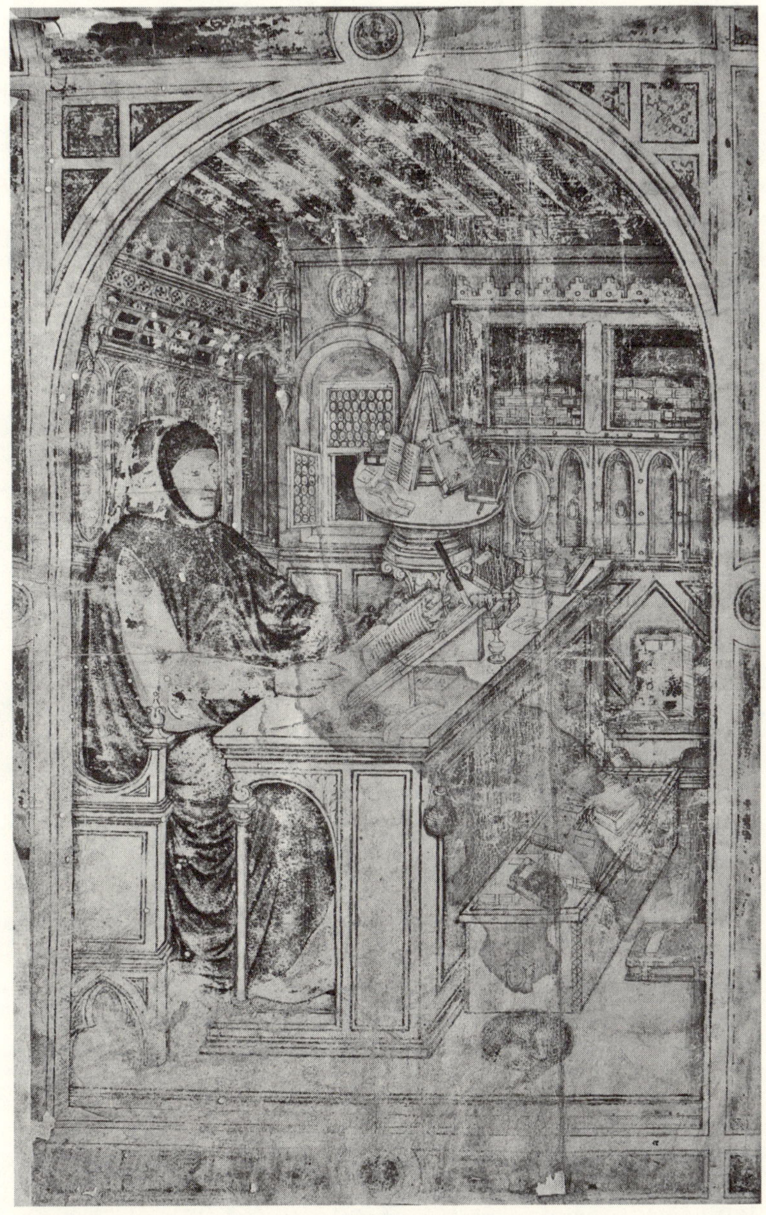

Figure I.4. Portrait of Petrarch in his studio, from Francesco Petrarca, *De viris illustribis*, ca. 1400 (Darmstadt, Hessische Landes- und Hochschulbibliothek, Hs. 101, fol. 1v).

the pagan poets (*City of God*, bk. 18) in a passage quoted by Petrarch, who shared the Church Father's conception of "history as a chronicle of human perversity that would perpetually frustrate the humanist aspirant."[15]

An earlier generation of historians dubbed Petrarch "the first modern man," both for the novel form of autonomous individuality he seemed to embody and for the bold line he drew between "ancient" and "modern" history. That gesture designated the long cultural epoch between the fall of Rome and Petrarch's own time as one of darkness (*tenebrae*) and rupture with the intellectual achievements of the past—a time of oblivion and loss, despite the Christian recognition that a "new light" had dawned in the era under grace.[16] More recent historians and literary critics have made the laureate an avatar of the postmodern self. "In Petrarch's poetry," writes Giuseppe Mazzotta, "time's ruptured dimensions (past, fleeting present, and expectation of future) are internalized within the self, and they are even identified as the constitutive, broken pieces of oneself."[17] Likewise for Gur Zak, Petrarch's poetic and philosophical program represents a sustained effort to "cope with the experience of fragmentation" and to recover the self, not as a "given presence" in the Romantic sense of authentic individualism, but as "a [virtuous] state of mind from which we are exiled."[18] Human excellence was deeply alienated from itself in his own age, Petrarch felt, a notion encapsulated in his famous complaint—recounted after his coronation as poet laureate, in a letter to the friar Giovanni Colonna in 1341—that contemporary Romans knew nothing about Rome or Roman virtue.[19]

So the pleasure of touching the optima of human experience, Petrarch sensed, is always accompanied by a painful apprehension of all that remains unachieved. Pain shadows pleasure in the very notion of perfection, which is always, to borrow from Frank Ankersmit, "the measure of its own success and of its own failure at one and the same time."[20] Though the prospects for perfection were "infinitesimally close" for the Renaissance humanist, they remained permanently out of reach, subject to a cruel fortune that no man could ever hope to master. Hope attaches itself to the future, as Petrarch wrote toward the end of the *Africa*, but should produce no illusions about the present. "My fate is to live amid varied and confusing storms. But ... [this] sleep of forgetfulness will not last forever. When the darkness has been dispersed, our descendants can come again in the former pure radiance."[21] Far more than the sorrows wrought by fortune itself, frustrated achievement in the present became, for the Renaissance humanist, a distinctive source of misery.

Remedies for Life

Now when Petrarch set about addressing the sorrows brought on by fortune, consoling himself and friends in the face of such ignorant and violent times, and providing for the miserable soul's remedy, he did not envision a cure so much as a down-to-earth regimen for ethical and spiritual training, a regimen grounded in reading and, for him, writing. Such a rhetorical therapy, aimed at restoring the soul to health through the prudent exercise of reason, was the goal of his great collection of 254 Latin dialogues, *De remediis utriusque fortunae* (On the Remedy of Two Kinds of Fortune), a work that earned lasting success as a popular "self-help book" into and beyond the Renaissance.[22] Building upon the vast tradition of medieval *speculum* literature as well as the wisdom of ancient Stoicism, *De remediis* was practical philosophy. Addressed to the tribulations of the inner man, its dialogues are not simply moral lessons, but exercises designed to mobilize the higher powers of the soul. Rhetoric had to be allied to philosophy in the care of the soul (*animi cura*), Petrarch understood, since their common aim was the cultivation of virtue and, through virtue, the correction of life and conduct (*vitam et mores*).[23] In transferring eloquence from the realm of moral philosophy and civic duty to the inward "care of the soul," Petrarch was largely following the lead of Seneca in his moral letters, where style and persuasion were meant to be transformative, awakening the listener's thoughts to the pursuit of virtue.[24] This effort was of a piece with Petrarch's effort to revive the ancient epistolary genre of *consolatio*, the consolation in times of grief and loss, and to innovate a philosophical therapy of the word, a tradition rooted in Socratic dialogue, Aristotelian rhetoric, and the Stoic training for life.

Petrarch's new mode of rhetorical healing announced in the *Secretum* and *De remediis* and the philosophy of life it advances will return as a key reference point later in this book, where I use it to take the measure of Dürer's therapeutic project.[25] Here we pause just long enough to register another of its key premises, that is, the

Aristotelian psychology it adopts for its model of a virtuous subjectivity. In the Hellenistic and Roman schools, all of which acknowledged a massive debt to Aristotle, philosophical training mobilized the higher powers of the mind—reason, will, and memory—in a way that would lead to the acquisition of *virtus*. Those powers allow the mind to combat effectively and eventually to overcome the pull of the lower, irrational faculties, or "passions," which bring the soul discord and confusion if left unchecked. For Petrarch, these irrational passions include not only fear and sorrow, our predictable emotional responses to misfortune (and not coincidentally, the key emotions targeted by tragedy, according to Aristotle in the *Poetics*), but also hope and joy, which are just as tightly bound to the experience of fortune. Only with a proper conversion to reason, a stoical inner training that would, in Pierre Hadot's words, culminate in a complete "metamorphosis of [the] personality,"[26] could the storm of the passions be calmed; only in this way could the swings of fortune, good and ill, be withstood. This was the Senecan ideal for self-care and the practice of wisdom, and it was one Petrarch recommended and sought to emulate. "I . . . request . . . O illustrious sir," the poet writes to a friend in one of his *Familiar Letters*, drawing on the classic Stoic precept of a "conversion to self" (*conversio ad se*), "that you subject your mind to your reason, or, to express it differently, you to yourself."[27] Inner virtue and intellectual discipline can be sustained only when reason reigns, when the passions are properly subdued, and when the way is cleared for the proper functioning of the higher faculties. For the scholar, the poet, and the artist—creative individuals prone to that particular disturbance of mind, body, and soul called melancholia—the stakes of "returning to oneself" were therefore even higher. Only from a state of equilibrium and calm could imagination and invention proceed; only in this way, according to eudaimonistic ethics, can humans flourish in the exercise of their natural abilities.

The revival of ancient Stoicism was such a powerful tendency in Renaissance thought that no less an authority than William Bouwsma could christen it, alongside Augustinianism, as one of the "two faces of Renaissance humanism."[28] Italian authors such as Petrarch and, following him, Northerners such as Sebastian Brant and Erasmus of Rotterdam (1466–1536) (figure I.5),[29] promoted the neo-Stoic view that reason, and the rational application of rules of the mind, would

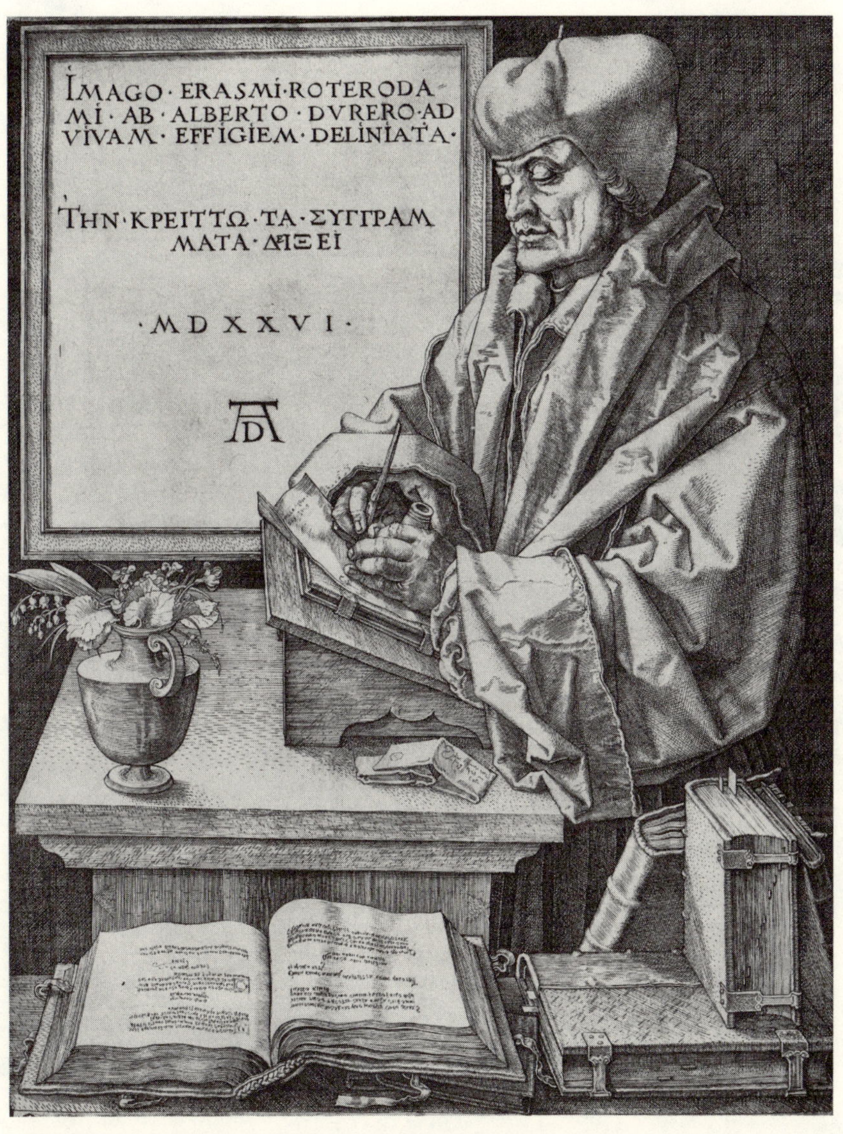

Figure I.5. Albrecht Dürer, *Erasmus of Rotterdam*, dated 1526, engraving, 25 x 18 cm, (Washington, D.C., National Gallery of Art, Rosenwald Collection).

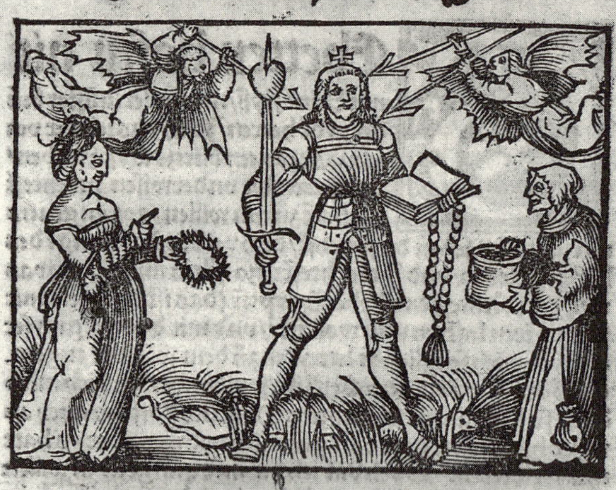

Figure I.6. Urs Graf, *The Christian Soldier between Virtue and Sin*, woodcut for Desiderius Erasmus, *Enchiridion, oder Handbüchleins eins christlichen und ritterlichen Lebens…* (Basel: Adam Petri, 1520), fol. xvi (photo: courtesy of Bibliothek Rotterdam, Erasmiana 2H22).

guide the soul toward perfection. Calming the passions had to be the first step. As a practical craft and therapy, philosophy meant forging rhetorical weapons to battle down the turbulent spirits that leave the mind vulnerable to attack. Only in this way can desires of the heart, among them the love of Christ and neighbor, find their proper order. Erasmus says as much in the conclusion to his widely read *Enchiridion milites Christiani* (Manual of a Christian Knight) (figure I.6), where he clarifies his purpose in writing about Christian virtue as a kind of inner training:

> This only was my desire . . . to show a certain manner and craft of a new kind of war, how one might arm oneself against the evils of the old life burgeoning forth again and springing afresh. Therefore, as we have done in one or two things [here in this treatise] so must you do . . . in everything, one by one: but most of all in the things wherein you perceive yourself to be stirred or instigated . . . whether it be through [the] vice of nature, custom, or evil upbringing. . . . [Against] these things some certain decrees must be written in the tablets of your mind, and they must be renewed now and then, lest they should fail or be forgotten through disuse, as against the vices of backbiting, filthy speaking, envy, guile, and other [such vices]: these are the only enemies of Christ's soldiers, against whose assault the mind must be armed long beforehand with prayer, with noble sayings of wise men, with the doctrine of Holy Scripture, with [the] example of devout and holy men, and specially [that] of Christ.[30]

It has been said that Erasmus spent the rest of his career as a reformer elaborating the principles set down in the *Enchiridion*. Vigilance in the face of ill-fortune, constant struggle against the forces of darkness, determination in the love of God and the practice of wisdom—these were the keys to fortifying and sustaining the Christian life. It was not hard for Dürer's greatest biographer and commentator, Erwin Panofsky (1892–1968), to detect a strong allegiance to Erasmian Christian philosophy in the earliest of the three so-called master engravings (*Meisterstiche*), the ominous *Knight, Death, and the Devil*, completed in 1513 (figure I.7).[31] Whereas Panofsky saw the luminous serenity of *St. Jerome in His Study* (see figure 2.1), completed in the same year as *Melencolia I*, as an allegory of the *vita contemplativa*, the steely determination of Dürer's famous knight, forging through the wasteland and heedless of the journey's dangers, seemed to embody the *vita activa*, outlined for all Christians by Erasmus in his little book of wisdom.

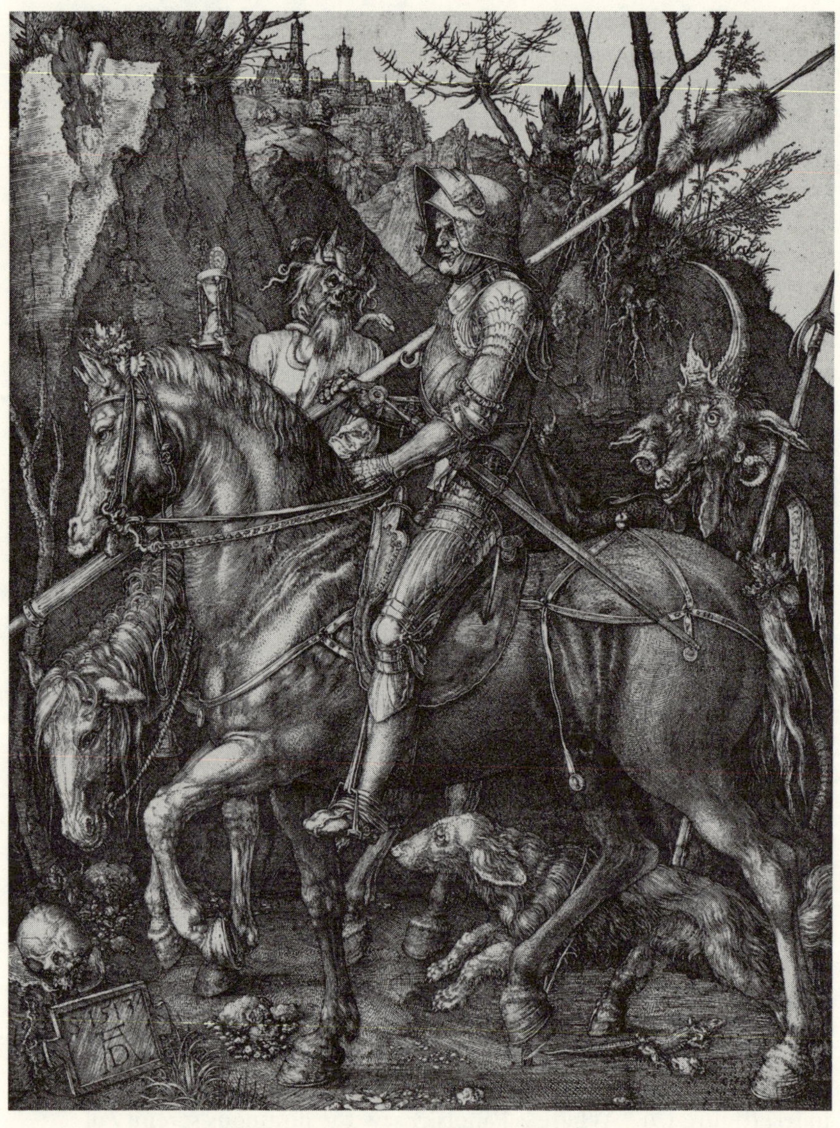

Figure I.7. Albrecht Dürer, *Knight, Death, and the Devil*, 1513, engraving on laid paper, 24.8 x 19 cm sheet (trimmed to plate mark) (Washington, D.C., National Gallery of Art. Gift of W. G. Russell Allen).

Melencolia I *and the Therapeutic Image*

Debate over whether the three *Meisterstiche*, Dürer's greatest achievements in the graphic arts, constitute a thematic program, an "iconographic trio" in which one informs the other(s), has been a constant feature in modern Dürer scholarship. For all the proposals and counterproposals, agreements and disagreements, few who have approached the problem, Panofsky included, have failed to appreciate the special difficulty of integrating *Melencolia* into any overarching allegorical scheme. *Saint Jerome* and *Knight, Death, and the Devil* more readily meet the requirement of being complementary opposites, respective expressions of Christian contemplativism and activism, as we just noted. Then again, it is not hard to see how *Melencolia* and *Saint Jerome* may team up to capture the polarities of creative thought: the gloomy disorientation that comes when secular learning reaches its limits, on the one hand, the radiant transcendence associated with divine wisdom, on the other.[32] None of the efforts to describe a programmatic unity among all three engravings, however, have yet proved persuasive. Nevertheless, the importance of the *Meisterstiche* as a group in Dürer's graphic oeuvre, and the signal moment their creation marks in his career, can hardly be overlooked.

Peter Parshall, one of Dürer's keenest observers, has recently drawn the *Meisterstiche* back into a coherent unity around Dürer's effort to come to terms with the vexing artistic and epistemological problem of imagination—its relation to mimesis, invention, verism, and certainty, and the dangers inherent in allowing it to wander beyond its proper bounds. These concerns play out in the different ways Dürer harnessed the descriptive technology of his medium to each of the three engravings' distinct themes. Whereas *Knight, Death, and the Devil*, in Parshall's words, "exploits the capacity of engraving to evoke hard and soft surfaces and to illustrate (as well as to exemplify) boundaries that cannot be transgressed," the *Saint Jerome* "captures the elusive, indeed unpicturable qualities of atmosphere, light, and temperature, allying these conditions with the ineffable movements of the mind."[33] Only *Melencolia*, a twilit scene whose luminary values seem to participate in both modes of pictorial description, without realizing either one of them fully, refuses accommodation to the conditions under which visual knowledge compels conviction about its sources; in other words, only in *Melencolia* does Dürer's representational practice seems to be less than up front about its motives. As we will see more fully in Chapter 2, structurally and optically, the engraving departs from the safe harbor of ordered perception and ventures into the dangerous depths of obscurity, confusion, and chaos—offering an experience of aesthetic and symbolic perplexity unknown elsewhere in Dürer's oeuvre. In Parshall's reading, the calculated sense of clutter yields "a space of mental and material disorientation, a circumstance in which hard facts resist assimilation and the possibility of spiritual transcendence is left profoundly in doubt."[34] This forces us to ask what kind of aesthetic value perplexity might be—what it might mean, in other words, for confusion and disorientation to be counted among the picture's resources and motives. We will consider the implications of this question more fully in the pages ahead.

Meanwhile, other features of the *Melencolia* distance it from nearly everything else in the artist's oeuvre, for instance, the presence of two light sources rather than one and, related to this, Dürer's conspicuously uncustomary use of direct lighting from the lower right side of the picture.[35] With its nocturnal messenger fluttering across the open sky, displaying the words "MELENCOLIA I" on outstretched wings (figure I.8), the image is also unique among the *Meisterstiche* in proclaiming its theme from within the pictured world—in fact, it is one of only two single-sheet graphic images to which Dürer ever affixed a title, the other being the large-format "Ercules" woodcut of ca. 1496 (see figure E.2). Further features that set *Melencolia* apart from the norms and conventions of Dürer's art, as well as from contemporary printmaking in general, will be encountered in the chapters that follow.

If Dürer's theoretical writings and artistic practice between 1512 and 1516—a period that in several respects marked the pinnacle of his career—are indeed characterized by a "suspicion" of imagination, as Parshall argues, and a strong reluctance to venture beyond the bounds of "plausible representation," the gambit he took in making a quasi-hallucinatory image such as *Melencolia* is all the more striking. The total atmosphere, with its weird airlessness and incantatory power, its surreal assemblage of unlike things, seems to evoke the kind of delusions to which physicians and churchmen thought morbid melancholics acutely susceptible. Luther called black bile, the humor responsible for melancholia, "the devil's bath" (*balneum diaboli*) for the way it poisoned the blood and lay the mind open to demonic interference, sinful fantasy, and carnal agitation.[36] Yet as we will see,

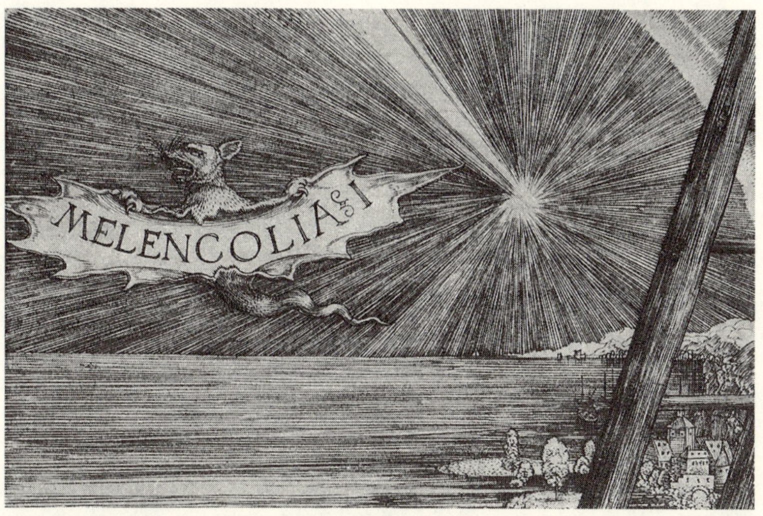

Figure I.8. Detail from Dürer, *Melencolia I*: bat with title on wings. (See figure 1.1 below.)

no single reading of the depressed mood of the scene—that it portrays Saturn's baleful influence, or diagnoses an unstable *duskrasia* in the organic systems of the body, or simulates a semidelusive state—satisfies; no single "explanation" knits together all the engraving's signs and symbols into a unified field of meaning. Chapter 1 considers the perpetual irresolution of efforts to discover something like a "Dürer Code" that would unlock this and other mysteries of the engraving.

Melencolia has been called the "image of images" for the enormous fascination it has exerted over its five hundred year history and for the heavy-duty knowledge production it continues to inspire among professional and amateur scholars, philosophers, humanists, scientists and mystics, code breakers and grail hunters of every stripe, and not least of all artists.[37] Barring the appearance of Dürer's ghost near the Tiergärtnertor, an unforeseen discovery in the Nuremberg archives or the Great Pyramids, to bring forth completely new information about *Melencolia* seems impossible today. However, this immanent crisis of interpretation is not without its own opportunities. Unlike previous projects of interpretation, we will not be bringing the engraving into relation with a particular text or testing alternative readings for competitive plausibility in order to deduce

Dürer's allegorical intentions. Throughout the book, I will be pursuing a different course, and this begins with the insistence that the "deep suspicion of the mind's operations" that Parshall convincingly attributes to Dürer's inventive processes and that may in fact constitute a central theme of the engraving should not be mistaken for, or transferred to, the *receptive* processes that his best work, the *Melencolia* perhaps above all, enables.

Those processes are by definition open-ended, and we will treat them as such. Although no text survives to document or prove Dürer's intentions to make the engraving function in a particular way, we will see in the first two chapters that the picture's visual order is marked by certain kind of aesthetic imperfection, a calculated retreat from harmony and order, a refusal of system, a structural incompleteness that gives the beholder's experience room for free play and growth. We will also see that this structural instability offers itself, in a sense, as the perfect visual counterpart to the "contradictoriness" of the engraving's symbolic program. On Hume's authority, Passmore has remarked that "some degree of aesthetic imperfection may be necessary if a thing is adequately to perform the task for which it was designed."[38] According to the theory put forward in this book, Dürer's print is singularly equipped to perform a particular task: to stimulate a certain kind of receptive process in the beholder. That process I will describe as therapeutic in nature—therapeutic in the Petrarchan sense, as a union of rhetoric and philosophy in the pursuit of virtue, and also in the "medical" sense, as a stimulant and balm for rebalancing the mind. Understood in these terms, *Melencolia*'s challenge to the beholder, we will see, takes on the quality of a cognitive exercise aimed at restoring and fostering health.

How Dürer leads us from the diagnosis of melancholia to its remediation will not be immediately obvious to longtime admirers of the engraving. In order to reach a clearer understanding of this therapy of the image, we will first have to show how the pictorial and allegorical programs Dürer deployed for *Melencolia* extended his understanding of the printed picture's capacity to serve as a focus for speculative thinking. This will be our work in Chapter 2: to show that it is by virtue of the engraving's perplexing visual structure and the artist's ingenious simulation of the delusive state associated with melancholia that the print could serve as a kind of a training ground for the natural human activity it mobilizes—speculation—and to which it offers free rein for the sake of rebalancing the mind. This activity is at once cognitive and emotional, spiritual and ethical, and is informed at its roots by ancient Stoicism's "attention to oneself" (προσοχή, *prosochē*), a "return to oneself" that counters the mind's vulnerability to fortune, its susceptibility to flux.

Those concerned with the care of souls in Dürer's time—poets and philosophers, physicians and pastors—understood the human person as a psychosomatic unity, and took health or illness to be a function of the "complexion" of substances and qualities encompassed by the individual. Dürer's attitudes in this regard seem to match those of the humanist elite with whom he was in close communication (Chapter 4), but may perhaps best be compared with those of Ulrich Pinder (d. 1519) from Nördlingen, who served Dürer's erstwhile patron, Duke Friedrich the Wise (1463–1525), as court physician before arriving in Nuremberg in 1493, where he soon came to be regarded as the city's *Achiatrus*, its chief medical doctor.[39] Alongside his medical practice, Pinder wrote and self-published several books of spiritual edification with titles such as *Beschlossen gart des rosenkrantz marie* (Enclosed garden of the rosary of the Virgin Mary) and *Speculum passionis* (Mirror of the Passion), several of them copiously illustrated with woodcuts by leading Nuremberg artists. For Pinder the Christian doctor, healing practices aimed at the body and the soul were necessarily imbricated, reflecting a belief that naturalistic medical remedies could affect the soul and, conversely, that spiritual medicine would benefit the body. Only by bridging them could the conditions necessary for ascending to a higher knowledge of God and eternal truths be met.[40] Dürer surely knew Pinder around the time he was at work on the *Melencolia*—whether personally or through common acquaintances such as Konrad Celtis is unclear—and would have shared his psychosomatic understanding of health and illness, as well as his belief in the need for multipronged therapeutic regimens. As we will see in Chapter 4, contemporary medical thought held melancholia to be a uniquely "contradictory" psychosomatic syndrome, one requiring a combination of therapies: pharmacological, psychological, philosophical, and, depending on the writer, magical as well.

Behind the very conception of *Melencolia*, I will argue, lies an imperative to mobilize precisely those mental faculties debilitated by an overheating of bile in the system—the most worrisome of the many clinical manifestations of the disease then known. Overcoming the pernicious "beclouding" effects of saturnine gloom, restoring the mind's equilibrium, and, with it, the health of the body, above all required moderate exercise, mental and physical. In providing such exercise, the print stands as a special and possibly unique remedy for a special malaise—Renaissance misery—and we will consider several kinds of evidence to show that Dürer, together with the intellectual aspirations he had for the print, conceived it as such.

To bring this possibility into historical focus, however, we must ask what our modern category, the therapeutic image, could have possibly meant to Dürer and his (mostly learned) sixteenth-century audience. Does such a notion deserve any kind of place in art history's lexicon of functional genres and image types? Chapter 3 takes up this problem in some detail, but here's a preview of what I think. In both its Greek origin and its Latin adaptation, the word "therapy" (θεραπεία, *therapeia*) encompasses notions of treatment, care, healing, and "attention." (The word *therapōn* [θεράπων] denotes an attendant.) Even a thumbnail etymology such as this reveals how vast a domain we will encounter when considering the therapeutic in the intertwined histories of healing and material making. European visual culture before the industrial era knew several long-standing therapies of the image. Art history has been aware of them, even if it has been unready to categorize them as such: the devotional image, which offered both emotional training and a kind of visual-sacramental therapy; the votive image, which functioned as a relay for securing the health of the body and the health of the soul through heavenly intercession and aid; the cult image, with its range of votive functions and an inherent, quasi-magical power of protection and cure; and the meditative image, the focal point for spiritual exercises of many kinds.

Within this rough taxonomy, I am proposing that we make room for a new conception of the *allegorical-speculative* image. This entails seeing the kind of cognitive-spiritual exercise that such an image makes possible not as a "stepping stone" to metaphysical truths beyond the sensible world, but as a practical and ethical therapy in this world, a remedy in the Petrarchan sense. Philosophy and rhetoric become allied in real time in the exercise of the mind, helping to move the soul of the spectator out of confusion and distress into clarification and health. This psychological movement toward well-being that the print's visual rhetoric encourages, the self-aware cognitive activity that it demands, spans the modern divide between psychological and somatic experience and is captured in a word with an equally complex pedigree: catharsis (κάθαρσις, *katharsis*).

In a daring conceit, Dürer has presented to the suffering soul a vital means for its restoration, a diagnosis it is the beholder's task to transform into medicine. That task, that labor, begins with an intensification of symptoms—brought on, we will see, by a certain structural disorder, an "impure harmony" offered to the beholder as a possible pathway, or itinerary (*ductus*), through the image.[41] What the engraving offers, I will argue, is not only an erudite portrayal of the peculiar misery that grips creative people, melancholia, but also an instrument for remedying it.

Each of the four chapters in the first part of this volume will furnish an essential building block for this argument. If I am successful in persuading the reader that a therapeutic impulse figures large in Dürer's conception of the print, we will not only have expanded our sense of what early modern works of art were empowered to do. We will also come to appreciate how the Christian-humanist artist could step into and transform a very "Petrarchan" role. Just as the poet, using eloquence and style as a means of awakening the rational soul to virtue, could claim the mantle of the *medicus animorum*, the physician of souls, so could the painter using the expressive means at his disposal. In the Renaissance rhetoric, poetry, painting, and medicine were each counted as an "art" (τέχνη, *technē*) with its own distinctive capacity for pleasing, persuading, and moving the subject. Rivalries and analogies between these arts formed an essential resource for educated humanists when evaluating the moral and aesthetic compatibility between the subject being addressed and the "style of speaking"—as a rhetorician such as Philip Melanchthon would put it—chosen for the address.[42]

Among the suffering subjects Dürer's medicinal art addressed was himself. Always prone to overwork; afflicted later in life with a "strange sickness" that sapped his energies; disturbed by dreams and premonitions; tested by the deaths of family members and friends; and acutely aware of his own mortality, Dürer's own miseries are well documented in word and image. So, too, are his varied auto-therapeutic responses to crisis and the slow advance of infirmity

(Chapter 5). More than any other work he produced, *Melencolia* may represent the culmination of the syndrome that caused Dürer, incapable as he was of following his own warnings about overexertion, the greatest of his own secular sorrows: the crisis of perfection. But this crisis, as is already clear, was hardly unique to him; it was, rather, a shared predicament. The sodality of creative men who considered Dürer the "Apelles of our age" (that is, the modern counterpart to the renowned ancient Greek painter) and whom Dürer called friends—an extended circle comprising scholars and poets, lawyers and scientists, churchmen and educators—stood in the same need of relief and restoration. So did the man who became Dürer's greatest patron during the middle third of his career, the German emperor and royal melancholic, Maximilian I (Epilogue). And so did his fellow Christians within and beyond the walls of his native Nuremberg. Addressing himself to the quality of their minds in the face of misery and misfortune, the artist presented himself as a healer trained by the experience of affliction. Behind the religious works examined in Chapter 6 is an ethos of care and a collaborative cultivation of virtue that recalls Petrarch's words to his friend Donato Albanzani in 1368, upon the death of his son: "so I succor and comfort you, dear friend, in what time there is, and to the best of my ability, and I comfort myself since we share everything: hopes, fears, joys, and grief. And so, as I have said, I combine our wounds in order to prepare the salves."[43] Like Petrarch, Dürer lived at the mercy of opposing forces, never achieving that "balance between the requirements of ancient humanism and of medieval religiosity," as Ernst Cassirer put it—never overcoming that "schism within his mind, that sickness of the soul."[44] Yet both men recognized, each in his own way, that the new art toward which they aimed their practice, and on which they staked their fame, would be born under the same sign as ancient philosophy and wisdom in both their pagan and Christian varieties: the injunction to care for the self, and to use one's gifts to call others to the same virtue.[45]

Figure 1.1. Albrecht Dürer, *Melencolia I*, dated 1514, engraving, 24.5 x 19.2 cm sheet (trimmed to plate mark) (Washington, D.C., National Gallery of Art, Rosenwald Collection).

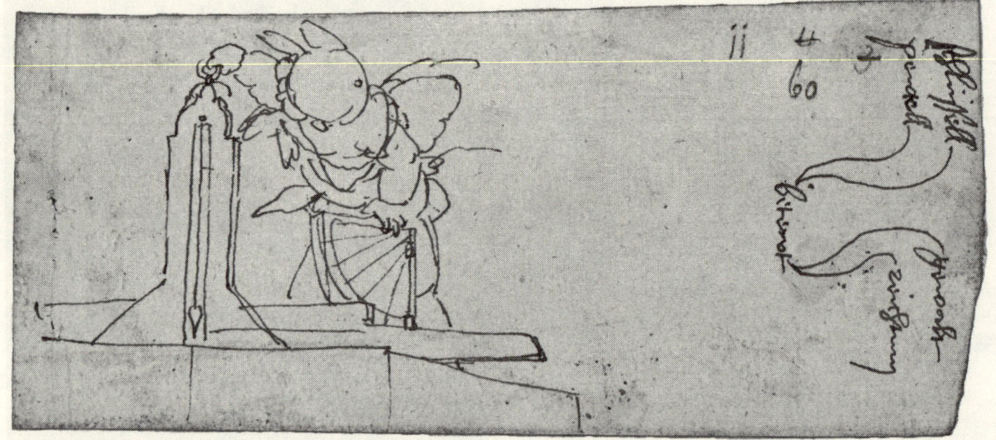

Figure 1.3. Albrecht Dürer, *Putto with Quadrant*, preparatory sketch for *Melencolia*, before 1514, pen and ink on paper (London, British Library, Add Ms. 5229, fol. 60r).

However we approach Dürer's engraving, whatever empirical or literary method we use to observe, catalogue, and describe its contents, we must cope with what the great German art historian Heinrich Wölfflin (1864–1945), over a century ago, called the "chaos of objects,"[2] a visual disorder that beguiles, perplexes, and perhaps even irritates the beholder, even as it charges and animates the gloom-filled space. That sense of a controlled chaos, pressing against the limits of optical and spatial coherence, imparts to the picture the quality of a *Vexierbild*, a puzzle picture, begging for a solution. But what could, what should such a solution consist of? Does each object contain or conceal a "meaning" we have only to identify correctly before the picture's ulterior purpose, its symbolic idea, can come into focus?

That Dürer possessed all the resources needed to craft a straightforward symbolic portrayal of melancholia is suggested by the notations he made on one of the handful of surviving preparatory studies for the engraving. The one shown here, now in the British Library, includes a winged putto with a quadrant and is inscribed with the words *Schlüssel—gewalt/pewtell—reichtum/beteut* (Keys mean power, purse means wealth) (figure 1.3).[3] Keys and purse are common

attributes of the German *Hausfrau*'s domestic authority—her budgetary discretion, her access to doors, cabinets, and chests—and they appear on another sheet featuring a hefty Nuremberg matron, a work regarded by some as a preliminary study for Dame Melancholy.[4] Purse and keys are also traditional symbols of melancholia and the planetary deity who rules over it, Saturn, but since that connection is absent from the London sketch, it's likely Dürer was merely jotting down what amounted to a received idea about them, something to retrieve for later use. Had we similar notes for every motif in the engraving, a breathtaking expanse of unnecessary scholarly labor might have been avoided. Or so one imagines. When we notice how loosely the keys hang from Melancholy's belt, how neglected the purse seems amidst her crumpled draperies, their status as symbolic attributes begins to blur. (Does she even *possess* them at all?) What appears as a straightforward passport to understanding the symbolic language of the print—delivered to us by Dürer's own hand no less—is already equivocal. In like fashion, nearly every other item in *Melencolia*'s catalogue of objects has defied efforts to tag it with a fixed meaning.

That the disorienting force of *Melencolia*'s "chaos," noted by many observers beside Wölfflin, was something calculated by Dürer the master geometrician is nearly beyond doubt. The peculiar visual effects his composition produces at the structural level will be the subject of the next chapter. Here we begin amidst the clutter itself, joining the great historical procession of those seeking meaning in the image, as well as those who have found in it something like a paradigm of meaning itself. The question is deceptively simple: to what end has Dürer sown such a confusion? Does the artist mean for us to find our way to a clarification? Does he expect we will actively construct a unity from the picture's scattered fragments, or has he anticipated our lapse back into perplexity, wherein we become, like Dame Melancholy herself, "incapacitated in the face of a neurotic need for knowledge"?[5]

That both the objects themselves and their placement in relation to one another are riven with ambiguities, if not outright "contradictoriness" (*Widersprüchlichkeit*),[6] was observed by the author of the earliest surviving analysis of the engraving, Dürer's friend and director of the Protestant *Gymnasium* in Nuremberg, the humanist Joachim Camerarius (1500–74). Camerarius recognized an essential absurdity in the symbolic objects such as the ladder, which seemed to point two ways at once:

Next to her we can see instruments belonging to the *artes*, books, rulers, compasses, squares and, besides, tools of metal and several of wood. In order to show that such [afflicted] minds commonly grasp everything and how they are frequently carried away into absurdities, he reared up in front of her a ladder into the clouds, while the ascent by means of rungs is as it were impeded by a square block of stone.[7]

Five hundred years later, Camerarius's ascription of a visual flight into "absurdities" has still not come undone, though not for lack of trying. As anyone who has waded into the ocean of erudite scholarship on *Melencolia* can attest, the assemblage of objects Dürer has packed into his enigmatic tableau have sustained a dizzying number of interpretations—all of them overlapping, many of them conflicting, quite a number of them diametrically opposed. Each one more elaborate and ingenious than the last, limited only by the erudition and imagination of their purveyors, such interpretations by and large aspire to be solutions to a puzzle of meaning. Treating the work of art as a special kind of rebus, that is, they aim to discover a hidden discourse behind the image. That discourse could be moralistic (for example, the symbolism of time, or death, or fortune); protoscientific or occult (the alchemist's vision of transformation, the astrologer's insights into the sublunary world); it could be aesthetic (in one view, it is Dürer's celebration of geometry, in another, his lapse of faith in rule-based art; in yet another, his quest for Platonic beauty through mathematics)[8] or strictly religious (the redemptive promise of Christ's Passion); or it could be epistemological (the stages of ascent to knowledge of God, the interpretive "undecidability" of the image, the labyrinth of meaning, and so on). Each interpretation that has taken its place in this grand procession has sought for a guiding principle behind or "inside" the work, and has therefore shared in the venerable project of understanding the picture as an enigma (from the Greek αἴνιγμα [*ainigma*], derived from αἰνίσσομαι [*ainissomai*], "to speak allusively" or in riddles). Once all its symbols, hidden or otherwise, are identified and all the abstract concepts behind them unraveled, the key to "unlock" the riddle, it is thought, can be found, its problem solved, and the engraving's real meaning interpreted.[9] Thus does the picture become comprehensible as something "other" than what it appears to be; it becomes an allegory (likewise descended from the Greek noun ἀλληγορία [*allēgoria*], related to the verb ἀλληγορέω [*allēgoreō*],

a compound word made from the adjective *allos*, meaning "other," and the verb *agoreúō*, "to speak"). Fully transposable to the domain of language, the allegorical image no longer flashes into our awareness as a materialized presence, but "demands to be laboriously decoded in time," as Michael Camille has explained it. Such a picture appears to its audience, in the words of our archtheorist of modern allegory, Walter Benjamin (1892–1940), "as a form of writing."[10]

Given the strong interest in hieroglyphs among the German humanists with whom Dürer associated and collaborated, and given their conviction that decoding this symbolic language could provide access to the *prisca theologia*, the unified theology embedded in all ancient religion and thought,[11] the scholarly default mode of interpreting *Melencolia* esoterically seems more or less justified. And yet the actual results, as we will shortly see, have been mixed. For the moment, then, let us set aside the recondite debates over symbolism—whether the rainbow, for example, is solar or lunar, whether the comet is meant as Saturn or actually shows Haley's Comet, whether the nails are thinly disguised *arma Christi*, and so on. Set aside all that has been exegetically discovered or demonstrated, and the ambiguities remain. They proclaim themselves, in fact, everywhere we look. Is it daylight rising on the horizon, or is that twilight descending upon the cluttered building site, and what exactly is the source of the scene's silvery illumination? Has the bat just fluttered into view, or has Dürer depicted him hastily departing the scene? Is it even a bat, or a batlike phantasm, or the demon of melancholia itself?[12] Where are the figures seated and situated? From where, and to where, if anywhere, does the ladder lead? And what kind of structure is behind them, a tower, or a temple, or a buttress, and how far does it extend beyond the frame of the picture?

To accept that these ambivalences and ambiguities, contradictions and confusions, were part of a deliberate strategy may help us understand the artist's expressive intentions. That is, it may help us appreciate Dürer's original objective in making "the visible representation completely answer to the invisible notion," as Raymond Klibansky, Erwin Panofsky, and Fritz Saxl put it in their incomparable compendium, *Saturn and Melancholy* (1964). For such an appreciation would reveal the artist, who was counted a melancholic genius by his friend Philip Melanchthon (1497–1560)[13] and certainly also in some sense by himself (see Chapter 5), as something of a master

diagnostician of melancholy's peculiar malaise: a profound sense of disorientation in the world, a haunting unreality that borders on the delusive. Such an appreciation would reveal Dürer, in other words, as uniquely capable of using his art to capture the pathology and to tell us, visually, that "melancholy is like this."[14] But is that the purpose of the engraving?

Inspired Hermeneutics

Developed over the course of four decades and three major publications, the interpretation put forward by the German art historian Erwin Panofsky (1892–1968) stands as the most enduring of modern answers to this question. Initially, Panofsky teamed up with his colleague at the University of Hamburg, Fritz Saxl (1890–1948), and took up where the unfinished work of Viennese art historian Karl Giehlow (1863–1913), an expert on the German humanists' discovery of hieroglyphics, had left off. Giehlow's preliminary reading of *Melencolia*, published as two long articles in 1903 and 1904, situated the work within the intensive interest in astrology cultivated among the intellectuals at Maximilian's court in Vienna; in the final analysis, he declared the rebuslike image to be an erudite summa of these interests, a comprehensive portrayal of the melancholic temperament, its positive and negative values held in perfect balance, its potential for "genius" suspended between divine inspiration and dark madness.[15] In the process, Albrecht Dürer was cast as a speculative thinker and iconographic innovator of the first order.

Accepting Giehlow's fundamental premise of a Renaissance reevaluation of the "saturnine" temperament, but dissatisfied with its restriction to the Vienna circle, Panofsky and Saxl embarked on a comprehensive archaeology of source texts and image types—they subtitled their project *ein quellen- und typengeschichtlichen Untersuchung*. The result was an encyclopedic account of the intellectual and pictorial background for Dürer's masterful allegorical synthesis.[16] Later, in 1943, the Hamburg team's elucidation of the engraving's symbolism was reprised in Panofsky's great Dürer monograph, which the emigré Jewish scholar composed in vibrant English while on the faculty of Princeton's Institute for Advanced Study. Finally, in 1964, the thesis was fleshed out in collaboration with Raymond Klibansky (1905–2005), a German-Canadian historian of philosophy who brought to the project a wealth of specialized knowledge in

ancient humoral theory and medieval psychology: the result was the monumental *Saturn and Melancholy*.

For these pioneers of iconological method, it was Dürer's bold stroke to transform the medieval imagery of *geometria* into an allegory of *melancholia generosa*, the "inspired melancholy" newly valued among Renaissance thinkers such as the Florentine Neoplatonist Marsilio Ficino (1433–99). This humanistic conception of melancholy saw it first and foremost as the temperament of intellectual and creative genius. Its personification appears in the extraordinary dark-faced spirit lost in contemplation, unable to realize in practice what theoretical reflection brings into view, a brooding figure Panofsky ultimately judged to be a "spiritual self-portrait" of the artist himself.[17] Surrounded by tools and measuring implements but immobile, poised on the brink of creative activity but despairing of the limitations of all human art, the protagonist of Panofsky's interpretation is a notably tragic figure, suffering something like the modern artist's failure of creative nerve, yet vigilant all the same.

The interpretation put forward first by Giehlow and then by Panofsky and his colleagues upended the traditional narrow association of the melancholic disposition with the "cold" and "dry" humor of black bile, from which Greek medicine derived the syndrome's name (μέλαινα χολή, *melaina cholē*). Integral to this older, negative conception were the ill effects of Saturn, most feared among the planets. Ancient medicine had correlated four planets with both the body's four organic "humors" and the four cosmic elements: Jupiter's influence prevails in blood and in air; Mars rules yellow bile and fire; the moon correlates with phlegm and water; and Saturn affects black bile and earth.[18] Medico-astrological diagrams explaining the interrelation of the four elements and qualities of the cosmos (*mundus*) with the four seasons (*annus*) and the bodily humors (*homo*) were important fixtures in medieval handbooks of learning such as Isidore of Seville's *De natura rerum* (seventh century), printed editions of which were popular with scholars in Dürer's Germany (figure 1.4).[19] Not all ancient and medieval sources regarded the saturnine temperament as the "lowest" (that is, the most earthbound) in the humoral system, however. Some, such as the Pseudo-Aristotelian compendium known as the *Problemata physica* (Problem no. 30), already pointed to the possibility that black bile, when sufficiently "heated" in the body, could produce an inspired frenzy, or *furor*, conducive to extraordinary achievement among scholars, artists, and statesmen.[20]

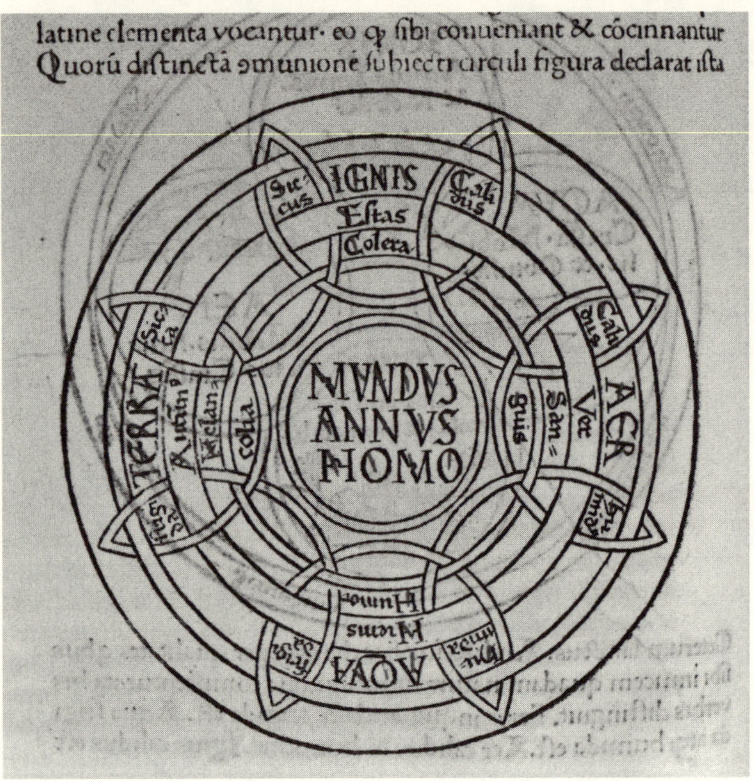

Figure 1.4. German, *Mundus—Annus—Homo,* hand-colored woodcut diagram in Isidore of Seville, *De responsione mundi et de astrorum ordinatione* (Augsburg: Günther Zainer, 7 December 1472), fol. 7v (New Haven, Beinecke Library, Mellon Alchemical +1) (photo: by the author).

This, Panofsky asserted, again building upon Giehlow's research, set the stage for a thoroughgoing reevaluation of melancholia among Renaissance Neoplatonists and occultists: Ficino, himself a melancholic, confirmed the *furores* associated with heated bile as the basis for creative genius in *De triplici vita* (1489), his treatise on the health of scholars.[21] So, too, did the German physician and occultist Heinrich Cornelius Agrippa von Nettesheim (1486–1535). In his *De occulta philosophia,* an important synthesis of ancient and medieval knowledge concerning ritual and astral magic, kabbalah, divination, numerology, angelology, and much more, Agrippa saw melancholia manifesting itself variously, depending on the cognitive faculty (*imaginatio, ratio,* or *mens*) most directly affected by atrabilious blood. It was this

broad effort to reinterpret melancholia not as a curse, but as a "gift" of Saturn—a fragile inheritance of creative geniuses whose endeavors, under the right conditions, would lift them closer than other men to the divine—that informs Dürer's scene, according to Panofsky and Saxl. "Like Melancholy, so too does Saturn, this demon of contradictions, on the one hand endow the soul with sloth and dullness, on the other, with the power of intelligence and contemplation; like melancholy, Saturn also constantly threatens those subjected to him . . . with the dangers of depression or manic ecstasy."[22] It was Dürer's genius alone to recognize in the allegory not only his own creative temperament, but his struggle as a *German* artist and humanist to reconcile theory (*Kunst*) and practice (*Brauch*), imagination and science, intuition and reason, at a time of Italian supremacy in the arts, on the one hand, and deepening spiritual uncertainty, on the other.[23]

Disseminated over vast areas of scholarship by a less than critical acceptance, reverently reprised and summarized in textbooks and exhibition catalogues too numerous to mention, Panofsky's brilliant solution to the enigma of the engraving has also found its challengers. Some have been content to pick around the edges; others have committed to a full assault. In 1978, Konrad Hoffmann of Tübingen University rejected the reading of the engraving's winged personification as an essentially ambivalent figure. Tracing the negative symbolism of the bat, a creature who shuns the light and who is shown by Dürer fluttering *away* from the comet and the rainbow, Hoffman places the full semantic weight of a dark, saturnine melancholy on the creature who, in the engraving, heralds it on outstretched wings (see figure I.9). In the seated genius, by contrast, Dürer gives us an antithetical personification of the melancholic temperament, one who is already protected from depressive astral influences by the numerological square above her head (see figure 4.13) and whose victory over despair is heralded by the rainbow, itself a kind of cosmic talisman against fears of a "second flood." (In the early sixteenth century in South Germany, astrophobic hysterias were periodically whipped up by journalistic predictions of planetary conjunctions and their impending catastrophes.)[24] Dürer's allegorical figure could not, therefore, embody the humanistic duality of genius and despair; the attribution of the bat's inscription, *MELENCOLIA I*, to the whole engraving collapses. In advancing this thesis, Hoffman also took aim at the strong link Panofsky had forged between Dürer's interpretation and

Agrippa's threefold division of melancholic genius. (In *De occulta philosophia*, as already noted, Agrippa explains that melancholia affects *imaginatio*, *ratio*, or reason, and *mens*, or intellect, in different "stages," unleashing different kinds of creative powers.) Not only is the assumption that Dürer consulted Agrippa's book prior to its 1531 publication far-fetched, Hoffman points out, but the allegorical portrayal of two kinds of melancholy, one dark and fully demonic, the other confidently creative and conscious of human mortality (the mysterious architectural structure can be seen as an "anti-Tower of Babel" and an attribute of *melancholia generosa*) does not need the Agrippan typology in the first place.

Roughly coincident with Hoffman's intervention, the renowned English scholar of Renaissance hermetic philosophy and Elizabethan literature, Dame Frances Yates, in a lecture given in Rochester in 1980, embraced the strong connection to Agrippa's occultism touted by Panofsky and his colleagues while also arguing that the authors of *Saturn and Melancholy* had missed the true import of that text for Dürer. That import resides, Yates argued, in Agrippa's engagement with kabbalah and the fascination with word-magic he shared with Christian Hebraists such as Johannes Reuchlin (1455–1522).[25] Tragic suffering for the sake of art falls away in the face of far greater forces. Transfixed within her "intense," nighttime atmosphere, so rich with saturnian allusions, Dürer's winged genius "is not in a state of depressed inactivity" at all, according to Yates. Invoking the astral powers of the higher planets and thereby lifted by a benevolent magic of angelic forces, freed from the disorder engendered by the senses (symbolized by the emaciated dog), the figure is depicted "in an intense visionary trance, a state guaranteed against demonic intervention by angelic guidance."[26]

Such a universalizing reading of the print's central figure strongly implies a visionary conception of the whole scene, and as we will see later (Chapter 4), there are otherwise good, unmagical reasons for connecting melancholia with both enlightened and pathlogical forms of visionary experience. Yates, however, did not pursue these insights beyond her own interests or into a fully worked-out reading of the engraving. (The defining purpose of her lecture was to show how Dürer's engraving and George Chapman's poem of 1594, "Shadow of the Night," elucidate each other.)

Nevertheless, the intervention by Yates laid bare something important about the interpretation of *Melencolia I* put forward by the

authors of *Saturn and Melancholy*, whose "Apollonian" vision of the Renaissance emphasized the rational heritage of antiquity, humanist revisions to the ancient links between humoral theory and iatromathematics, Dürer's philosophical and spiritual struggles, and so on. To the degree that these authors, all of whom enjoyed close ties with the Warburg Institute (which opened in Hamburg in 1926), suppressed the elements of theurgy, magic, kabbalah, witchcraft, and the occult as factors in Renaissance philosophy and psychology, they were turning against a key dimension of the institute's legacy. For it was precisely these preoccupations with the irrational, demonic, and "Dionysian" forces in European culture that had guided the institute's founder, Aby Warburg (1866–1929), in the conclusion to his great study of pagan prophecy and divinatory magic during the early Reformation, which appeared in 1919.[27] In that profoundly empirical and imaginative synthesis, Warburg, who once defined himself as an "image historian, not an art historian," had already recast Giehlow's ambivalent personfication into an avatar of postmedieval man's spiritual victory over astrological fate. Dürer's creative, indeed, optimistic gesture in fashioning an image that could empower and console the melancholic mind as it confronted Saturn's influence made the engraving, in Warburg's phrase, a "humanist's consoling image" (*humanistische Trostblatt*), a token of spiritual self-liberation and a resource for dispelling the darkness wrought by the malevolent dark planet.[28]

In advancing their Apollonian interpretation of inspired melancholy, the Warburgians under Panofsky parted company with Warburg, whose aphoristic *Denkbild*, "Athen will eben immer wieder neu aus Alexandrien züruckerobert sein" (Athens must be wrested back, over and over again, from Alexandria), made the painful struggle between reason and unreason, civilization and barbarism, the center of a research agenda in which they developed their thought.[29] Acknowledging the "sagacious argumentation" of Giehlow and Warburg, Panofsky and Saxl averred in a footnote, "perhaps Dürer's sheet could be better designated a 'warning image' [*Warnungsblatt*] than a 'consoling image' [*Trostblatt*]."[30] Conversely, when Yates reenvisioned the engraving, for all the points of agreement with Panofsky's "romantic" interpretation, she did so in a thoroughly Warburgian spirit,[31] and many of the questions Hoffman would later answer were first asked by Warburg. A similar interest in Renaissance magic and the "immanent polarity" Giehlow discovered in the astrological

idea of Saturn drove Walter Benjamin's dialectical engagement with *Melencolia* in the 1925 book on German Baroque tragedy, where he ventured that the engraving "anticipates the baroque in many respects" and that the "images and figures presented in the German *Trauerspiel* are dedicated to Dürer's genius of winged melancholy." Failing as a *Habilitationsschrift* at the University of Frankfurt, the book, despite the high praise it extended to the Warburgians, was summarily dismissed by Panofsky after he received a copy from Benjamin's friend and benefactor, the poet Hugo von Hofmannsthal.[32]

Much more could be said about the contrasts and contradictions of these interpretative programs, as well as about the clashes and rivalries of their authors, and in due course, the reader will learn why I come down in favor of this or that position—why, for example, Warburg's idea of a "humanistische Trostblatt" holds so much interest for my own effort to recover the therapeutic efficacy of Dürer's image. What should be emphasized now is something that easily escapes notice when the exegetical intricacies and respective merits of particular interpretations hold our focus—and that is the outlook they fundamentally share.

Except for Benjamin at his most dialectical, what they all share, in a nutshell, is a commitment to reading Dürer's picture as a unified statement, a symbol in the sense articulated by Panofsky's mentor, the neo-Kantian philosopher Ernst Cassirer (1874–1945). For Cassirer, the work of art by definition should not "appear as if put together of its parts, but as if it itself is the source of its parts and the grounds of its concrete determination."[33] This principle guided Panofsky's efforts to capture the "symbolic form" that works of art instantiate and to systematize iconology as a method for reaching this level of meaning; traces of Cassirer's doctrine can therefore be detected in nearly every interpretative run taken at *Melencolia* ever since. Each in its own way is an archaeology of meaning; each assumes that the engraving's accumulated object-signs all point beyond themselves, to something mysteriously "contained" by the work, as if gestating there, awaiting the hermeneutical act that will liberate it and bring it into the light of day. Once successful, such an act will show the whole work to be a synthesis of these revealed meanings. Vulgar allegorists and popularizers, by contrast, are usually satisfied to unearth one tantalizing piece of codework from the matrix and make it transmit its

"secret" meaning to the whole, as if Dürer had devised the engraving as an elaborate encryption device.[34] One author has gone so far as to regard the blazoned theme of the engraving, melancholia, as itself a "disguise" for the image's ultimate layer of esoteric significance, a significance lost to posterity once Dürer's circle of initiates had passed away.[35]

To put a fine point on it, we can say this: by definition, all the great interpretations of *Melencolia*, with the possible exception of Warburg's,[36] and even those that see a strategic ambivalence built into the picture's own mode of signifying (*Bildsinn*),[37] share in the insistence that Dürer's engraving must be an *allegory of something*, whether that something is the duality of aspiration and failure in the humanist enterprise, the divine inspiration of the melancholic artist, the mobilization of angelic forces against darkness, the limits of human knowledge, the consciousness of mortality, the victory over apocalyptic fear, the Platonic search for beauty, or some other thematic yet to be discovered.

Viewed from a lofty height, the history of all these hermeneutic confections is a colorful one. For good reason, *Melencolia* has been dubbed the "image of images"—an inexhaustible resource for exegesis, speculation, and debate.[38] Such an unruly sprawl of thought and writing has been generated that it requires periodic indexing, turning the critical analysis of *Melencolia* discourse into a discourse unto itself.[39] One might narrate its ebb and flow as a parable for art history's aspiration to become a modern human science, or as a self-reflecting poetics of cultural work turned melancholy, as more recent views would have it.[40] Measured by its power to tempt the tender sympathies of psychiatrists, physicists, mathematicians, curiously credentialed symbologists, and grail hunters of every stripe, *Melencolia* certainly holds its own against the *Mona Lisa* or the Sistine Chapel. Any complete history of its many (mis)interpretations could be read as a cautionary tale about academic hubris, the dangers of amateurism, or too much cross-disciplinary traffic. Those who believe they are harboring the next great theory about the engraving—*the one that will change everything*—are patronized with knowing smiles at cocktail parties and in academic corridors. Sensible students of German Renaissance art regard the print as an inescapable masterpiece, but also as something of a third rail. Little about this situation is ever likely to change.

Beyond the "Dürer Code"

Fortunately, the intellectual prospects for a reevaluation of *Melencolia* are more promising than today's jaded experts might suspect, and it is crucial for my own purpose to narrate how this came to be. In 1991, the German scholar Peter-Klaus Schuster published the most comprehensive study to date: *Melencolia I: Dürers Denkbild*, a two-volume monograph weaving together nearly every strand of existing research into a totalizing picture of Dürer's singular "image of images," its humanist context, its receptions, and its afterlives. Schuster's labor in synthesizing all that remained valid in the work of founding fathers Giehlow, Warburg, Panofsky, and Saxl must be admired, and his energy envied, but his conclusion that *Melencolia* is an elaborately wrought allegory of virtue (*Tugendallegorie*), structured through an almost diagrammatic opposition of virtue and fortune, fell short of proposing anything conceptually new.[41] Nor has his proposed resituation of *Melencolia* within a four-part cycle devoted to the temperaments—a project Dürer allegedly abandoned—found much acceptance among Dürer experts.[42]

A herculean undertaking of iconographic research in a discipline no longer convinced of iconography's validity, the inner contradictions of Schuster's project are evidence of a turning point, one with unintended consequences. Consider the declaration of the engraving as a *Denkbild* in the study's title: with this term, the author invoked a genre of aesthetic writing favored by the theorists of the so-called Frankfurt School (the Institute for Social Research, founded in Frankfurt am Main in 1923), men such as Walter Benjamin and Theodor Adorno. This was a telling choice, for the term has a double meaning: it denotes both a "thought image," in the sense of a Platonic ideal form, an object of contemplation available only intellectually, and also something like an "image of thought" itself, in which the form thought takes becomes its content. For Gerhard Richter, who has studied the genre closely, the *Denkbild* is the quintessential "philosophical miniature."[43] And indeed, integral to *Melencolia*'s reception history has been its enlistment as a "tangible stimulus to philosophical reflection," for example, in Benjamin's *Trauerspiel* book, where it served, in Camille's words, as a "constantly changing object for [the author's] own melancholy immersion."[44] Curiously, although Schuster acknowledged the conundrum imposed on scholarship by the immense historical accumulation of contradictory meanings,

and was acutely aware of Benjamin's reflections, he never engaged the term directly or clarified its applicability to Dürer's print.[45] To produce a fitting double monument to Dürer's masterpiece and the immense exegetical labors it has inspired, to write an impossible summa of all that has ever been thought or said about the engraving, only a conservative attitude will do.

Readers may already suspect what happened when the edifice so painstakingly constructed by a collective labor of scholarship, and then monumentalized in Schuster's work, exposed itself as an accumulation of fragments, an allegorical "ruin" in its own right. Schuster's super-interpretation of *Melencolia I* inadvertently revealed the possibility that there was, after all, no "Dürer code" to break, no master key to discover, no puzzle awaiting a solution. Had *Melencolia*'s inventor brilliantly, knowingly, set out to foil the grand expectation his own work sets in motion—the expectation that we can read the objects together allegorically, as units of sense in a discourse? Did he know the print would steer its exegetes into a "labyrinth of meaning," as Hartmut Böhme characterized the work's power to lead and mislead thought?[46] Ideas and symbols of geometry, astronomy, medicine, theology, and art theory mingle and collide in cluttered confusion in the engraving, but no sum of learning ever becomes possible—none, that is, that is not already a mirror of the thought that conjures it into being.

The most eloquent spokesman for this proposal is surely Joseph Leo Koerner, who has called the print "an occasion for thought." In his far-reaching monograph on Dürer's self-portraiture—published two short years after Schuster's work—Koerner casts *Melencolia*'s opacity, its stubborn resistance to penetration, as the dialectical other of an "abstract" inwardness characteristic of modern subjectivity itself:

> Instead of mediating *a* meaning, *Melencolia* seems designed to generate multiple and contradictory readings, to clue its viewers to an endless exegetical labor until, exhausted in the end, they discover their own portrait in Dürer's sleepless, inactive personification of melancholy. Interpreting the engraving itself becomes a detour to self-reflection, just as all the arts and sciences whose tools clutter the print's foreground finally return their practitioners to the state of mind absorbed in itself.[47]

In a sense, such notions have been present all along in art history's grappling with Dürer's vexing *Vexierbild*. Heinrich Wölfflin, with the multiple modes of scientific and artistic knowledge invoked by the

engraving in mind, had already in 1905 referred to it as an "allegory of deep, speculative thought." Unlike Koerner, however, he doubtless maintained some faith that the multiplicity harbored a unity, that the puzzle would someday yield a solution.

With the rise and fall of so many recondite interpretations, and a dawning recognition of the internal "contradictoriness" of Dürer's symbolism as a structural fact of the engraving, some scholars from the early 1980s onward began to pronounce this faith illusory. Martin Büchsel, for example, declared the unbridgeable divide between intention and result in the intellectual effort demanded by *Melencolia* a negation of the *melancholia generosa* extolled by Ficino—a failed, or "wrecked" (*gescheiterte*) version of the power of divine insight that black bile bestowed upon men of genius.[48] Others have detected in Dürer's chaos of objects a deep philosophical uncertainty, if not a bona fide skepticism, about the powers of human sense perception and reason to participate in the fulfillment of divine wisdom, let alone lead to a knowledge of God.[49] By ensuring the defeat of even the most learned efforts to master the code, the argument goes, Dürer's engraving exposes the folly of trying to transcend reason's "natural" limits. Less a prism for a penetrating speculation, then, the picture becomes a stubborn surface that turns back efforts to peer into its depths, exposing the folly of those who try. In this respect, *Melencolia* would seem to take its place among the sixteenth century's most ambitious critiques of secular learning, a complex emblem of *vanitas vanitatum*.[50] Others have argued—rightly, I believe—that the "undecidability" of symbols, thus the impossibility of ever arranging the parts into a cohesive and meaningful whole, should be understood as a deliberate effort by Dürer to convey the *feeling* of melancholic distress, to simulate the disorientation that attends a particular state of mind. As we will see in Chapter 4, it is but a short step to read the scene as a surreal delusion of the kind associated with extreme forms of depression and psychosis (though this may already be taking things too far).

By Dürer's time, Renaissance humanism, after more than a century's work applying the tools of critical philology to every human invention, had indeed come face to face with the contingency and unreliability of language and symbols—the *res signa* of the world—and thus the limits of speculative reason. "One of its results," explains William Bouwsma, was a "diminished confidence in the intellectual competence of human beings, and thus in the comprehensibility of

nature." Such epistemological doubts were already redirecting the search for authoritative truths—those necessary for reforming an imperfect world—away from antiquity and classical learning per se and back to Scripture.[51] Dürer, who later in his life turned decisively for consolation to the spiritual leadership of Martin Luther, may have shared this sense of contingency and the loss of a center, especially at the time he was working on *Melencolia*, a time of personal grief over the deaths of his mother and several close friends in succession (see Chapter 5). Mournfulness as a "pathological state," Benjamin wrote, the increasing "distance between the self and surrounding world," transfigures the most ordinary object into "a symbol of some enigmatic wisdom because it lacks any natural, creative relationship to us." Like the "utensils of active life" lying at the feet of Melancholy, the everyday thing we encounter in the midst of mourning fixes itself as "an object of contemplation," resistant to any closed meaning.[52]

Whatever we can ultimately make of the artist's intentions or the degree to which Dürer projected his own anxieties about creative achievement and perfection into this great "image of images," there can be little doubt that the calibrated contradictoriness of *Melencolia*'s signs and symbols signaled to contemporaries the imminent danger of depleted meanings, the futility of human grasping toward certainties. From this perspective, the perplexity of the winged genius seated among objects whose meanings have been reduced to absurdity (*in absurda defferentur*) becomes a lament over the doomed search for a unified knowledge of the world.

Let us suppose we have reached a tenable conclusion about the strategic "undecidability" of things that structures *Melencolia*—what then? Are we content to call the image an allegory of indeterminate meanings? Do we retreat into the fashionable notion of an "empty center," giving interpretation over to the endless recursivity of the *mise en abyme*? The latter, of course, runs the risk of turning the image into a reflection on epistemological problems that Dürer and his contemporaries would scarcely have recognized. (This is not to say there were no epistemological problems one *could* recognize and explore as a sixteenth-century artist, only that they were different than ours.) A cul-de-sac of a different sort, equally anachronistic, comes with Benjamin's dialectical opening out of Dürer's picture into a

self-mortifying object, an allegorical ruin that, like the Baroque trag-edy, is marked for death by the very criticism that engages it.[53] How might we avoid such end-game propositions, in which undecidabil-ity, emptiness, or even "absurdity" constitute their own, sufficient sources of value, while at the same time coping with the engraving's ingenious play of opacity, ambiguity, and indeterminacy?

Suppose we can answer the challenge of the image by putting it to a different use. Productive avenues for doing this open up when we turn our attention to the *form* of thought that the engraving occa-sions, without, however, mistaking it for the *content or condition* of that thought.[54] Wölfflin called the form of thought that *Melencolia* allegorizes "speculative," and in the next chapter, I return in a new way to that founding intuition. A different picture of the engraving's value for thought appears when the consolations of closure that earlier generations of interpreters expected are allowed to fall away. We must pay careful attention to the cognitive activity *Melencolia* mobilizes and try to understand why it finds its most productive outlet on the surface of things, not in their depths—in an open-ended *kinesis*, not a closed *allegoresis*. To regard Dürer's print as both allegorical *and* speculative requires, in short, a different conceptualization of both terms, one that allows us to capture the full potential of the image, its unique capacity to jump the tracks of established genres and functions. Put another way, I am proposing that we maintain the engraving's allegorical iden-tity without asking it to conform to the classical rules of allegory, in which "people, animals, plants, and objects form an intellectual puzzle, a specific rebus to puzzle out."[55] How do we refrain from requiring the engraving to be a container for something hidden, an allegory of this idea or that, and at the same time take seriously its claim to mobilize our cognitive energies in a way that produces results?

Looking toward ideas about the therapeutic efficacy of such cog-nitive work is one way we can do this. Understood in psychosomatic and somatopsychic terms as a kind of hydraulics of the soul's higher and lower faculties, the dynamic cognition sparked, sustained, and exercised by Dürer's print was, we will see, the common concern of Renaissance painters, poets, rhetoricians, and physicians: a "move-ment" of the soul from one state to another, a return of the self to itself, a therapy of the passions aimed at the restoration of balance and health.

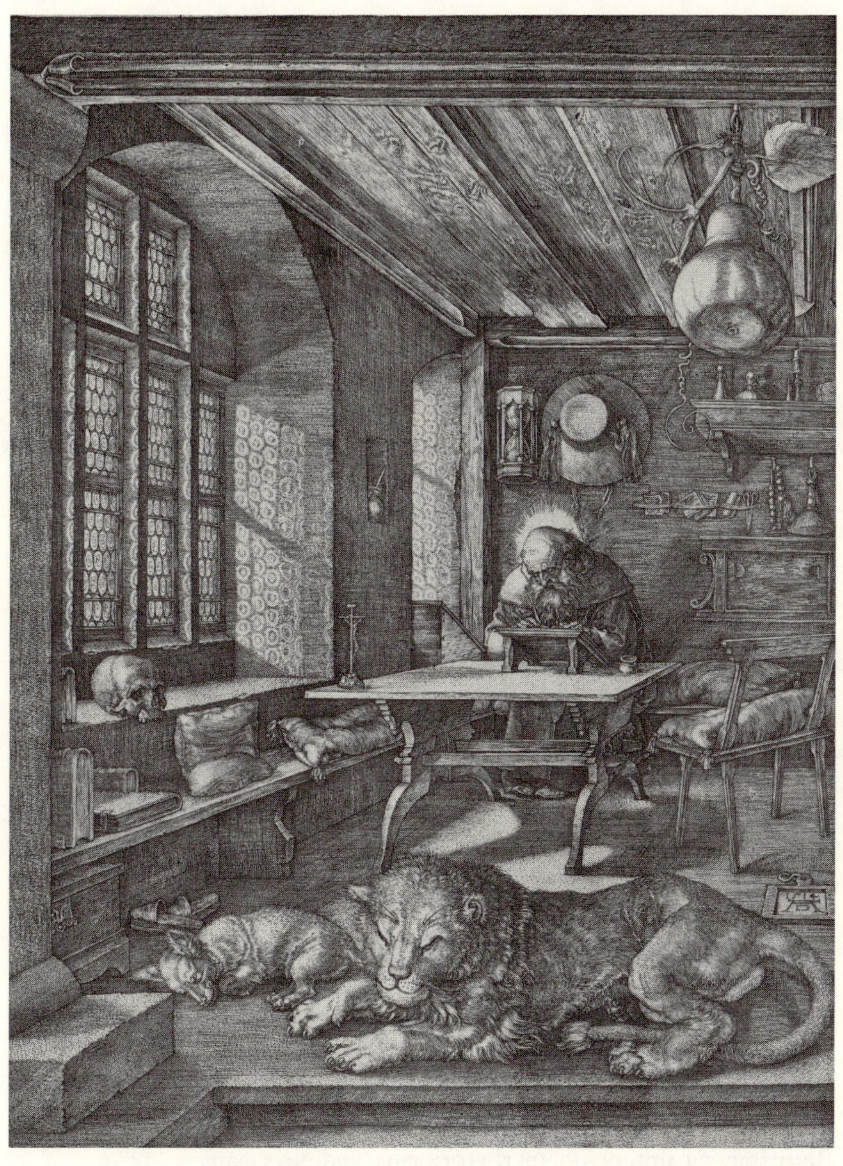

Figure 2.1. Albrecht Dürer, *Saint Jerome in his Study*, 1514, engraving, 25.4 x 19 cm (sheet trimmed to plate mark) (Washington, D.C., National Gallery of Art. Gift of R. Horace Gallatin).

Restless Eye, Active Mind

Indetermination is the choice springboard for artistic revery and imagination because it is the necessary passage for determination, the vacant site where new forms take shape. At this stage things do not yet exist, their shape is not fixed, their genesis is still a pure project. . . . This vagueness, which paralyzes the geometric spirit, stimulates the creative imagination.

—Michel Jeanneret, *Perpetual Motion: Transforming Shapes in the Renaissance from Da Vinci to Montaigne*

An "Impure Harmony"

Stepping back from the "chaos of objects" and looking at Dürer's composition as a whole, we can not help but sense a certain kind of spatial unrest, an optical shiftiness that disrupts the harmony of the perspectival view. Vision is challenged to draw order from confusion. This is a calculated effect and, one suspects, a stylistic conceit, the intentionality of which can be brought into focus by comparing *Melencolia*, as many writers have done previously, with two other engravings from the same year. The first of these is the luminous image of *Saint Jerome in his Study* (figure 2.1),[1] one of the three *Meisterstiche* whose thematic relatedness, as remarked in the Introduction, has remained an open question among scholars for over a century. That Dürer conceived the *Saint Jerome* as a kind of loose conceptual pendant to *Melencolia* is pretty safe to say: they are of nearly equal size; his travel digest (*Tagebuch*) of the Netherlands journey (1520–21) informs us that he distributed the two engravings together on at least four occasions, more than he did with any other pairings; and we know the two images were discussed in tandem among Dürer's learned patrons.[2] All that has been remarked about the two prints as emblems of theological and secular learning respectively may be set

aside for the moment, however, in order to attend to their striking formal differences.

Employing an orthodox method of geometrical perspective in the *St. Jerome*, Dürer has conjured a lucid architectonic space for the scholar's wood-paneled *studiolo*, creating a vision of order in which the location of every object is logically subordinated to the whole, where everything finds its natural place of repose, like the interior of the great philologist's mind. An ardent admirer of the Italian approach to perspective (as he found, for example, in the work of Andrea Mantegna, Antonio Pollaiuolo, and Jacopo de' Barbari) and a strong believer that art attains perfection only with the aid of measurement (*Messung*), Dürer devoted himself to the study of geometry, proportion, and perspective throughout his career, but at no time more intensively than in the decade preceding the master engravings, when he was reading Vitruvius's *De architectura* (ca. 30–15 BCE), among other sources on ancient art, and laying the groundwork for his two geometrical treatises, *Instruction in Measurement with the Compass and Straightedge . . .* (1525) and the *Four Books on Human Proportion*, which was not published until after his death in 1528.[3] In the *Saint Jerome* that effort has already borne extraordinary fruit: the coordinated convergence of orthogonals that define ceiling beams, window moldings, furniture edges, and the like is so rigorous that it seems a didactic display of illusionistic prowess. "The whole [composition] gives the impression," writes Wojciech Bałus, "of being influenced by a magnetic field passing through the [saint's] cell and arranging all the objects along the lines of force."[4]

No such force grips the objects assembled around Melancholy, and there are several reasons for this. Although Dürer did employ linear perspective in the *Melencolia*—its vanishing point is located on the line separating the sea and the sky, just below the bat, which would, along with the sphere at Melancholy's feet, be cut in half by any line bisecting the horizon at this point[5]—the whole composition lacks a predominant vertical, horizontal, or diagonal line, and no visual center holds. Lighting contributes powerfully to this effect. That the rainbow is visible at all means the sun has not yet set and is probably in the west, the direction from which we look;[6] in addition, Dürer has placed a second, dominant light source outside the frame to our right (a conspicuously atypical choice for him), and accordingly, highlights are set low.[7] Illumination is not concentrated, but

divided and distributed in such a way that every object is touched by a fiery, flickering light suggestive of astral radiance. Chiaroscuro effects merge imperceptibly with more sharply registered forms, transporting the whole tableau into an airless, dreamlike space. In the *Saint Jerome*, by contrast, Dürer has mostly confined shading to the middle range; light does not so much strike objects as bathe them in a warm, dappled glow, wondrously metaphorical of the "ether of spiritual tranquility" in which the saint's mind is immersed.[8] This is not to say that the composition of *Melencolia* lacks any kind of structure. In a remarkable set of design investigations, Luigi Toccacieli has managed to tease multiple layers of superimposed geometry from the print (figure 2.2), although some of his derivations are less convincing than others.[9] To the extent that such embedded geometries shape the beholder's experience of the work, they do so as silent subversives, arousing our expectation of optical uniformity without ever satisfying it. We can think of them as brilliantly overdetermined gestures toward artificial perspective, elements of a visual-rhetorical *ductus* both arousing and frustrating.

Another kind of dynamism is imparted to the scene by the displacement effect of all those scattered objects. Two in particular introduce special instabilities and deserve our close attention. The first is the wooden ladder rising up past the cornice of the stone building, where it evidently comes to rest on its vertical edge—ascending "into the clouds," as Camerarius described it in his 1541 account of the engraving.[10] A closer look reveals that its feet are likewise out of sight, planted somewhere below the elevated terrace on which the figures sit (see figure 2.10). Heinrich Wölfflin was the first to draw attention to the ladder's ambiguity, and he credited it with infusing the whole composition with an "impure harmony."[11] We will return to the ladder shortly.

The second agent of instability is the large polyhedron planted in the middle distance (figure 2.3). An otherworldly presence amongst mundane things, the monolith is placed so conspicuously before the vista that, according to Wölfflin, "the eye cannot avoid it." Camerarius, in whose view the hulking form specifically impedes our view of the ladder, and thus the path of metaphorical ascent thematized in the engraving, referred to the monolith—with a "certain willful vagueness," according to William Heckscher—as a square piece of rock (*saxum quadratum*).[12] Though the form is directly level with

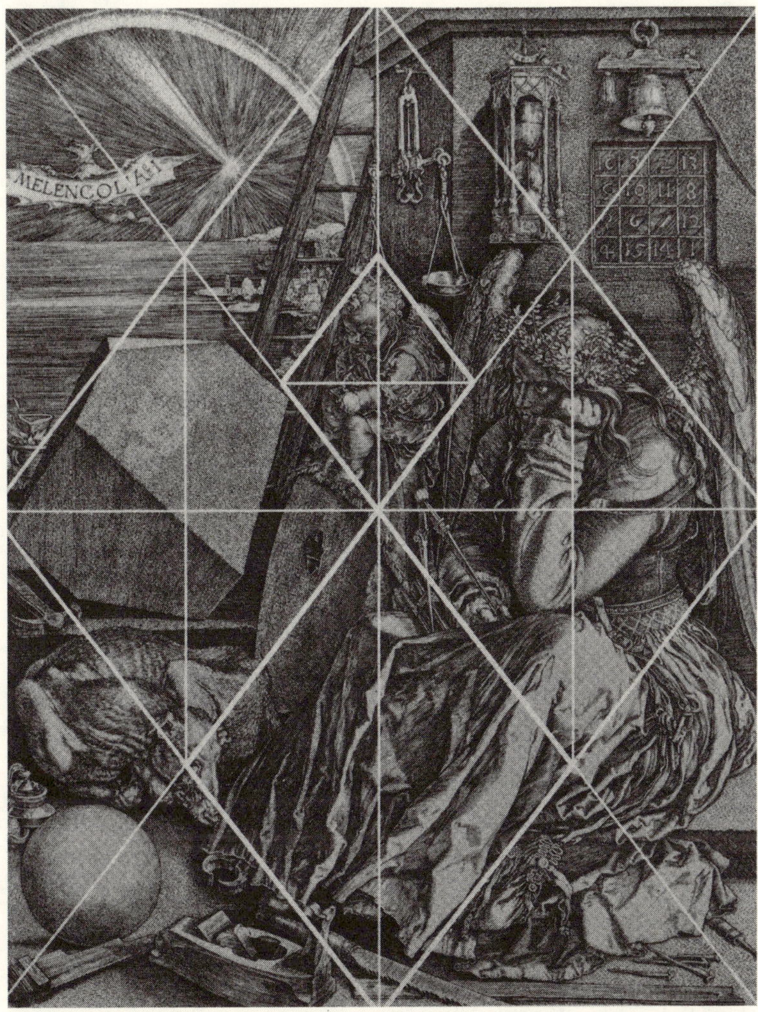

Figure 2.2. Figure from Luigi Toccacieli, *Melencolia I di Albrecht Dürer*, 2008, plate 9.

Melancholy's upper body and the line of her gaze, it's clear she takes no notice, but looks well past it. Just how much visual disruption the strange object brings to the engraving can be gleaned from the smaller, but compositionally almost identical *Virgin and Child Seated by a Wall* of 1514 (figure 2.4).[13] Here, despite the fact that the intersection of the horizontal platform and the vertical rise of the tower is obscured by the massive seated figures, the continuity of space from the most

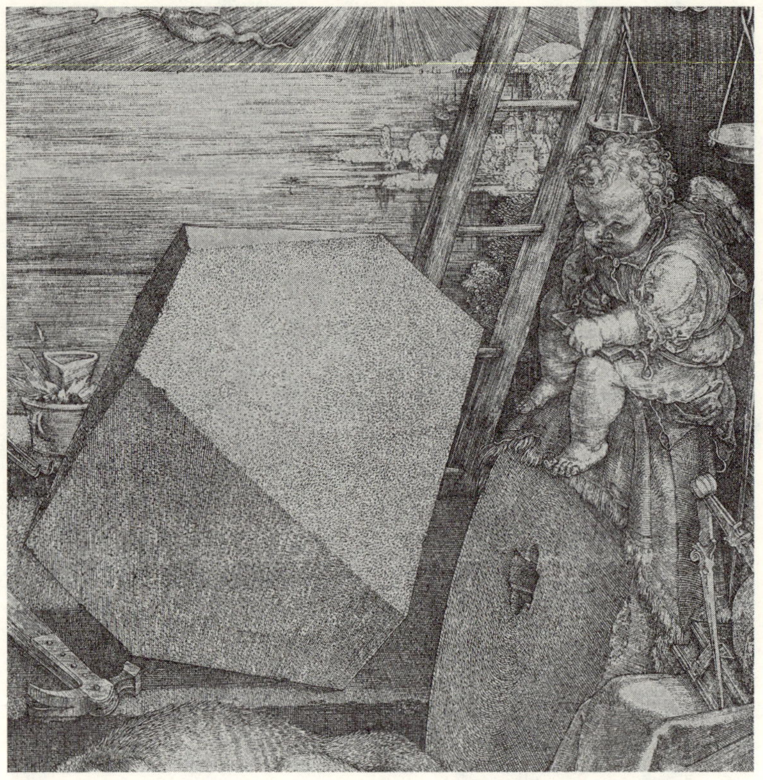

Figure 2.3. Detail from Dürer, *Melencolia I*: rhombohedron. (See figure 1.1 above.)

distant to the nearest point is pleasing and clear. Thus does the *ductus* of the work, the itinerary set out for the beholder's vision, befit the subject's dignity and grace. In the *Melencolia*, by contrast, the eye's free passage into the distance is blocked, causing it to circle back into the chaos of objects, where it finds no obvious place of repose. Together with the penumbral gloom that enshrouds the left half of the image, the monolith foils our "ingrained habit (or perhaps biological predisposition) to enter visually from the left," as Peter Parshall has related it.[14] Visual *ductus* as a governing element of style breaks down here, as if corrupted or short-circuited. Optical movement through the accumulated objects and bodies takes on the quality of an agitated restlessness, giving way to a sense of claustrophobic unease.

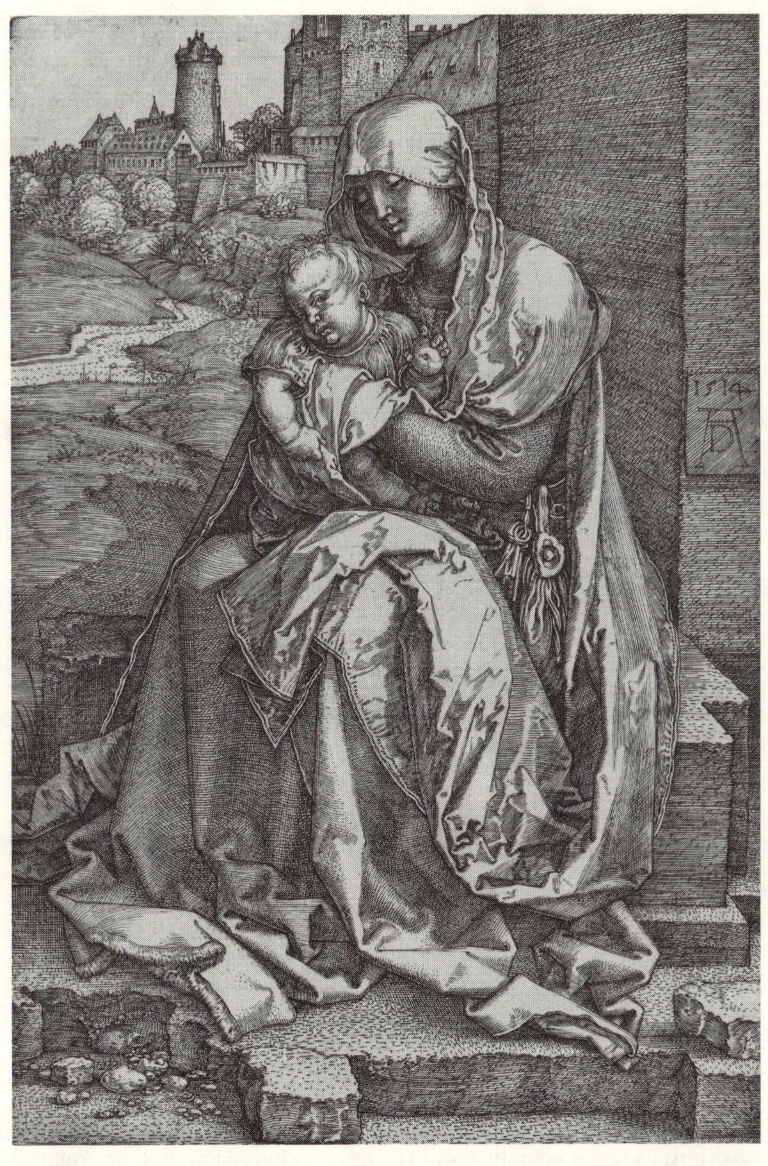

Figure 2.4. Albrecht Dürer, *Virgin and Child Seated by a Wall*, 1514, engraving, 14.8 x 10.0 cm (Washington, D.C., National Gallery of Art, Rosenwald Collection).

The monolith contributes to this spell of agitated confusion in other ways. Dürer could have contrived any kind of large object, a form of virtually any shape, simple or complex, to occupy the stage space at the platform's edge if all he had sought to do was obstruct the eye's passage into space. The choice of this highly irregular polyhedron and its strategic placement are therefore especially telling. In describing such a form so accurately, Dürer doubtlessly sought to place his command of perspective drawing on display, offering a striking attribute of "geometry gone melancholy" (*melancholia artificialis*), which Panofsky famously declared the winged genius to personify.[15] After all, the representation of polyhedra was considered in Dürer's time one of perspective geometry's greatest challenges.[16]

How the artist met the challenge in this instance is a question worth pausing over. After experimenting with the different methods he knew, Dürer evidently settled on the "Brunelleschian" technique, named for the architect Filipo Brunelleschi (1377–1446) and also known as *costruzione legittima*. Complex forms are plotted according to the intersection of two grids derived from plan and elevation, respectively. Guided by the systematization of this technique by another Florentine, Leon Battista Alberti (1404–72) in the treatise *Della pittura* (1436), Dürer would later experiment with perspective machines, which allowed him to plot the points of projected forms directly onto a grid—surrogate for Alberti's notional window—set up between the object and the eye, fixing both in space to certify the visual angle (figure 2.5). Knowing from experience that a strictly rule-bound geometry was no panacea for aesthetic problems, however, Dürer altered the results of his "legitimate construction" of the polyhedron, shaving a little here, a little there.[17] Clearly, the form is not a cube, as Camerarius was the first to claim, nor is it one of the five Platonic solids—based on Euclid—whose construction Dürer outlined in the *Instruction in Measurement*.[18] Rather, Dürer has rendered in projection a modified type of rhombohedron: a solid figure whose sides are six equal rhombuses in which opposite corners are sliced off to produce two more sides that are equilateral triangles. (It is on one of these triangular sides that Dürer has the form precariously balanced.) Among the many fascinating things about the invention is its geometric affinity with the "magic square" of Jupiter (*mensula Iovis*) on the wall behind Melancholy, about whose symbolism more will be said later. As Terence Lynch has shown, the irregular pentagons

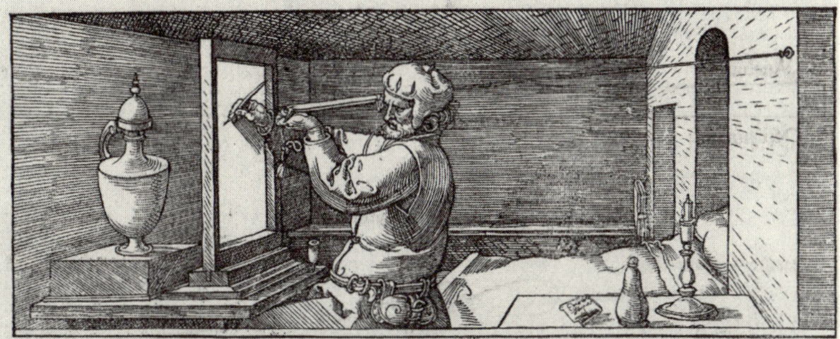

Item noch ein anderen brauch zu Conterfeten/dardurch man eyn yeliche Corpus mag grösser oder kleyner abconterfeten wie vil man wil/deshalben nutzlicher dañ mit dem glas darumb das es freier ist/ Darzu soll man haben ein ram mit einem gitter von starckem schwartzen zwirn gemacht/die lucken oder fierungen eine vngeferlich zweyer finger breyt/ Darnach soll man haben ein abfehen oben zugespitzt/ also gemacht / das man es höher oder niderer richten mag / das bedeut das aug mit dem. o. Darnach leg hinaus in zimlicher weitten dz corpus so du conterfeten wilt/ rucks vnd peugs nach deinem willen/vñ gee al weg hindersich vnd hab dein aug zu dem abfehen.o. negst daran/vnd befich das Corpus wie es dir gefall/ vñ ob es recht nach deinem willen lig/ Darnach stell dz gitter oder ram zwischen dem Corpus vnd deinem abfehen also/ wilt du wenig lucken oder fierungen begreiffen/so ruck es dest neher zu dem Corpus/darnach befich wie vil dz corpus im gitter lucken begreuf nach leng vñ breyten/ darnach reiß ein gitter gros oder klein auf ein bappir oder tafel darein du conterfeten wilt/ vnd sich hin vber dein aug.o. des spitz am abfehen auf das Corpus/ vnd was du in yder fierung des gitters findest/ das drag in dein gitter das du auf dem bappir hast das ist gut vnd gerecht/ Wilt du aber für das spitzig abfehen ein löchle machen/dardurch du sihest ist eben so gut/solcher meynung hab ich hernach ein form aufgeriffen.

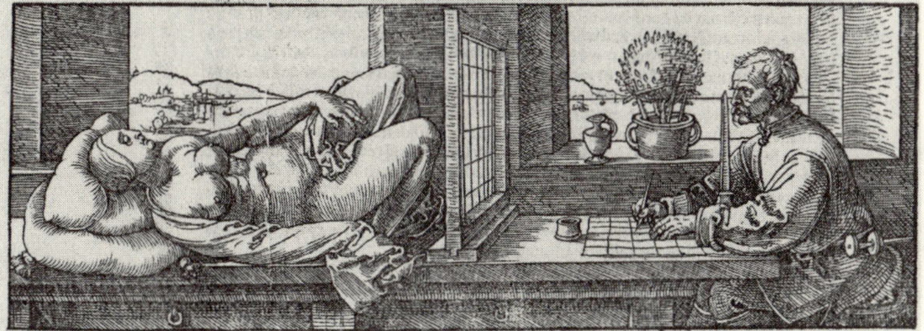

Figure 2.5. Albrecht Dürer, *Artist Using Perspective Devices*, page from *Unterweysung der Messung...* (Nuremberg, 1538), 31.9 × 21.5 cm (New York, Metropolitan Museum of Art. Gift of Felix M. Warburg, 1918) (photo courtesy of the Metropolitan Museum of Art, www.met museum.org).

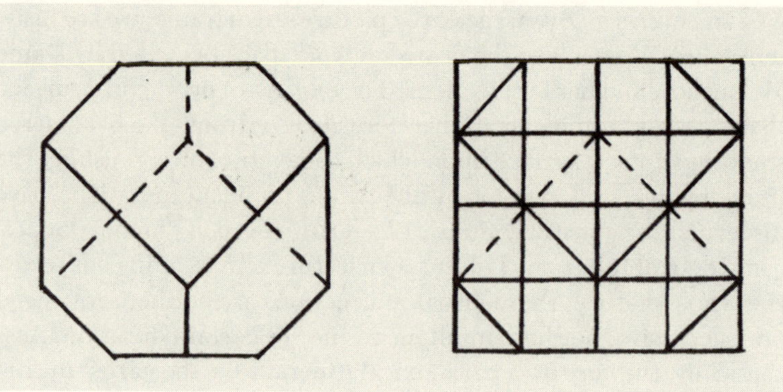

Figure 2.6. Figure from Terence Lynch, "The Geometric Body in Dürer's Engraving *Melencolia I*," p. 228.

formed when the rhombuses on the form's six sides are sliced off fit perfectly as mirrored polygons overlapping inside a square of sixteen equal cells (figure 2.6).[19]

Beyond the geometrician's bravura, Dürer seems to evince here an interest in making optical unease a reverberative effect of form. Immobile mass that it is, the polyhedron seems weirdly possessed of an inner torque, a kinetic potential that makes its planar components seem to rotate away from the central axis. This instability lends the form an almost uncanny agency in steering the eye's activity around within the composition, setting up a peculiar optical experience of the engraving. It was Bałus who first noted the especially arresting quality of the form's edges, which, he correctly observed, allow "the sides of the polyhedron, running in all directions, [to] focus the viewer's attention, then make him follow their different courses."[20] Like a prism refracting light in several directions at once, the polyhedron serves the beholder's probing vision as a relay, as it were, sending the gaze out and into the scene's diverse (and disconnected) volumes of space and returning it to the objects that occupy those spaces: the hammer and sleeping dog below the sloping front face of the polyhedron; the ignited brazier adjacent to its dark, leftward-facing side; the fluttering bat and the comet's burst reflected upon its slender top surface; and the ambiguous void past which one leg of the ladder can be seen descending and rising, faced by the side of the polyhedron

we can't even see. By virtue of the picture's own frame, we are insistently brought back to the crowded workspace occupied by Dame Melancholy and her companions. The expansive pentagonal surface that faces and frames them therefore also confronts the beholder: a smooth, stippled surface upon which some observers, relishing the freedom imparted to vision by nighttime's luminary mutations, have discerned the ghostly contours of a death's head, a graphic doppelgänger possibly bearing Dürer's own features.[21] Spreading out across the whole picture, these visual redirections are neither sequenced nor successive, neither simultaneous nor of certain duration. Aesthetically, they create a paradoxical itinerary for the gaze—in rhetorical terms, an *antiductus*. Such intuitions find another kind of confirmation in the investigations of Toccacieli, whose diagrams conjure a virtual geometry of bodies, optical zones, and lines of force out of Dürerian space (figure 2.7).[22]

Ponderously immobile, the planar form would, in any other phenomenal field, stand as a perfect antithesis to the sphere at Melancholy's feet. In Dürer's glimmering dreamworld, however, the rhombohedron makes a parallel allusion to the "passion-propelled agitation" traditionally associated with the sphere, especially in the iconography of Fortuna, where it symbolizes the fickleness of the world (figure 2.8).[23] Precariously poised, the cubic form even appears as if it might careen forward onto the sleeping dog. Stasis belies a kind of dynamism—the form disturbs visual activity inside the virtual space of the image and at the same time directs it across its surface, where forms interact. Whatever visual fascination the rhombohedron might compel by virtue of its uncanny, quasi-anamorphic appearance and its mysterious affinity with the "magic square" of Jupiter, whatever fixed concentration it might otherwise invite—all this is immediately dispersed, sending the eye back into its restless movements in and out of the scatter of things. In sum, whatever the rhombohedron may denote (symbolically), and whatever it may demonstrate (artistically), Dürer has given it a radical phenomenological role to play in the experience of the engraving. That role imposes a demand on the beholder—a demand not to "solve" a puzzle (for no solution is possible) or to "resolve" chaos into order (no regular structure is available), but to exercise one's powers of discernment and interpretation in an open-ended fashion. To engage in speculation. But to what end?

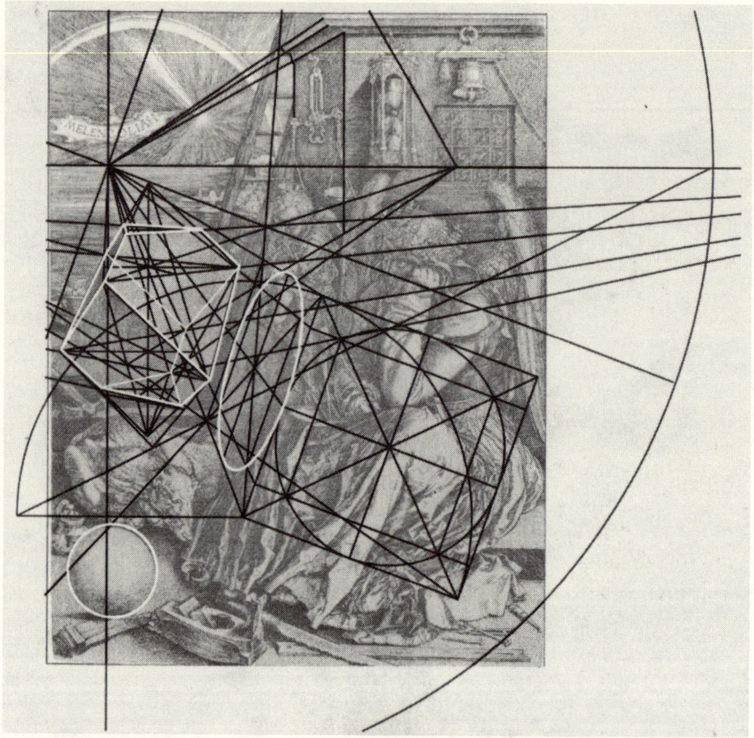

Figure 2.7. Figure from Luigi Toccacieli, *Melencolia I di Albrecht Dürer*, 2008, plate 5.

Obstruction and Reflection

So far we have described how the beholder of *Melencolia* could be incited by the print's stylized chaos to experience a perplexity of vision and use it as an occasion for quasi-meditative exercise, for speculation. Now the second part of that claim requires closer treatment. What would "speculation" consist of in this context, and how does its incitement betoken therapy? Let us take these questions in reverse order.

A comparison drawn from the image cycle accompanying the German edition of Petrarch's *De remediis* can help draw out the therapeutic logic of pictures that perplex. Published in Augsburg in 1532, the new edition, *Von der Artzney bayder Glück des guten und widerwärtigen*, was furnished with woodcuts designed by the

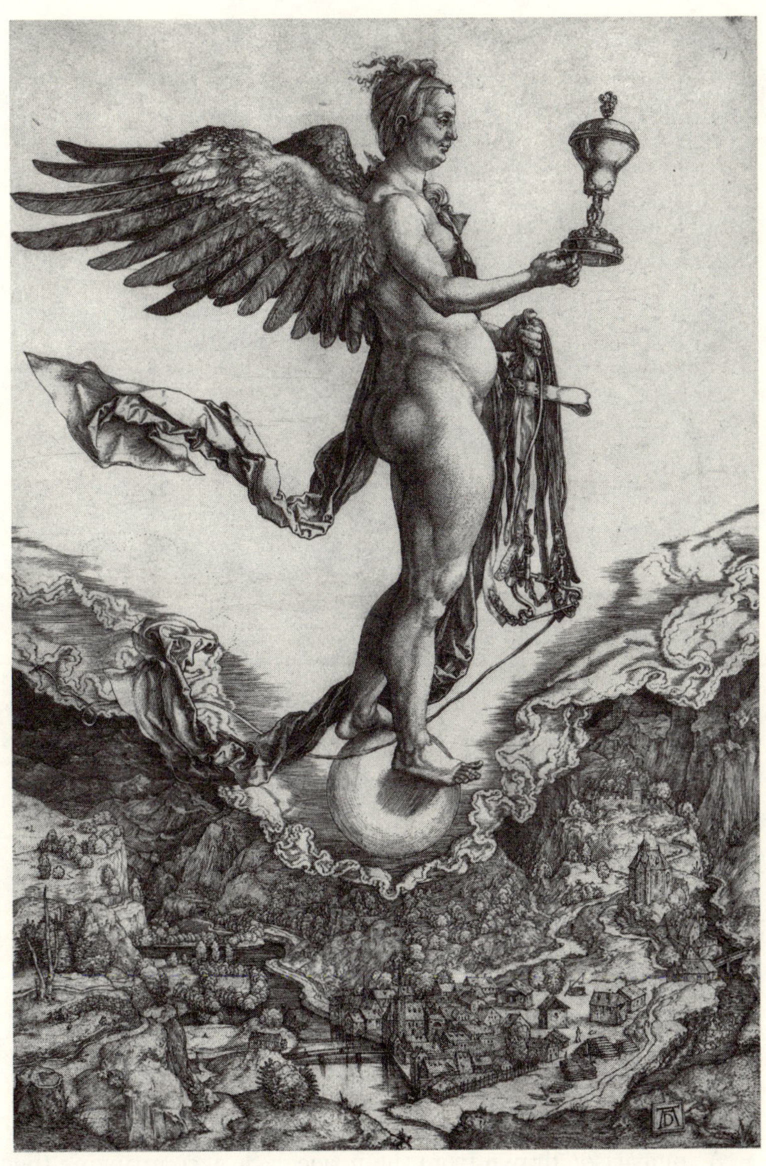
Figure 2.8. Albrecht Dürer, *Nemesis ("The Large Fortune")*, ca. 1501–1502, engraving, 33.5 x 23.3 cm (plate) (Washington, D.C., National Gallery of Art, Rosenwald Collection).

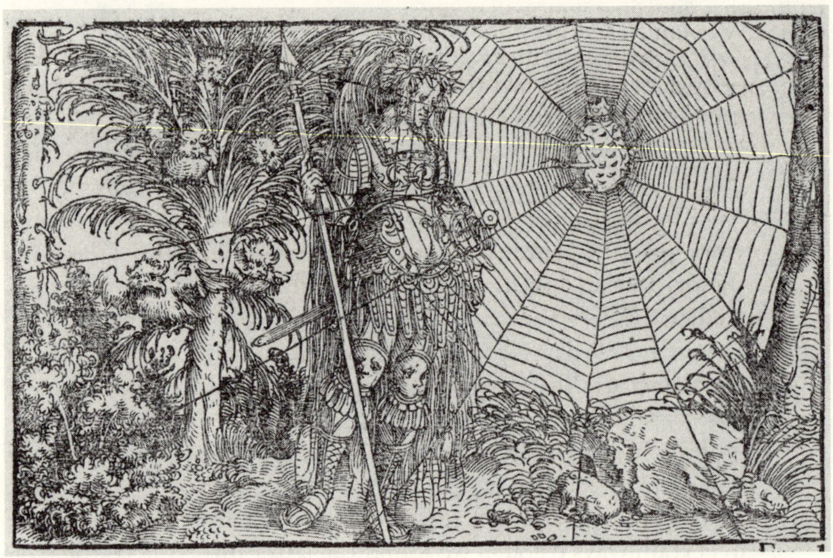

Figure 2.9. Petrarch Master (Hans Weiditz), *Von Verstand*, woodcut from Petrarch, *Von der Artzney bayder Gluck...* (Augsburg, 1532), bk. 1, ch. 7, fol. 7r (Washington, D.C., National Gallery of Art, Rosenwald Collection. Anonymous gift).

so-called Petrarch Master (probably Hans Weiditz the Younger).[24] The woodcut heading up chapter 7 in book 1, titled "Von Verstand" (Of reason), shows a rather disconsolate figure of Pallas Athena, personification of wisdom, standing before an exotic tree in whose foliage nest a number of owls, attributes of the goddess (figure 2.9). Overtaking the wide interval between Athena and the right edge of the composition is a giant web and, at its center, a sickeningly large spider. Petrarch's text makes accounting for the creature easy enough: in antiquity, Reason tells us, it was said that Wisdom was antagonized by the spider because of the cleverness and subtlety with which it spins its web—even though, in their fragility, such webs were no match for Reason's sharp sword. Here, as elsewhere in the book, Petrarch is making no secret of the low opinion in which he holds sophistic argument, the epitome of false reasoning.[25] What is remarkable, however, is the way the web threatens the dominion of Reason that the text proclaims. Spreading over the visual field and nearly flush with the picture plane, its radial threads reach every corner of the space, one of them even appearing to pierce the eyes of the goddess, while three others seem to trace the

orthogonal lines by which the *contrapposto* of the figure is composed. Engulfing the expanse of white surface between the goddess and the tree at the right, the web fractures space and creates a mesmerizing, chiastic depth. Going beyond metaphor, it not only obscures the clear "sight" of reason, it stimulates and maps the beholder's speculative work with the print. As Reindert Falkenburg explains, "the visual rhetoric of the image is directed at a play of shifting, sometimes contradictory, perspectives in the mind of the beholder and reader."[26] Cognitive free play is paradoxically enabled and threatened by a pictorial rhetoric that holds "the mind captivated in a web of visual obstruction."[27]

From its privileged place upon the membrane between pictorial space and the space of the reader, the Petrarch Master's web refracts vision. This operation parallels the effects of Dürer's rhombohedron in certain ways (though we found the latter directing traffic from the heart of the engraving's stage space, rather than its surface). Each motif is metaphorical, but also generative of a receptive activity aimed at breaking the spell of obstruction.

Each motif in its own way, therefore, proclaims its respective picture to be a speculative image. By guiding us toward an alternative, even transformed, way of seeing to which thinking must adapt; by coaxing forth the effort to impose order on chaos, even as that visual order collapses back into disorder, obscuring what had just been clarified, speculative imagery of this kind offers more than an occasion for thought—it holds out the promise of "remedying" the viewer by exposing the contingency of perception and (often false) consolations of belief, casting the beholder back upon his or her own inner resources, training the self to return to itself, to reason.

To describe it more precisely, we might say that this kind of speculation therapy entails the conjoining of two challenges for the beholder: one ethical, the other, for lack of a better term, phenomenological. In the spirit of Petrarch's philosophical-rhetorical project for the care of souls (see the Introduction), Falkenburg sees the Petrarch Master's woodcuts exercising the beholder's ethical judgment in a particular way, "by letting him take the medicine of insight against the illness of quick and superficial judgment regarding good and bad fortune, to which mankind is inclined to succumb."[28] No simple antidote for sorrow is to be found in its opposite, joy, nor could despair ever be remedied by a strong dose of hope: rhetorical therapy

in the Petrarchan mold maintains that the "medicine of insight" works instead by fortifying reason against the illusions wrought by the unfettered rule of the passions and the seductions of the world. Speculative imagery exercises the mind's own natural efficacies, as it were, mobilizing antibodies in the battle against ungovernable attachments and desires.

At another level, the exercise such imagery provides is phenom-enological (in something close to our modern sense of the term). It imposes novel sensory challenges to which cognition must respond, alongside the novel cognitive challenges that reorient perception in turn. In John Dewey's classic formulation from *Art as Experience* (1934), "What is done and what is undergone are . . . reciprocally, cumulatively, and continuously instrumental in each other."[29] Speculation exercises the soul (*anima*) and the mind (*animus*), but never loses touch with the sense perception that sets it in motion in the first place.[30] A con-joining of two modes of therapeutic action, perceptual and ethical, is the common property of all speculative imagery, the foundations and functions of which we will explore further in Chapter 3.

Returning to *Melencolia*, we are better prepared to analyze the second operational motif of visual disturbance to which I alluded earlier: the ladder (figure 2.10). Emerging ambiguously from below, it rises, just as ambiguously, "into the clouds." Recall first our discus-sion of Dürer's polyhedron and the twofold virtuosity—the art of geometry and the science of perspective—that made its subversive effects possible. A perfectly described geometric form that under-mines the certitude of vision is ironic, to say the least; it also shades into the pathological, at least as far as description goes. Does the action of blocking the eye's access into deep horizonal space and refracting it back through the closed circuit of objects express what William Heckscher calls a characteristically "Saturnian preoccupa-tion" with the "dimension and weight as well as [the] quantity and measurement of things"?[31] That is a question of symbolism we can let others decide. Here, we need only establish the visual-rhetorical effect of the ladder.

When Camerarius referred to the object's ambiguous directional-ity and described a figurative reach "into the clouds," he was invoking the whole medieval exaltation of verticality—the religious ego's per-fection, the spirit's purification, the soul's ultimate union with divine wisdom—as well as Neoplatonism's "general picture of a graduated

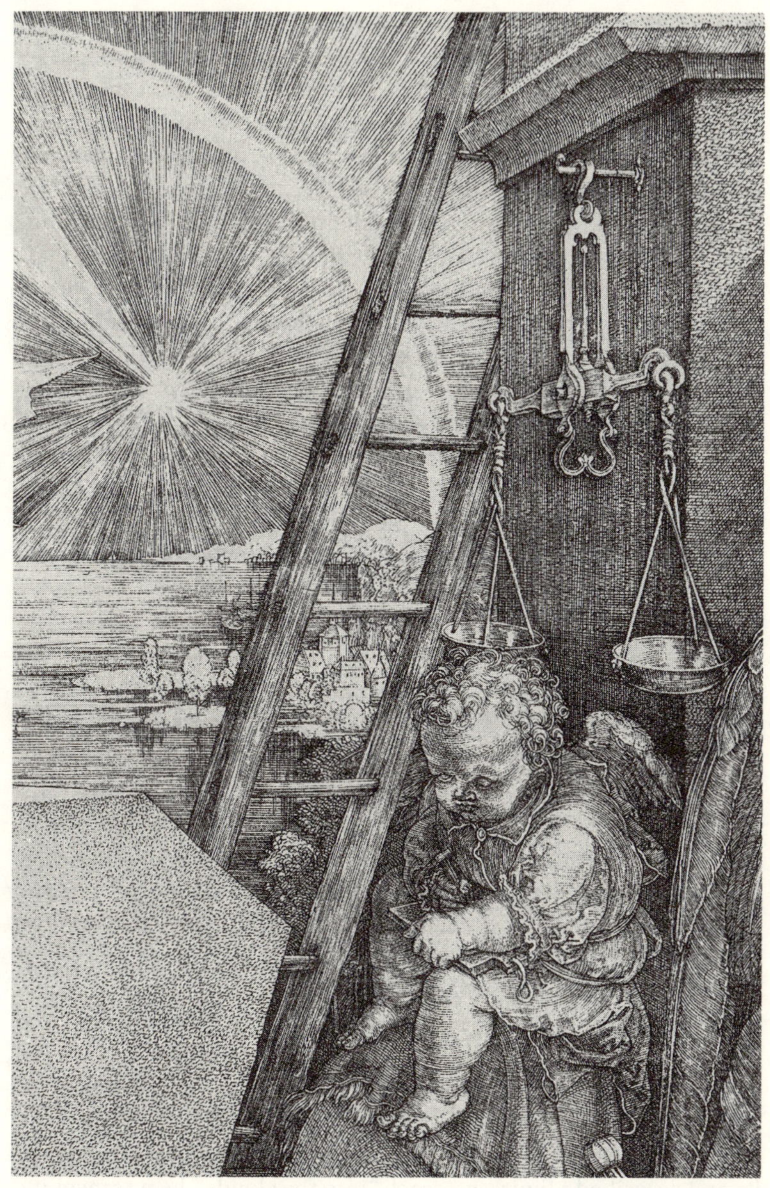

Figure 2.10. Detail from Dürer, *Melencolia I*: ladder rising "into the clouds." (See figure 1.1.)

cosmos," on which all metaphysical speculation depends.[32] At the same time, Camerarius ascribed to Dürer a desire to harness the vertical motif to a diagnosis of "the unrestrained and often disastrously absurd flights of which melancholic minds are capable," as Heckscher has surmised.[33] We have already observed the ladder's ambiguity and recalled Wölfflin's perception that the fragmentary object infuses the whole with an "impure harmony." Both symbol and structuring device, the ladder's special role in troubling vision consists in its strong allusion to an idealized movement, an ascent—the eye and the soul's freedom of passage. Raised to heaven but reaching nowhere, it elegantly condenses the obfuscating chaos of the whole ensemble of tools and implements, each one silently hinting at a creative aspiration that has, by implication in the whole, been rendered useless, "reduced to absurdity."[34] This makes it emblematic of the print's subtle subversion of *ductus* as a metaphorical pathway to conviction.

Such a conclusion would seem to return us to that reading of the print that sees everywhere a critique of intellectual, scientific, and artistic vanities, as if the truest allegory of melancholia would of necessity pathologize all knowledge, including knowledge of itself. But would Dürer—or Camerarius, for that matter—have left the aspirant so bereft of options, so mired in gloomy irresolution? Is melancholy an irrevocable curse, a pathology without a cure, a syndrome beyond remedy? A fuller discussion of melancholia, its identity as both humoral predisposition and mental illness, each with its own "narrative" of onset and intensification and remission, will occupy us in Chapter 4. For the time being, we can work our way into the problem by recalling Heckscher's insight concerning the spiritual striving toward transformation that united medieval and Renaissance spirituality and that fed the Christian humanist concept of perfection: "The path of . . . purification (*Läuterung*) knows, generally speaking, two fundamental possibilities: horizontal and vertical, pilgrimage and ascent."[35] Medieval aesthetics likewise recognized two fundamental pathways for experience: vertical and horizontal, anagogical (mystical) and rhetorical (ethical). By despairing of the attainment of perfection or the beautiful through the mathematical disciplines,[36] and foreclosing on the prospects for a "vertical" enlightenment through earthbound speculation, might Dürer have been urging his audience to attend better to the "horizontal"—to philosophical and creative action for the sake of cultivating virtue in the

here and now, to an open-ended engagement with words and images that amounts to a spiritual exercise, to a therapy of the passions? That Dürer's twilit tableau seems to glimmer with the hope that creativity will resume, that the path toward perfection has not been permanently cordoned off, has been suggested by several commentators.[37] The spark of dawning recognition discernable in the bright eyes of Melancholy—piercing the darkness that envelopes her face, symbolic of the black gall dominating her complexion—already suggests this. But it is, above all, the speculative labor the print demands and almost imposes on its viewer that provides the clearest evidence that a path toward restoration is open.

Speculation and Refreshment

V. A. Kolve has written, "In the Middle Ages to be audience to an 'image' (whether verbal or visual) implied activity, not passivity. It called one to thought, to feeling, to meditation."[38] This is an admirably concise way of reminding us that, in Dürer's time, images meant something only after they instigated something in the beholder—an emotion such as sorrow or joy or pity, the "prick" of conscience that led to an examination of self, the performance of a prayer for help or thanksgiving, and so on. Images also instigated certain kinds of mental activities—chains of associative thinking and memory work, meditative itineraries forged and pursued—activities that could be valued as much for the therapeutic effect of their performance as for the salvific benefit attached to their goal.

With Dürer's print in hand and the allusive clutter of objects and bodies spread before us, we beholders are called upon to work the allegorical puzzle picture as a kind of intellectual-cognitive exercise. Its controlled chaos structures a restless, indeed turbulent movement across the surface of things seen, a movement that mirrors the turbulence of a psyche as it faces the challenges of experience: hardship and loss, misfortune and misery, illness and death, all of which required remediation and consolation through reason.[39] Attracting and repelling the gaze, each object in *Melencolia*'s arsenal invites associations with the human arts, excites expectations about the meaning of things, satisfies learned associations here and there, even as referentiality remains in flux, returning us again and again to "the literal sense of the picture."[40] As we described in the first part of this chapter, movement around the visual field of objects

and bodies in their allusive relationships to one another provokes a virtual movement into the semantic field of symbols and characters—from surface appearance to interior substance—a movement that is ultimately frustrated. The beholder's activity concentrates itself in "working it over" without the requirement of ever quite "working it out." Proposals and counterproposals emerge, but any certification of the whole remains elusive.

To describe the reception process instigated by *Melencolia* in this way makes it clear that we are not dealing with a straightforward instance of an "exchange built on an anticipation of viewer response" for which the medium of prints, in particular, has been credited.[41] Anticipation of response in a general sense is one thing; shaping the rhetorical *ductus* of an image to enable a collaboration between external seeing and mental imaging, cognition and memory, interpretation and inference, is another. What *Melencolia* stimulates and sustains is closely akin, I submit, to what Latin theologians of the Middle Ages called *speculatio*, a natural-philosophical mode of seeing that would, in the course of the fifteenth and sixteenth centuries, become integral to humanist ethical education, Christian naturalism, and secular science.[42]

No summary of the history of speculation in European thought will be attempted here, but it is important to recall its double roots in theological thinking (in particular, the exegesis of Romans 1:20, a tradition effectively inaugurated by Augustine) and German mysticism (here, the most exemplary figure may be the Dominican Heinrich Suso). As Jeffrey Hamburger has shown, both faces of medieval *speculatio* entailed a rejection of dichotomies.[43] Sensory versus suprasensory perception (alternatively described as "seeing" versus "vision" or corporeal versus spiritual sight) is one of these dichotomies; visible nature versus supernatural reality, creation and creator, *signum* and *res*, inner and outer, are others—we need not decide which is primary. The key thing is that speculation always "occupies an intermediary position," according to Hamburger;[44] it traverses these rigid categories and in doing so opens productive pathways for perception, wonder, discovery, and knowledge. This can encompass knowledge of the created world, its plethora of natural phenomena, and its interlaced hierarchies; it may concern knowledge of the moral order underlying human affairs, knowledge of the endless *psychomachia* of opposing forces in the soul (*anima*) and the mind (*animus*), or knowledge of God. When the created world is grasped as a *speculum*,

a mirror of eternal realities, all knowledge, including knowledge of the self, becomes accessible to human perception, but only obliquely. Our grasp of eternal realities, according to Paul in 1 Corinthians (13:12), is enigmatic because of our fallen state. Before the return of the Lord, when we will finally see "face to face," all our knowledge of God and creation will necessarily be "seen through a glass darkly" (*Videmus nunc per speculum in aenigmate*).

All of this makes *speculatio* something like the sine qua non of privileged witnessing in medieval thinking about human sense perception, the receptive intellect, and the limits of both. An imperfect, fragmentary counterpart to the eternal and holistic viewpoint occupied by God in the "the lofty watchtower of his providence . . . embracing the infinite spaces of past and future," as Boethius (ca. 480–524) wrote in the *Consolation of Philosophy*,[45] speculation becomes an Archimedean point that *human* knowing, despite the limits placed on it, could properly hope to occupy. It would therefore come to serve scientific-philosophical method as a technique for reflecting on hidden significances by way of sensory perception, metaphor, symbol, and interpretation, and as a "primary framework" for "reflection on the epistemology of mystical experience and on the place of nature, perception, and vision within Christian soteriology."[46] Finally, something like it became, in the hands of ambitious poets and painters, an interpretative activity with reflexive, ethical-spiritual aims, both lofty and down-to-earth. Speculation prompted by the poetic or visual work of art could aim toward to higher knowledge, for example, in the experience of anagogical ascent attested by many monastic writers. At the same time, as a method for comprehending the incomprehensible, for coping with complexity, speculation might be valued as an occasion for the exercise of mental faculties. "Obscurity announces a particular sort of meditation game," Mary Carruthers writes about the medieval attraction to the aesthetically difficult. "Like all games, it is to be enjoyed for its own sake and also—since conferring a benefit helps to license one's enjoyment—for the salubrious exercising and strengthening of one's wits."[47]

Given this complex history of the term, to speak of the "speculative" character of *Melencolia* or any work of art (see Chapter 3), presents several dangers of misunderstanding, so let me be clear what I am *not* arguing before closing this chapter. I am not arguing that the engraving invites the beholder to penetrate the symbolic-allegorical

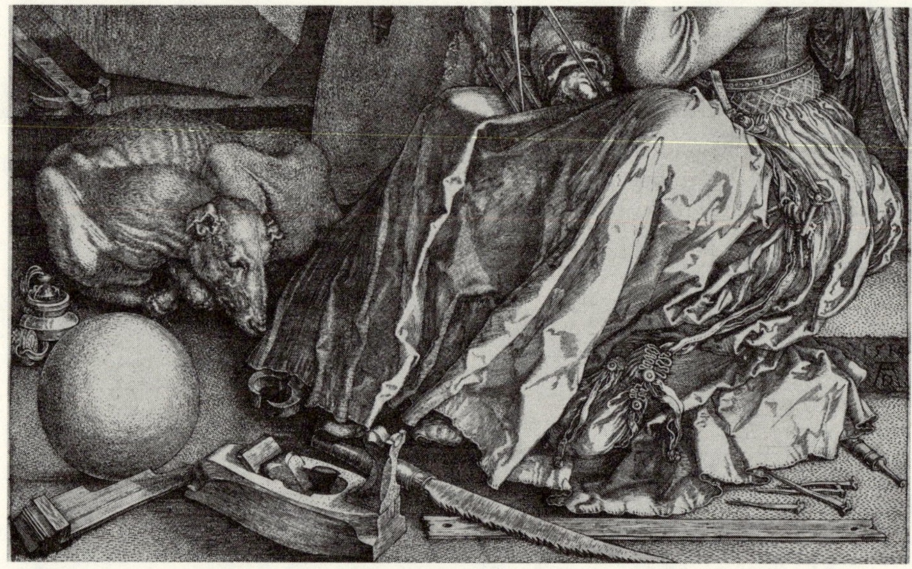

Figure 1.2. Detail from Dürer, *Melencolia I*: tools at the feet of Melancholy. (See figure 1.1.)

almost forgotten; half hidden beneath Melancholy's robe, nearby some nails, is a syringe, or perhaps it is the tip of a bellows? Other things are deposited in the little interstices between the larger forms: a template for making moldings is visible in the picture's lowest left corner, then an inkpot, and then a hammer (figure 1.2). On the far side of the monolith sits some kind of ceramic brazier, possibly a smelting crucible, with another vessel nesting in it, surrounded by flickering flames. And there's still more to the clutter! A ladder rising from somewhere out of view is propped against the windowless building, of which nothing can be seen above its cornice. Hanging from a bracket secured to the wall is a balance, while an hourglass crowned by a sundial and a bell are secured to the cornice itself. Below the bell, set into a shallow niche in the wall above Melancholy's head—her wing seems to reach toward it—appears a square numerical chart, divided into sixteen equal cells. Over a seaside town in the distance a rainbow arcs across the horizon, while a celestial body—some see a comet, others the planet Saturn—blasts its radiance in every direction.[1] From out of nowhere, a bat flutters into view. On outstretched wings, it heralds the theme of this dreamlike tableau and offers up the picture's ostensible title: *MELENCOLIA I.*

An "Allegory of Deep, Speculative Thought"

"Dürer is symbolically perfect," Langdon was saying as they followed the trail of illuminated EXIT signs. "He was the ultimate Renaissance mind—artist, philosopher, alchemist, and a lifelong student of the Ancient Mysteries. To this day, nobody fully understands the messages hidden in Dürer's art. . . ."

Katherine stopped abruptly and looked at Langdon. "Robert, *Melencolia I* is here in Washington. It hangs in the National Gallery."

"Yes," he said with a smile, "and something tells me that's not a coincidence."

—Dan Brown, *The Lost Symbol*

A Chaos of Objects

A collection of objects and beings has come to rest in a place both intimate and strange, a stone construction platform at the base of windowless structure, the whole installation perched high above a darkened seascape (figure 1.1). There sits a brooding winged genius in thick, luxurious dress, her bright eyes piercing the shadows that envelope her face, her head crowned with a leafy garland and pressed against a clenched fist. A closed book lies in Melancholy's lap, and, next to it, a compass barely gripped, nearly robbed of its purpose. Next to her, seated on a millstone, a putto is writing or carving with a tool of some sort; head bowed, he concentrates on the tablet he holds in his lap, while a lanky hunting dog curls in fitful slumber at their feet. Around the three companions are a scatter of implements and contrivances, tools, and devices: a sphere that seems to have just rolled from the lap of the despondent genius, and on the opposite side of the dog, a strange monolith carved of stone—or is it crystal?—set precariously on its narrowest edge. Then the sprawl of tools: a ruler, a handsaw, a plane, and pincers, all lying discarded,

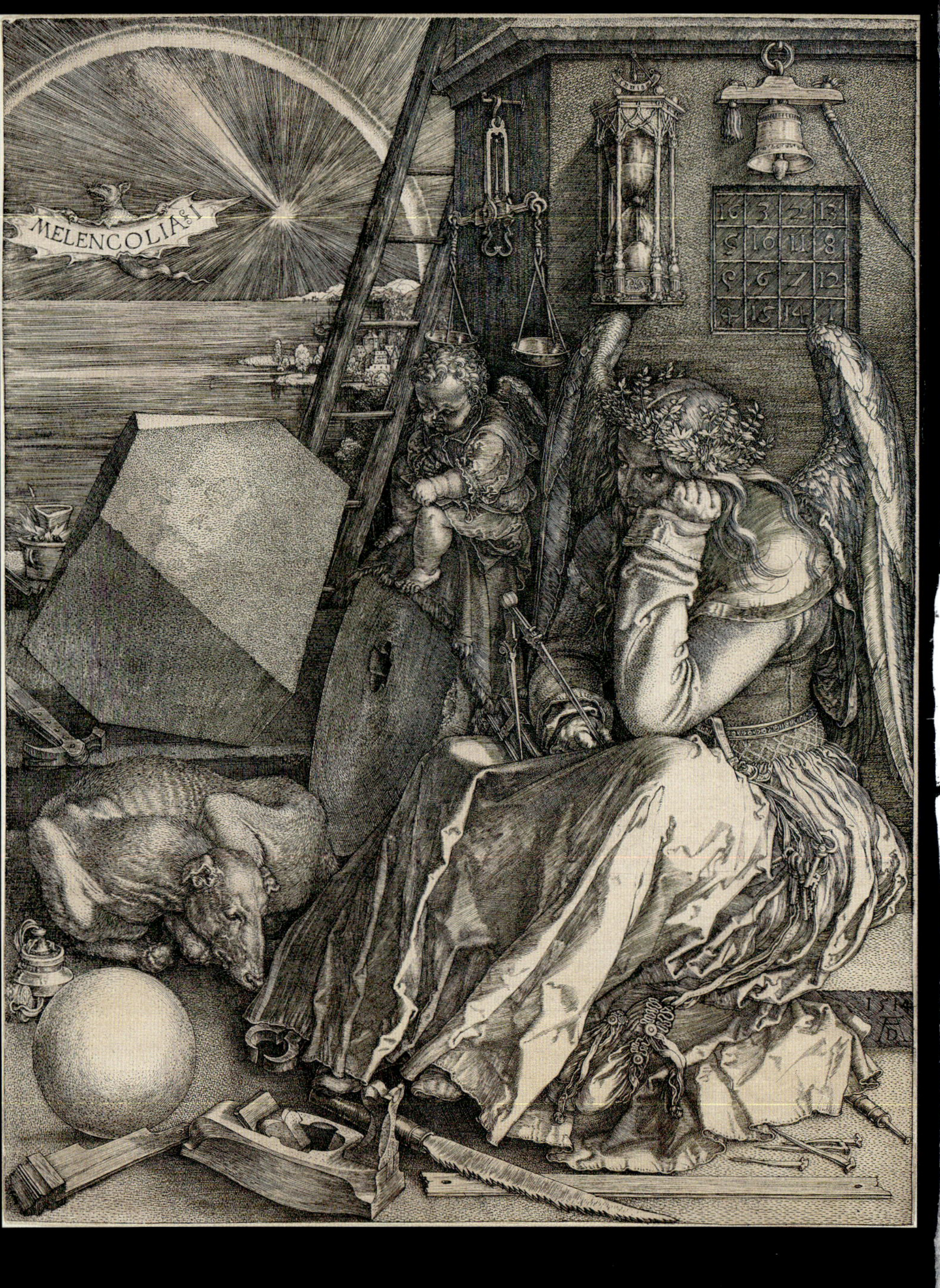

MELENCOLIA § I
16 3 2 13
5 10 11 8
9 6 7 12
4 15 14 1
1514

surface in order to arrive at a comprehension of higher realities, hidden significances, and mutual affinities. Unless I am completely wrong about this, the beholder is not being called upon to enact a Neoplatonic ascent from the sensible world to the sphere of the intelligible, from the visible to the invisible (*per visibilia ad invisibilia*), nor are we being asked to recognize the picture as a "symbolic form" in the Cassirean sense. Iconographical scholarship on our engraving has been there and done that, ad nauseum, leaving Dürer's masterpiece not simply worse for wear, but colonized by cliché, "historiographically ravaged," as a fellow traveler once confided.[48] Speculation as an interpretative activity is more protean than all that. Like the medieval work marked by an often perplexing diversity and *varietas,* or the paradigmatic "unfinished" Renaissance work, perpetually in motion, the speculative image is as inherently open-ended as the human mind is constantly active. And herein lies its potential for refreshment, its capacity to assist in rebalancing and bringing about a "cure." As the Benedictine Peter of Celle (d. 1183) once reminded his readers, no doubt with the ancient identification of melancholia with *acedia,* or spiritual apathy, in mind: "if the soul is thus compassed about with such a harmonious variety, it will avoid boredom and receive its cure."[49] As an instrument and an exercise, speculative imagery as we are describing it here was too invested in its own operations to rest satisfied with fixed meanings wherever they might appear, too suspicious of the vision of a "stable, compartmented world"[50] to conform to the classical rules of allegory (see Chapter 1). If speculation carries thought toward recognition of an order within the fertile chaos of things, that vision of order will always be provisional, its power to illuminate always probationary.

Taking this in a postmodern spirit and describing speculation as a technique of knowing doomed to indeterminacy would be misleading, however. This is the second thing I'm not arguing. All disciplinary therapeutics—magical, medical, moral, penitential, and so on—share a belief that the syndromes they treat are in fact treatable, that the subject can be "moved" from one state, defined as illness or imbalance, to another, defined as health or proper functioning. So it is with speculation as spiritual-ethical exercise. Just as crucial to realize is the fact that for Renaissance humanists from Petrarch onward, the salutary effects provided by even the best moral and rhetorical therapies were never permanent. One always had to make do with "certain modest steps... toward health," as Petrarch put it in his dedicatory letter to Azzo da Corregio that prefaces *De remediis*, and simply keep at it.[51] And it bears repeating that for Renaissance artists, too, for men such as Dürer and Leonardo, "indeterminacy" (had they even a word for it) was not about condemning the beholder to endless wandering in the labyrinth of meaning, bereft of all purpose. It was, rather, to call attention to the inexorable flux of time and things, to permit the "vagueness" of semiexistence to spur the creative imagination (see the epigram for this chapter); to let perception itself become the spark that sets things in motion. This view was a natural correlative to the humanist effort to overcome the medieval antagonism of the *vita contemplativa* and the *vita activa* and to replace it, as the authors of *Saturn and Melancholy* argued, with a conception of intellectual inquiry as constituting its own form of activity: "vita contemplativa sive studiosa."[52] Humanism brought with it "a fundamentally altered way of living... the ideal of the speculative life, in which the 'sovereignty of the human mind' seemed to be most nearly realised; for only the 'vita contemplativa' is based on the self-reliance and self-sufficiency of a process of thought which is its own justification."[53] To enter upon the kinesis of speculative labor is therefore to affirm reason and imagination's *ethical* roles in the cultivation of virtue as a search for spiritual truths. Practicing discernment as an end itself would bring the passions under control and exercise the higher faculties, pointing toward the restoration of healthy functioning, thus flourishing.

Our effort so far has been to reconceive Dürer's great "enigma" as an allegorical image that, for all the learning poured into it, defeats the best efforts to stabilize any particular form of disciplinary knowledge or art to which it may refer. In this sense, *Melencolia* may be counted among those cultural documents attesting to a generalized "crisis of allegory" in the Renaissance.[54] We have taken this insight further, however, in seeing the refusal of symbolic closure as a deliberate strategy to keep speculative activity going, wherein this natural human activity becomes a form of ethical-spiritual exercise—a good in itself—so long as the print remained, so to speak, in the beholder's hands. In different ways, the chapters that follow will pursue this conception of *Melencolia* as representing a new genre of Christian ethical art directed toward therapeutic ends.

Some of these therapeutic expectations are metaphorical, while others, we will see, are undeniably concrete and practical. For melancholia, as a "physically-conditioned sickness of the soul" (Klibansky, Panofsky, and Saxl), was a syndrome with a complex and fugitive identity, resistant to straightforward diagnosis and requiring a flexible regimen of combined therapies to combat it: medical, psychological, and magical. Later, we will see the importance assigned to a modulated exercise of the cognitive faculties among the various prescriptions medical writers, ancient and medieval, offered for treating melancholia in both its morbid and milder forms (Chapter 4). The promise of an emotional and intellectual "clarification"—in a word, a type of *katharsis*—embedded in the engraving's germinal narrative will also come under scrutiny. For only when the suffering soul experiences itself *in time*, in the flow between memory, presence, and anticipation of the future, can a "return to self" and a remedy of melancholy be envisioned. Following that discussion, we will be considering the evidence that Dürer, the self-styled Christian-humanist painter, poet, and preceptor of the arts, was uniquely motivated among his peers to assume the mantle of the Petrarchan *medicus*, to draw upon the medical analogy and cast the vocation of the Christian artist in similar terms and therefore to see his imagery as a kind of medicine, efficacious when properly applied (Chapters 5 and 6).

Ultimately, when we return to *Melencolia*, we will see it more vividly as a kind of alternative to the traditional Christian "meditative image," one that is not devotional, strictly speaking, but speculative—geared toward self-examination and self-transformation, offering a kind of homeopathic treatment by proxy for the suffering soul. This notion of a therapy by proxy, critical to my argument, must be set within the full constellation of therapeutic expectations and meanings in which Dürer's art became intelligible in its own time. Mapping that larger constellation is the task of the following chapter.

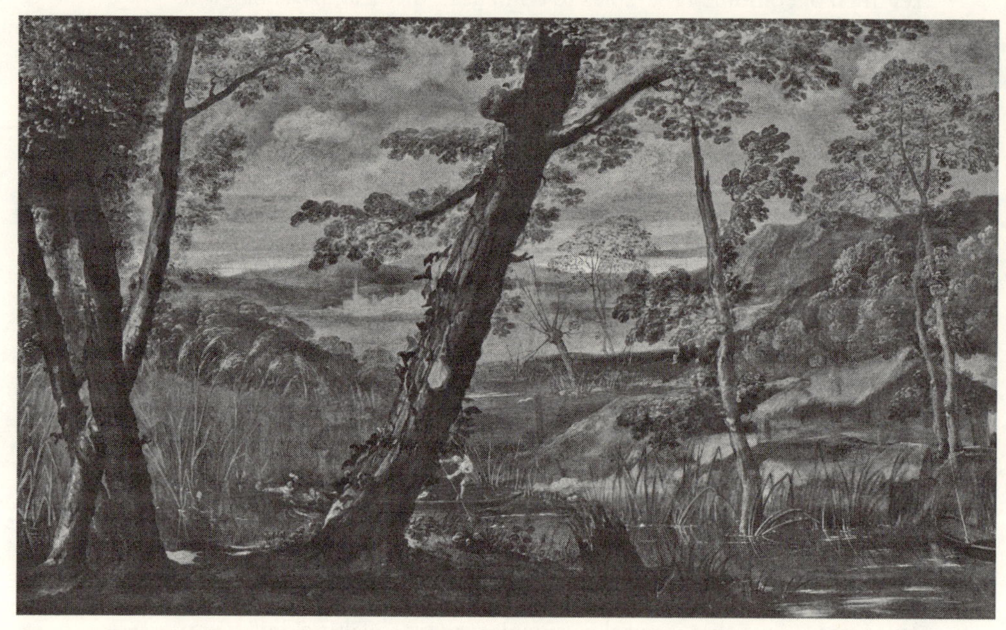

Figure 3.1. Annibale Caracci, *River Landscape*, ca. 1590, oil on canvas, 88.3 x 148.1 cm (Washington, D.C., National Gallery of Art, Samuel H. Kress Collection).

Therapies of the Image
in the Age of Dürer

Now of all motions that is the best which is produced in a thing by itself, for it is most akin to the motion of thought and of the universe, but that motion which is caused by others is not so good, and worst of all is that which moves the body, when at rest, in parts only and by some agency alien to it. . . . And this holds also of the constitution of diseases; if anyone regardless of the appointed time tries to subdue them by medicine, he only aggravates and multiplies them. Wherefore we ought always to manage them by regimen, as far as man can spare the time.

—Plato, *Timaeus* 89a–d

To trace the changing relationships between the imaginative arts and the wide array of practices and pursuits that have counted as therapies for the body, mind, or soul would be too great a task for a single study, let alone one chapter. Material evidence bearing on the *historical* problem of the therapeutic image as a functional category within the domain of the visual includes such a diversity of artifacts, contexts, and situated behaviors that the question of appropriate models and categories for analysis begins to look quite vexed, even when we narrow our focus to the uses and efficacies of images in the world Dürer and his patrons inhabited. What do we mean when referring to a picture, or any other kind of visual representation, as "therapeutic"? Are we always, necessarily, speaking metaphorically, as when a philosopher refers to a persuasive argument as "medicine"? Have we already stepped irrevocably into the vast territory of magical thinking and behaviors, expectations of efficacy that cross the divide of natural and supernatural worlds?[1] Or can we find therapeutic expectations attaching themselves to aesthetic objects in patently unmetaphorical and unmagical ways? How are such expectations to be distinguished from one another? Are there particular genres of art that deserve to be called therapeutic, and what interpretive advantages come with describing them so?

Before casting back to the long cultural history of the therapeutic image before Dürer, we might consider one telling chapter in this history that unfolded during his lifetime, with no small contribution from the Nuremberg master himself: the emergence of landscape as an independent genre of art, and its concurrent use as a therapeutic resource. Art historians tend to discuss the invention of landscape in terms of Renaissance perspective and the optical conquest of space; the protoscientific description of natural phenomena; the growth of artistic specialization in cities such as Antwerp; the effect of Italian art theory's terms and categories on scene painting; or changes in cartographic representation.[2] Less well examined are the ways early landscape painting could be enlisted within practical regimens aimed at health and hygiene. The art historian Frances Gage has recently called our attention in this regard to the writings of the Sienese physician Giulio Mancini (1559–1630), who during his career served as personal physician to several cardinals in Rome. An energetic advocate of the works of the Caracci (figure 3.1) — writing about them for benefit of Italian collectors — Mancini also espoused a lifelong admiration for the works of Dürer. Both his connoisseurial and medical advice were aimed at aristocrats. Building on predecessors such as Marsilio Ficino, who recommended music and figural art as sources of comfort to melancholics,[3] Mancini in particular promoted the benefits of outfitting private galleries with landscape paintings as an alternative method for exercising the natural coordination of body, eyes, and mind. This recommendation extended his belief in the health benefits of open-air walking, both in nature and through architectural passages. In Gage's considered view, Mancini's therapeutic conception of beholding landscape represented "a major force in the development of princely art collecting in the sixteenth and seventeenth centuries."[4]

Mancini's recommendations were anything but idiosyncratic for his time; Robert Burton (1577–1640), for example, in his encyclopedic *Anatomy of Melancholy* (1621), advised the melancholic who wished to be "eased of his griefe" to visit "those well furnished Cloisters and Galleries of the Roman cardinals, so richly stored with all moderne Pictures, old Statues and Antiquities."[5] Such prescriptions are choice expressions of what Gage calls a "pre-Cartesian philosophy of the unity of the body and soul that provided a foundation for the belief that the exercise of the mind produced somatic effects, and that the viewing of art might be therapeutic."[6] In the course of this chapter, we will come to better appreciate how the image could be reckoned a distinctive resource for alleviating the disturbances of the soul, the mind, and by extension, the body—indeed, the "whole nature of man" as it was understood by Christian natural philosophy.[7]

Yet it is also crucial to see that landscape could become such a therapeutic resource—and this is my key point—only where it was engaged under specific conditions of viewing, as an instrument in an overall practice or, to use Michel Foucault's term, a technology of the self. Landscape enlists the beholder in a form of virtual exercise by virtue of both its consoling subject matter—trees and other greenery, clear-running streams and pools —and its immersive visual structure. When properly exploited for the curative properties of what it showed and the restorative possibilities of what it invited, landscape became, in other words, a natural extension of other forms of hygiene, self-cultivation, and training for life. In Mancini's world, in courtly life especially, that training meshed with the ideal of an upright physical comportment, the proper alignment of spine, shoulders, neck, and head necessary for skillful equitation and fencing. This body image was advanced not only as a moral ideal of civility (that is, "rectitude") and graceful appearance, but also as a matter of health and optimal functioning.[8]

The idea of the landscape image as a virtual space for meditative renewal, thus an occasion for mental and spiritual hygiene, was likewise not altogether new in Mancini's time. In discussing the categories of imagery proper to the decoration of buildings and interiors, Leon Battista Alberti, in his *Ten Books on Architecture* (ca. 1450 and first published in 1486), called special attention to the cheering effect of "the sight of paintings depicting the delightful countryside, harbours, fishing, hunting, swimming, and games of shepherds—flowers and verdure." Venturing further in the same chapter, he offers up the landscape painter's vision for its restorative, psychosomatic effects, prescribing natural imagery for fever, dryness, and insomnia:

> Those who suffer from fever are offered much relief by the sight of painted
> fountains, rivers and running brooks, a fact which anyone can put to the test;
> for if by chance he lies in bed one night unable to sleep, he need only turn his

imagination on limpid waters and fountains which he had seen at one time or another, or perhaps some lake, and his dry feeling will disappear all at once and sleep will come upon him as the sweetest of slumbers.[9]

Between the time of this passage and Mancini's medical recommendations, the symbolic interpretation of nature painting and its thematization as an arena for spiritual self-cultivation had already gained ground among landscape specialists and their patrons. In the work of Antwerp artist Joachim Patinir (ca. 1480–1524), called "the good landscape painter" by his close friend Dürer,[10] wending roads and virtual pathways through geographic space updated the medieval topos of a "pilgrimage of life" through a sinful world, and thereby offered flexible opportunities for "mental pilgrimage" and related spiritual exercises (figure 3.2).[11] Sixteenth-century and seventeenth-century heirs to this tradition developed these associations further. Jan Brueghel's (1568–1625) allegorical images of sea voyages and rural traffic, for example, have been persuasively linked by Leopoldine Prosperetti to a neo-Stoic ideal of speculative retreat, an imaginative *otium* that promised spiritual regeneration.[12] Here again, we find the tasks given to landscape imagery by painters and patrons not confined to representing nature, symbolizing the cosmos, or even merely simulating outdoor experience, but functioning in an open, creative interaction with other practices, meditative, philosophical, and hygienic, to offer their users an alternative, and renewable, therapeutic resource. Ethical-spiritual introspection, speculative free play with the endless *varietas* of God's creation,[13] the exercise of one's natural faculties, release from worldly attachments and the pull of the lower passions, the return of the self to reason, to human flourishing and "happiness" (Aristotle's εὐδαιμονία, *eudaimonia*)—these kinds of benefits could be unleashed with the right kind of attention "within" the landscape image, an attention to *world* that merged with an attention to *self*.

This conception of the image as a virtual space of speculative movement and spiritual exercise parallels the mode of therapy we have attributed to Dürer's *Melencolia*. When actively taken up by its beholders—and one class of beholders in particular, as we will see in the following chapter—the therapeutic image instigates a practical activity, provokes a change in thinking, effects a shift in perspective, removes blockages, and opens new pathways to health. How far back can we trace such notions? Are they confined to the higher echelons of learned

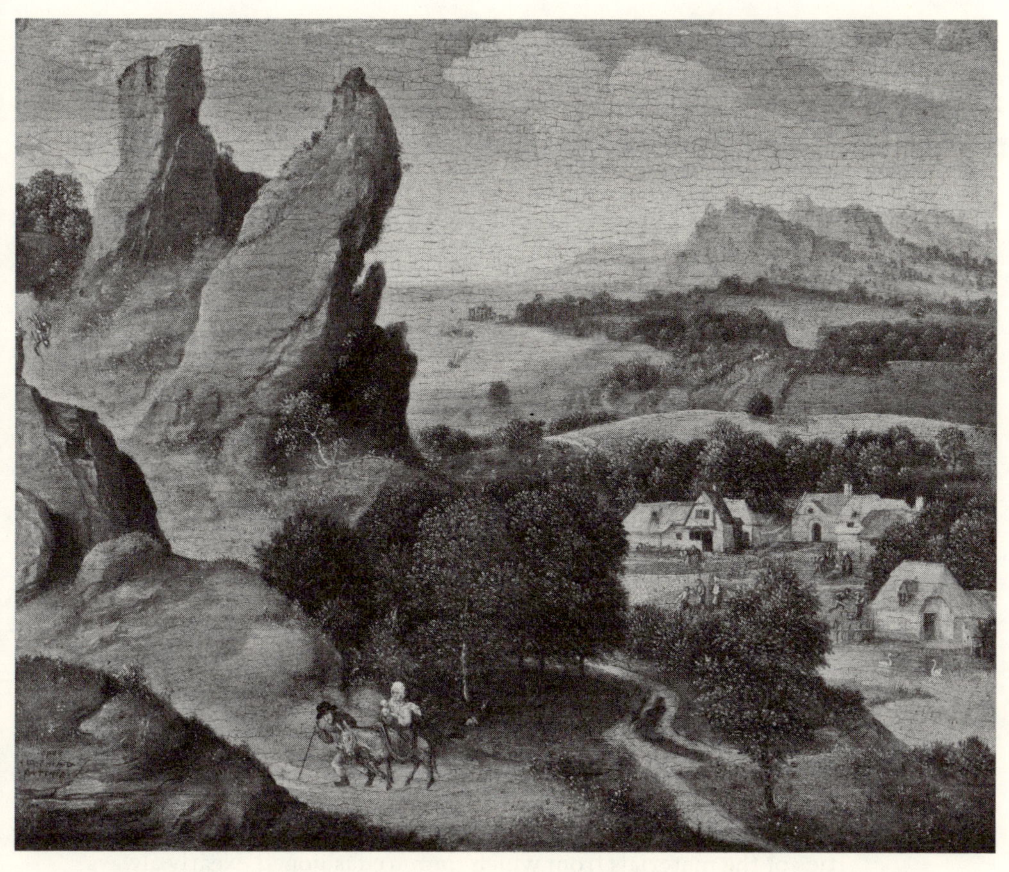

Figure 3.2. Joachim Patinir, *Flight into Egypt*, ca. 1510–15, oil on panel, 29.3 x 33.3 cm (Antwerp, Koninklijk Museum voor Schone Kunsten/Royal Museum of Fine Arts, inv. 64) (photo: Scala/Art Resource, NY).

culture? When Burton needed support for his contention that melancholics might find relief in the beholding of pictures, he appealed to the first-century philosopher Dio Chrysostom (ca. 40–after 112), who attributed a medicinal efficacy to the works of the sculptor Phidias: "if any man be sickly, troubled in mind, or . . . cannot sleep for griefe, and shall but stand over against one of . . . [his] images, he will forget all care, or whatsoever else may molest him in an instant."[14] Collective perceptions of the efficacy of images is ancient, and the *longue durée* of its history defies summary, so we must begin with a more limited question: What kind of efficacy are we talking about?

Inherent Efficacies

The intimate connection between the treatment of human suffering and material making, the making of images specifically, constitutes an enduring theme in the history of religion and culture.[15] Ancient societies took for granted the therapeutic efficacy of certain kinds of crafted objects and counted on their power, alongside natural forces, to bring about health and protection when properly applied—much as we trust in the properties of our favorite analgesic, taken in the correct dosage, to alleviate a headache or lower a fever. Anthropologists and medical archaeologists can cite hundreds of parallel examples of protective amulets, wands, talismans, and fetishes across the globe—from red coral necklaces worn around the neck to *mezuzot* posted on doorposts—whose power to banish disease and ensure health depends on word magic, image magic, or the natural properties of the materials from which they are fashioned. Nearly always some form of human agency, some ritual performance, is required to mobilize an object's natural healing powers or to invoke supernatural assistance in order to produce the desired effect.

The mobilization of mimetic images to secure benefits—for example, the banishing of illness—has long presented a special problem to researchers, who differ on the question of whether the "likeness" struck between the affliction's cure and its cause is what ensures the better kind of magic, whether the essential logic is sympathetic ("like cures like"), antipathetic (cure by the law of contraries), or amuletic (protective, from the Latin *amulētum*). A stone pendant plaque from Mesopotamia, dated to around 700 BCE and today in New York, was once the focus of this kind of imitative image magic (figure 3.3). With crisply carved contours and incised lines, it depicts

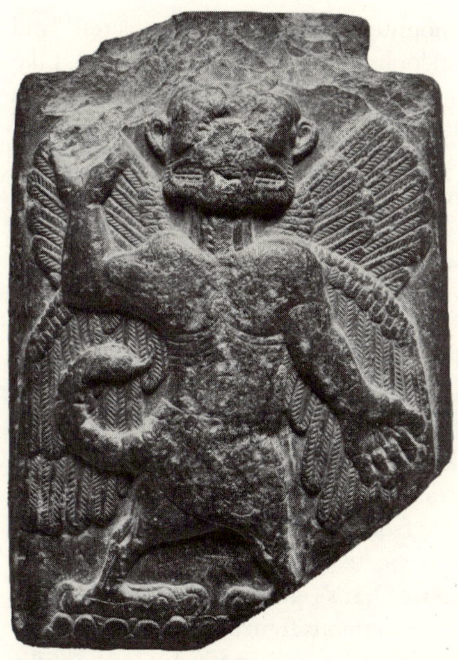

Pazuzu, hybrid king of the wind demons, whose image provided powerful protection against disease-bearing winds from the west, which were associated with the malevolent demon Lamashtu. Pregnant women were the special targets of Lamashtu's wrath. In ancient Near Eastern cultures, this wrath was imagined—millennia before the modern understanding of disease contagion—as a malevolent airborne attack. By invoking the protective deity and welcoming his presence, images such as this offered a magical prophylaxis, ensuring reproductive health and hence survival.

Even those ancient cultures that disavowed the use of cult images and attributed all healing power to God found ways to affirm the power of images, allowing that representation could become medicinal. Complaining of thirst and hunger in the desert and doubting their deliverance, the Israelites were punished, according to the story told in Numbers, with "seraph serpents" sent by God to afflict them (Numbers 21:4–9). When Moses prayed and God answered, the therapeutic solution was image-based. A bronze effigy of the self-same serpent was to be mounted on a pole, God instructed, "and if anyone who has been bitten looks at it, he will recover" (21:8). Like cures like (*similia similibus curantur*)—the source of healing stands in the closest possible relationship to the natural form of the affliction. Interpreted typologically by the evangelist John (3:14–15), who declared the brazen serpent to be a figure for the Crucified who rescues the faithful from death ("And as Moses lifted up the serpent in the desert, so must the Son of man be lifted up: That whosoever believeth in him, may not perish; but may have life everlasting"), the Old Testament legend deposited a sympathetic power at the heart of the mimetic image—both for Judaism, which abhors the enchantment of material images, and Christianity, which embraces it.[16]

A more complex mode of efficacy for ensuring women's health was offered by objects such as the carved amulet from Byzantine Egypt (sixth to seventh century), also in New York (figure 3.4).[17] An inscription running across the entire front surface and concluding on the reverse excerpts the story first reported in Mark's gospel (5:25–34), and then reprised in Luke (8:43–48), of Jesus's encounter with the woman "under an issue of blood" (an anonymous figure enshrined in medieval legend as the *haemorrhissa* and variously associated with the saints Martha and Veronica). Emerging in relief amongst the carved words, Christ is shown making a blessing gesture over the woman depicted at the moment she "fell down before him," there to testify that merely touching his garments had stopped her hemorrhages. On the reverse side, we see a female figure—perhaps the sanctified patient, perhaps the amulet's intended owner, in a sense, both—who stands upright in thanksgiving and prayer. Precisely how the amulet was used, how word and image might have been ritually activated to transfer healing virtue to the object's owner, remains a matter of conjecture, but two things are clear. First, a type of Graeco-Roman magical amulet used to aid the womb (ὑστέρα, *hystera*), a type that often juxtaposed a central face radiating serpents with an inscription and produced in a wide variety of materials, has here been updated and Christianized.[18] Second, the physical matrix of the object contributed something of its own efficacious charge. The gemstone heliotrope (aka bloodstone), a variety of jasper with inclusions of reddish hematite, was extolled by ancient writers such as Pliny the Elder (d. 79 CE) and medieval commentators such as Albertus Magnus (d. 1280) for its special virtue in preserving vitality and youth.[19] These writers understood that blood

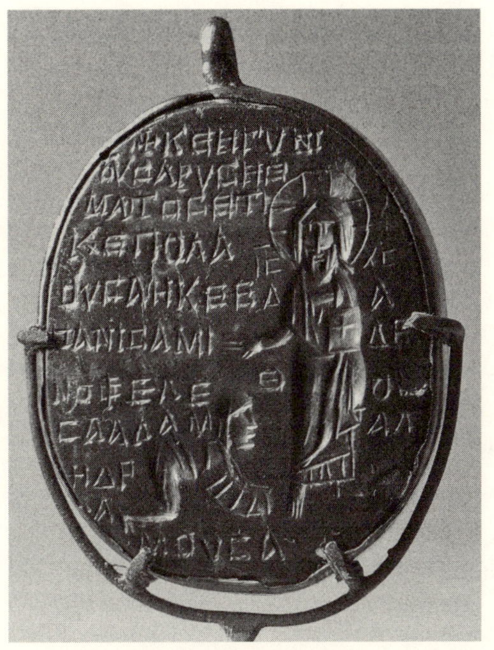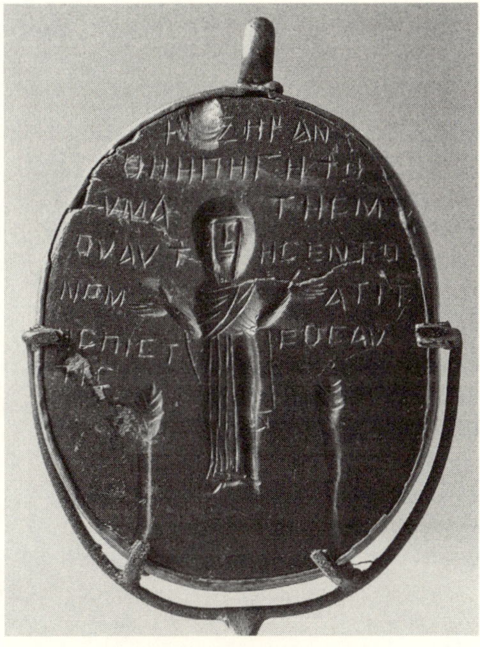

Figure 3.4. Byzantine Egypt (Coptic), amulet with Christ and the woman with the issue of blood (obverse) and orant figure (reverse), sixth–seventh century, carved hematite with silver mount, overall dimensions 5 x 3.7 x 1 cm (hematite portion: 4.8 x 3.6 x 1 cm) (New York, Metropolitan Museum of Art. Gift of J. Pierpont Morgan) (photo courtesy of the Metropolitan Museum of Art, www.metmuseum.org).

diseases found effective treatment in hematite because of its appearance and because, according to Pliny, it "gives off a blood-red smear" when rubbed (correlative to the healing power attributed to rust, the *antipathia* of iron, the metal whose "death" brings it into being).[20] Thus did perceptions of the amulet's magical matter, together with its incantatory legend and its image of Christ in his role as *medicus*, ensure its overall, we might say its holistic, therapeutic effect.

Protection, aid, blessing, cure—the wide range of efficacies ascribed to late antique gems is expressed in the inscription so many of them bore: *sphragis theou*, which carried the double meaning of "god's seal" and "god's medicine," according to Véronique

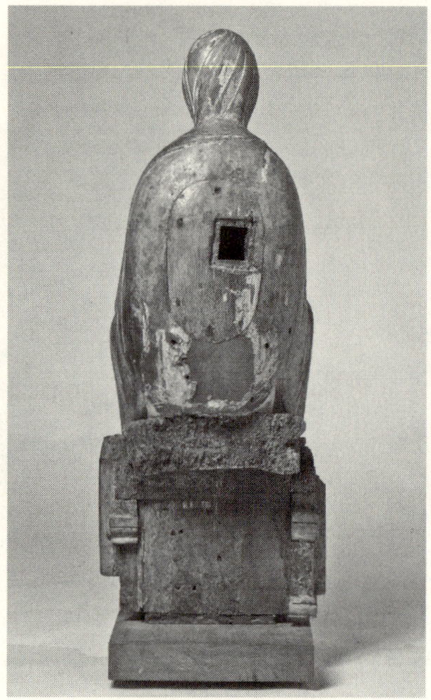

Figure 3.5. Ottonian, *Madonna of Bishop Imad of Paderborn*, reverse side showing depository for relics, ca. 1051–58, limewood, oak, and traces of polychromy and gilding, 112 x 45 x 52 cm (Paderborn, Erzbischöfliches Diözesansmuseum Paderborn) (photo: Ansgar Hoffmann).

Dasen.[21] The practice of fixing amulets to the body—expressed in the Greek terms *periammata* and *periapta*, likewise the Latin *ligatura* or *alligatura*, meaning "what's attached around"[22]—did not change when saints replaced pagan gods as the guarantors of heavenly medicine.

In premodern Christianity the most potent reserves of healing power were earthbound and accessible at particular cult sites, shrines, or "holy places" (*loca sancta*), whose reputations were spread by the pilgrims who journeyed to them, regionally and transregionally, for cures.[23] At such places, homeopathic thinking joined hands with collective perceptions of supernatural agency in effecting miraculous remedies. Pilgrims encountered an array of sanctified objects at the shrine and learned a variety of ways to access their inherent powers. Like the tomb or reliquary *châsse* of a saint, a cult statue of the Virgin Mary that housed relics in its body—our example is the eleventh-century *Imad Madonna* now in Paderborn—was believed to be suffused with a healing potency (figure 3.5).[24] Such

86

virtues could be accessed directly through human touch or transferred and made portable through various media. Cloths might be wiped over holy objects and carried away as "contact relics" (*brandea*); water, oil, or wine poured over them might be consumed or carried away in small vessels as another kind of "blessing" (*eulogia*).

A broad category of cult images lent themselves to a therapy that was quasi-sacramental in nature. Certain devotional images, especially those replicating famous relics such as Veronica's sudarium (figure 3.6), offered salvific benefits that could be accessed through touch or just as directly through vision. To describe the belief in the magical efficacy of looking at holy things, an earlier generation of German researchers coined the term "salvific seeing" (*heilbringende Schau*) and named the mode of piety that privileged it "visual devotion" (*Schaudevotion*).[25] Visual touching not only brought the supplicant closer to the sources of power, they argued, it actualized pious desire, and this desire was thought capable of accessing divine presence wherever it inhered in material things. What cult images provided was a visual equivalent to the Eucharistic bread, an "efficacious sign" that offered the carnal senses, over against their inherent limitations, something like a foretaste of the perfect heavenly manna enjoyed by the Blessed in eternity. To call the consecrated bread and wine "medicine of the soul" was no mere metaphor. "Vision meant incorporation and eventual self-transformation," explains one recent study of sacramental healing through images, and "seeing in such a manner implicated the psychosomatic unity of the person."[26]

Holy matter of all kinds, not the Eucharist alone, was felt to be charged with distinctive healing properties; such notions were easily transferred to the most inventive and colorful of folk *sacramentalia*. A charmingly literal type of Eucharistic substitute is the sheet of engraved *Schluckbildchen*, or "little image tablets," from seventeenth-century Bavaria, small engravings printed on the reverse side of a decorative mélange of blossoms, fruit, and birds, signed by the Master I. E. (figure 3.7). Believed by some folklorists to be intended for sick cattle, these detachable, swallowable, mix-and-match miniatures of the Holy Mantle of Christ (venerated at Trier), Veronica's image-bearing sudarium (a Roman relic), Charlemagne's ivory hunting horn (Aachen), and the icon known as the "Mother of God with the Inclined Head" (a *Gnadenbild* worshipped in Landshut), were surely deemed therapeutic for humans as well.[27]

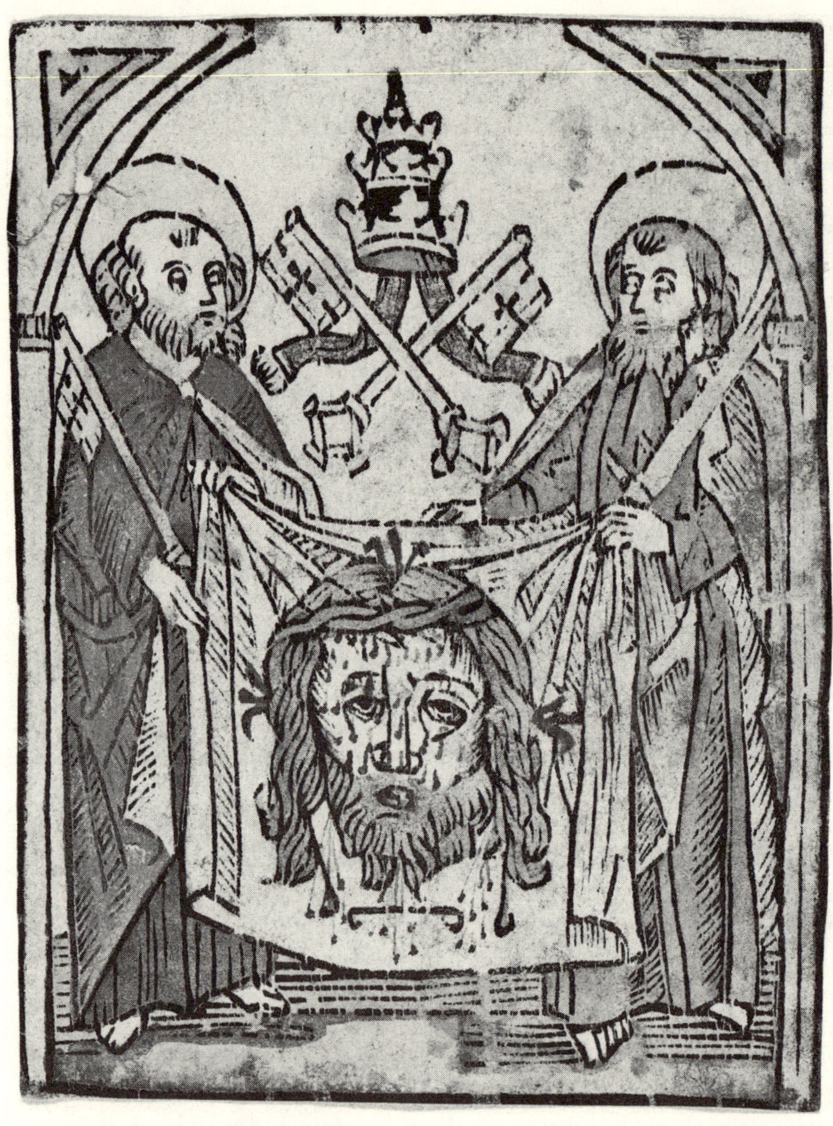

Figure 3.6. German, *Saints Peter and Paul Displaying the Sudarium Relic*, ca. 1475, hand-colored woodcut (Washington, D.C., National Gallery of Art, Rosenwald Collection).

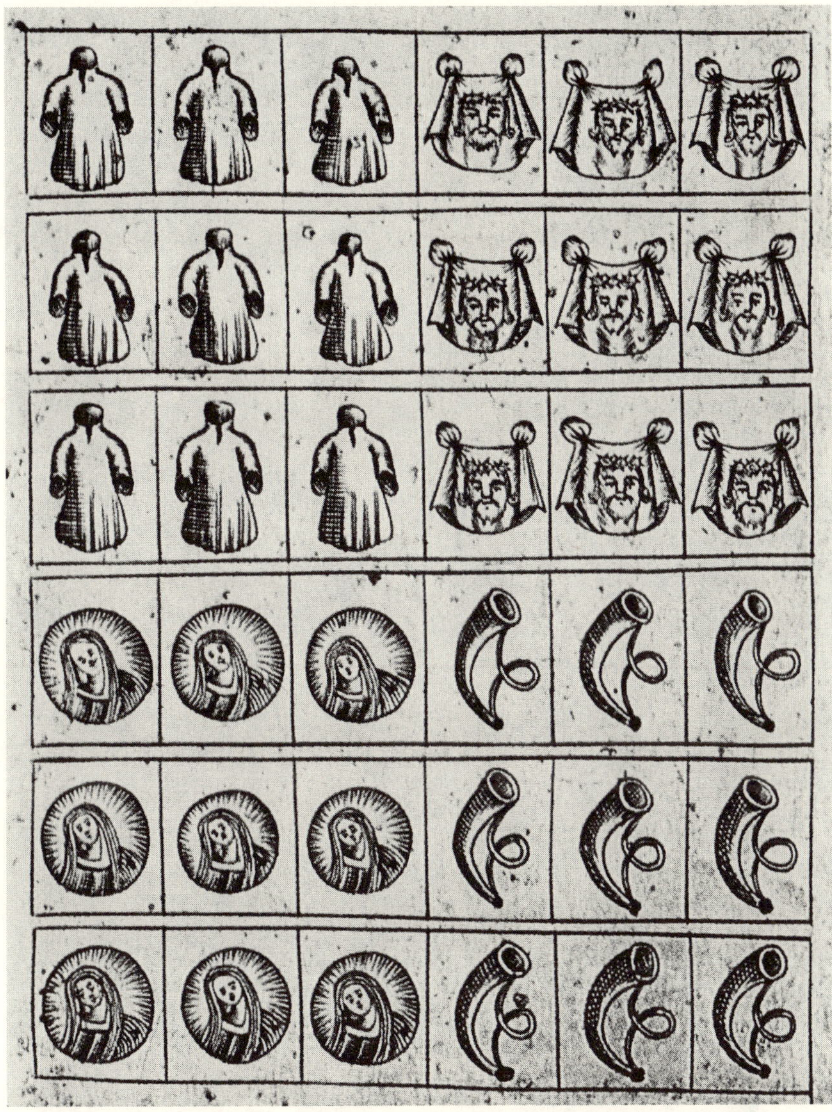

Figure 3.7. German, sheet of image tablets, seventeenth century, engraving, 6.8 x 10.4 cm (Landshut, Ursulinenkloster St. Josef, Plattensammlung) (photo: Franz Niehoff (ed.), *Maria allerorten: Die Muttergottes mit dem geneigten Haupt 1699–1999. Das Gnadenbild der Ursulinen zu Landshut—Altbayerische Marienfrömmigkeit im 18. Jahrhundert*, exhibition catalogue [Landshut: Museen der Stadt Landshut, 1999], p. 344).

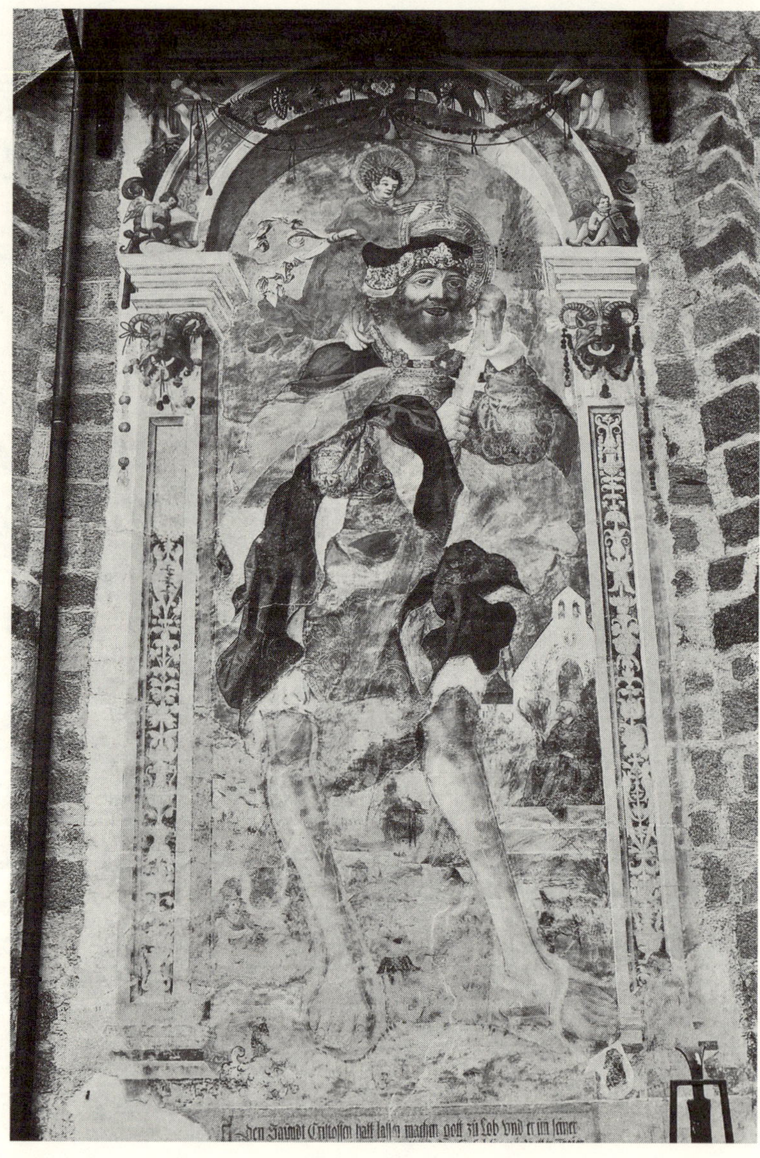

Figure 3.8. *St. Christopher with the Christ Child*, 1519, mural on southwest exterior corner, Church of St. Sigmund, Trentino-Südtirol (Italy) (photo: by the author).

Legend and custom imbued certain holy personages and their images with an apotropaic power that was also accessible visually. At a time when the most terrifying personal health crisis one could imagine was meeting an unexpected death far from home, an end bereft of sacramental ministrations (*mors improvisa*), a half-magical, half-supernatural "inoculation" could be had simply by looking at the image of the legendary giant St. Christopher, patron saint of travelers, shown ferrying the Christ child across a raging river. Monumental murals painted on the sides of churches broadcast the saint's image for the convenience of those hurrying to work (figure 3.8). Images that served as more personalized relays for supernatural assistance—healing miracles, rescue, protection—form the preeminent type of votive object studied by art historians and ethnologists of religion. Documenting a vow (*votum*), the votive could be a thank-offering for a benefit already received, but just as often functioned prophylactically, as a guarantee of heavenly assistance in case of insecurity, misfortune, affliction, or tribulation. Pilgrimage ex-votos across the Catholic world place the fulfilled contract between earthly patient and heavenly physician on display for all the shrine's visitors to see.[28] In Catholic teaching, the power of miraculous healing came solely from God; issuing, fountainlike, from his heavenly throne, it flowed through the hands of his saints, whose virtue and mercy as intercessors privileged them to pass it along to their votaries (figure 3.9).[29]

Finally, mention must be made of the range of images that were coordinated with indulgenced prayers. Prominent in this category was the devotional icon known from the late fourteenth century onward as the *imago pietatis* (later called the "Man of Sorrows") and its narrative counterpart, the Mass of St. Gregory (figure 3.10), which depicts the suffering Christ of the Passion, paradoxically alive in death, appearing on the altar. Both image types allowed ordinary Christians to leverage the vast storehouse of penitential merit accumulated by Christ and his martyrs and held under lock and key by the heirs of St. Peter—the so-called Treasury of Merits.[30] Acquired in sufficient quantity, indulgences inoculated the patient against excessive future suffering in purgatory.

Considering the endless variety of folk remedies, popular sacramentalia, and healing paraphernalia known from across the Christian world, the reader will appreciate that we are looking at the tip of the iceberg only. What this quick procession of examples reveals,

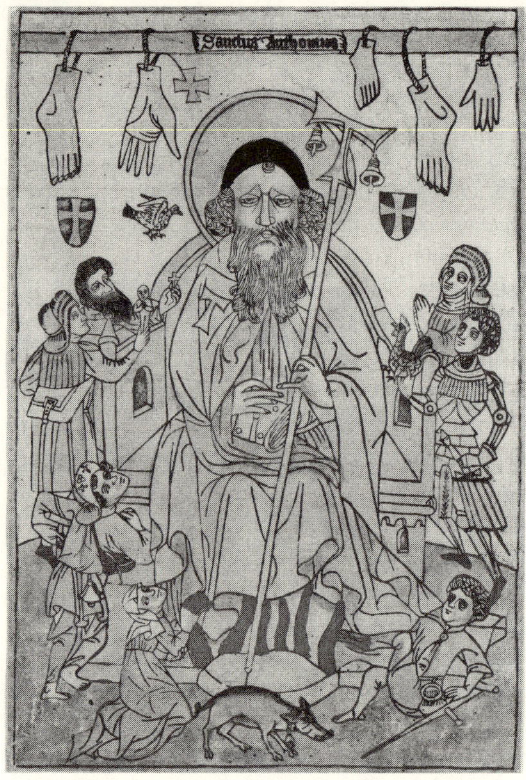

Figure 3.9. South German (Augsburg?), *St. Anthony Abbot*, ca. 1440–50, hand-colored woodcut, 37.6 x 25.6 cm (Munich, Staatliche Graphische Sammlung).

however, is that within the sacramental economy uniting the late medieval church with folk practices and magical beliefs, consecrated objects, their form and substance, could legitimately be seen as efficacious. And that efficacy was perceived as somehow inherent in the object, in its imagery, or in its very physical substance. Though supernatural in origin, the healing virtues of consecrated or holy objects were seen to operate *in* the natural world, and *with* the natural world.

From the Care of Souls to Care of the Self

A positive reliance on images—as aids to instruction, prayer, and remembrance, as conduits to heavenly assistance, healing, and protection, as sacramental surrogates or stepping stones to mystical contemplation—permeated Christian devotionalism in the two centuries before the Reformation, despite the occasional worries of churchmen. Across the divides of aristocratic, bourgeois, and everyday cultures,

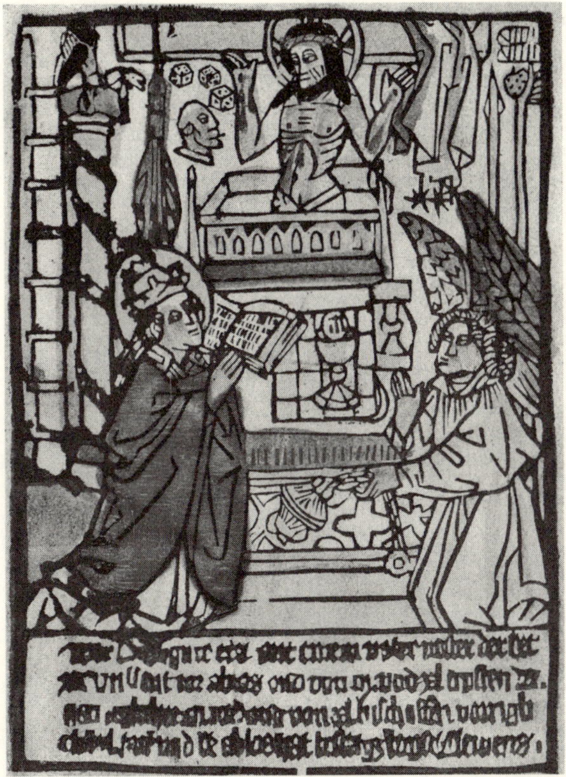

Figure 3.10. German, *Mass of Saint Gregory with Indulgence*, ca. 1470, hand-colored woodcut (Washington, D.C., National Gallery of Art, Rosenwald Collection).

Christian images were given multiple and often dynamic roles to play in the individual's attention to moral, ethical, and spiritual hygiene. Over the course of time, these forms of self-care seem to have intensified, especially as the burden of penitential record keeping was progressively transferred to individuals.[31] Even so, the pastoral "care of souls" (*cura animarum*) of the medieval church, with its elaborate, clerically guided regimentation of sacramental confession and penance, continued to play a major role in people's lives and formed a critical point of contact for the therapeutic use of images. Parish priests or mendicant friars wielding crucifixes or small devotional panels (called *tavoletti* in Italy) were fixtures of public life; we see them pictured in countless death-bed scenes. Likewise were the sick attended with images in hospitals, or the condemned criminal at the place of public execution, where penitence was urged upon the sinner and consolation offered at the moment of death. Images proffered in this way formed a vivid reminder that the ultimate antidote to human pride is humility—the principal virtue Augustine and other patristic writers attributed to the savior Jesus in his role as *medicus humilis*, the doctor who heals with his own humility.[32] Even the most strictly "didactic" images in the church,[33] in their admonitory address to carnal man, participated in the cure of souls. Their purpose was to guide the faithful back to obedience to God, back to the promise of his Word, just as the biblical sages once did with "stiff-necked" Israel,[34] providing aid and comfort against the "sting" of death. Eloquent in providing consolation as well as exhortation, official imagery in the church continued an ancient tradition of rhetorical healing.

Altarpieces and mural programs commissioned specifically for hospital sanctuaries often combined these discursive and devotional functions. Caregivers and the afflicted alike understood them as therapeutic resources that could comfort and console, channel heavenly assistance, feed the craving for spiritual nourishment, and counteract the "poison" of sin that threatens spiritual health—even promote healing simply by stimulating the senses therapeutically.[35] "To heal and be healed," writes Marcia Kupfer in her excellent monograph on Romanesque hospital chapel decoration, "was to enter into an economy of redemption in which the exchange of gifts and services, suffrages and sacrifice, cross the boundary between material and spiritual planes," while "the very act of looking at images opened a way into the circulation of grace."[36] Hospital altarpieces, in particular, anchored the social-therapeutic bonds forged between their donors, the institution, its wards, and the artist behind the commission. Dürer himself entered into one such association with his work on the so-called *Landauer Altarpiece* of 1508–11, one among several works that reveal the painter's self-understanding as a physician of the soul. (See Chapters 5 and 6.)

Images designed to foster contemplation and to focus religious ardor, especially in the setting of private devotion, deserve special mention here. *Andachtsbilder*, or "devotional images" (the term is still preferred by art historians, despite being borrowed from postmedieval Catholicism) are less a fixed set of iconographic themes or image types than a constellation of image functions characteristic of late medieval piety; together they form a key domain of sacramental, spiritual, and ethical therapy that has, in a sense, never been recognized as such. Barring an unnecessary overview of a familiar subject and putting it rather too neatly, we can say that devotional images conjoined in their function three distinct forms of therapy. We have already invoked the sacramental dimension of images, wherein a form of salvific contact—vision or touch as sublimated forms of incorporation—unleashes something of the object's immanent sanctity; and below we will examine a second, meditative dimension, wherein contemplative immersion in the image is interwoven with self-examination, the regulation of the passions, and the cultivation of virtue. Here, we pause to consider a third, different efficacy of the late medieval devotional image: its power to provide consolation (*consolatio*).

After Panofsky's groundbreaking 1927 study of the "image of pity" formula and its mutations,[37] the most compelling account of the appearance of a new class of images after 1250 has come from Hans Belting, who traces the transformation of an older, Eastern type of cultic icon—based on ancient models and styled for the Greek liturgy—and its adaptation to new devotional needs in the West.[38] Just as the form and iconography of the old icons were styled for rhetorical effect, so did the newer devotional types make their address to the beholder with greater and greater force. Exhortations to pity, compassion, joy, and gratitude are integral to this rhetorical function; so, too, is the way they foster a sense of communion and dialogue. Offering consolation as a therapy for the sorrowing soul, their insistent focus on the human dimension of Christ's suffering during the Passion (*humanitas Christi*) and on Mary's compassionate sorrow oriented religious thought and feeling for centuries.

Frontal presentations that directly acknowledge beholders, turning them into participants; rotated perspectives that thematize the Virgin Mother's compassionate perspective on her son's sufferings; the introduction of narrative "gaps" or voids into which spectators might imaginatively enter—these were common strategies in the devotional image's consolatory address.[39] Theatrical elements that heightened the reality effect of painted and three-dimensional images—real hair on crucified Jesus, real clothes on baby Jesus—closed the distance between the devotee and God's loving presence and did so in a way that often simulated visionary appearance, the type of miracle that offered the most profound reassurance. In visionary unions with the lactating Virgin or the suffering Christ, such as those attributed to the mystic Saint Bernard of Clairvaux (1090–1153), tactile sensation takes over (figure 3.11).[40] Bodies draw together in tender embraces

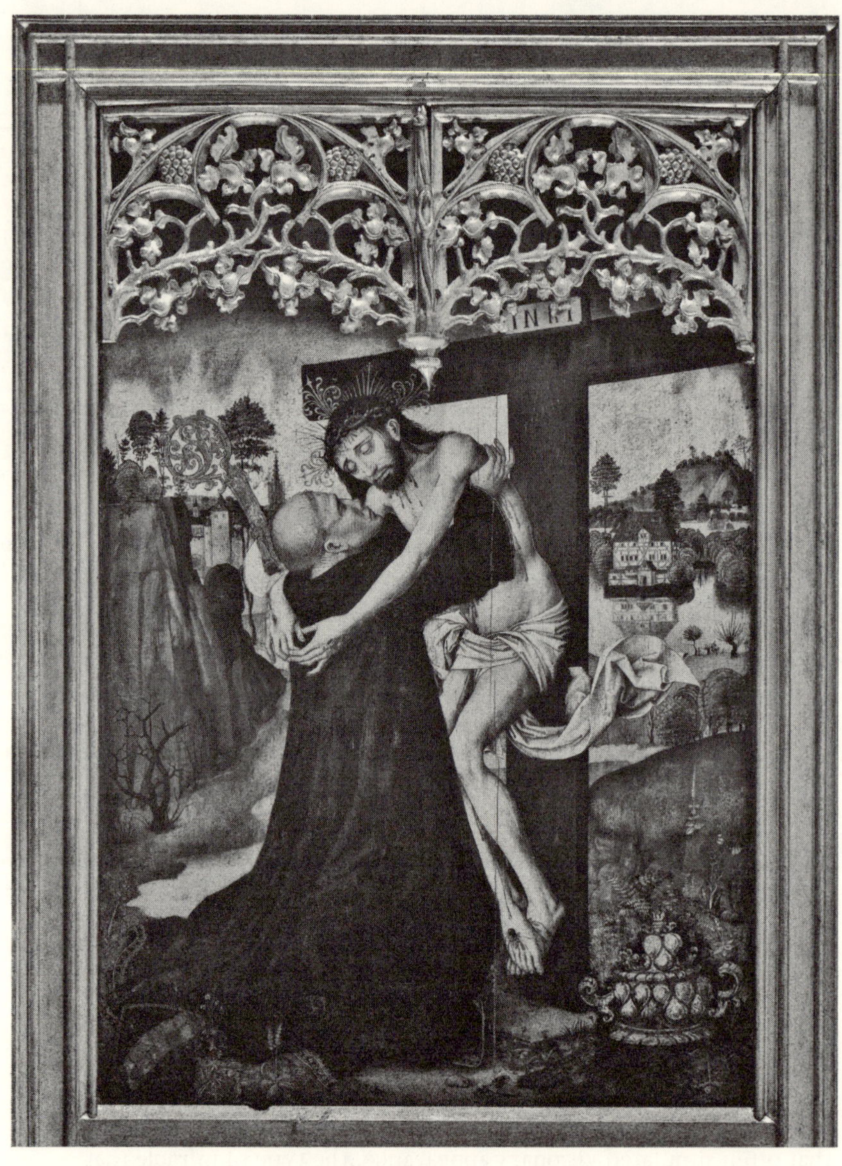

Figure 3.11. Master of the Augustiner-Altar, *Mystical Union of St. Bernard and Christ* (panel from former high altar, Augustinian Church, Nuremberg), 1487, oil on fir panel, 135 x 90 cm (Nuremberg, Germanisches Nationalmuseum).

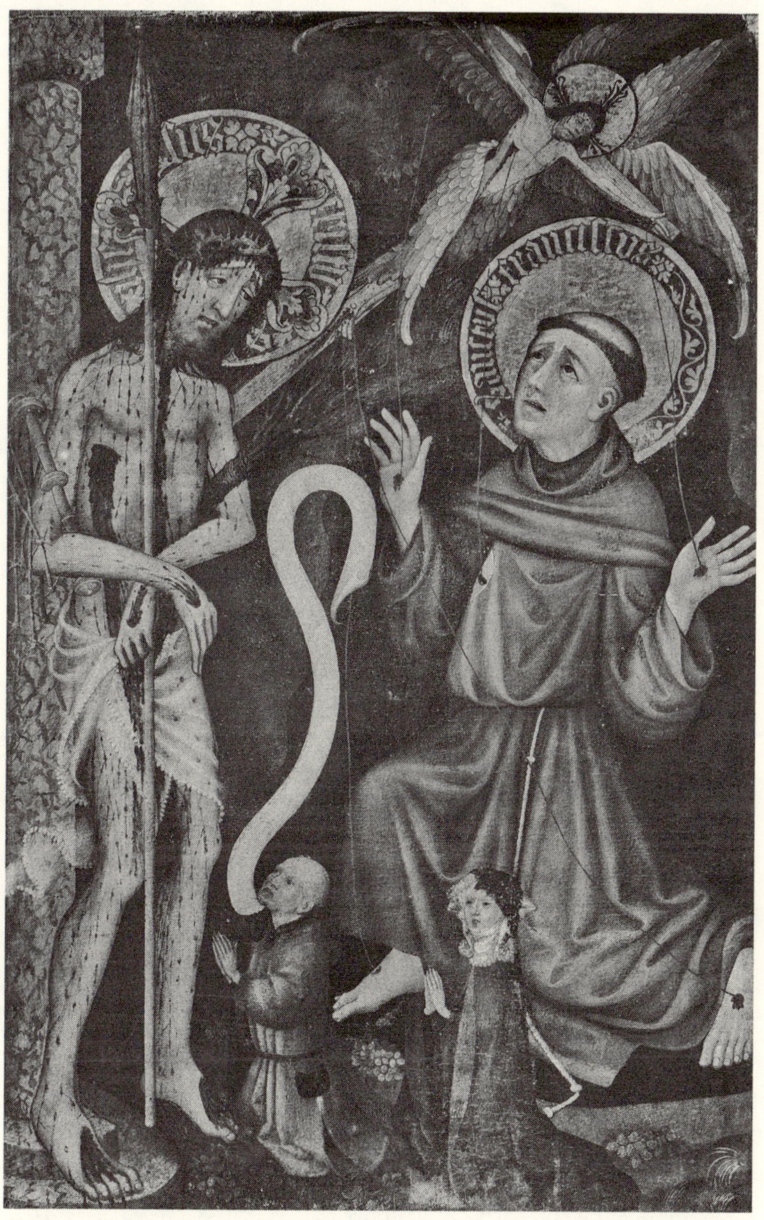

Figure 3.12. Master of the Lindau Lamentation, *St. Francis and the Man of Sorrows*, first quarter of the fifteenth century, oil on panel, 111.5 x 68.5 cm (Cologne, Wallraf-Richartz Museum) (photo: © Rheinisches Bildarchiv Köln).

that intimate the "spiritual wedding" of *sponsa* and *sponsus*, the soul and her divine bridegroom. In such images, the mutual consolation of sufferers swells with devotional ardor. Complex votive formulas, such as we find in a panel by the Master of the Lindau Lamentation (figure 3.12),[41] visualized and then fostered chains of mimetic identification inside and outside the image. Here, Francis of Assisi and the flagellated Christ confront one another in a tense circuit of suffering solace that is poignantly reflected in their rhymed facial expressions. A kind of free-flowing penitential therapy of the emotions is unleashed, an *askesis* at once purgative and renewing as it motivates and guides the beholder's own identification.

Here again we have had to make do with a compressed survey. Still, we can discern from it something of the contours of a great family of therapeutic images, spread across several distinct genres and functional categories of the Christian image. This tradition within European art presented the painters of Dürer's generation, perhaps more than any other before, with a deep well of resources for rethinking the potential of the devotional image as well as the necessary challenge to update it.

Up to this point, we have described, on the one hand, a cluster of inherent efficacies that premodern people attributed to images as well as to other types of sacramental, consecrated, or enchanted objects. By definition, these stemmed from the natural properties of matter, properties that lent objects a healing virtue, or the ascription of supernatural powers on the basis of a saint's *praesentia,* or a mystical identity with the body of Christ. On the other hand, we have a cluster of efficacies that are better described as the effects of human agency. These agencies might be played out in ritual or rhetorical performance, in natural or supernatural communication, or some combination of these. We have also suggested that devotional images, in particular, by combining a sacramental-spiritual hygiene with a consolatory address to the suffering soul, could straddle the line between inherent and rhetorical effectiveness. Now we cross that line and turn decisively to a third mode of efficacy. In the absence of inherent powers, this mode is to be understood in terms of bridging the raw receptiveness of the "sensitive soul" and the workings of reason that take place in the "intellectual soul."

Rhetorical persuasion was ancient philosophy's model for this bridging. Chapter 2's discussion of speculation began this investigation of a therapy that arises from the mediating power of images in the sense theorized by classical rhetoric—the power arising from communicative agency, directly analogous to the persuasive power of the word and its action upon the soul of the listener. This action of the word upon the soul was said to depend as much on the character (*ethos*) and disposition (*diathesis*) of the listener—itself understood as the product of a unique "blend" (*krasis*) of organic matter and spiritual animation (*pneuma*)—as it did on the eloquence or authority of the orator or the style of speaking. Rhetoric's imperative to tune into the receptiveness of the listener's soul was often explained via the medical analogy: as the physician takes into account the humoral "complexion" of the patient before prescribing treatments, so must the speaker or artist who intends to compel the beholder's attention, arouse an emotion, and produce an effect.[42] When we turn more decisively to the Renaissance artist's self-conception as a practitioner of a therapeutic art (see the Prologue to Chapters 5 and 6), this rhetorical model will help us see that the transfers between painting, poetry, and medicine were, in Dürer's time, more than metaphorical.

What remains for the present discussion is to consider more closely the place where efficacy and agency intersect. Examining this intersection can help us make better sense of the many linkages that exist between somatic and spiritual treatments, between biological and psychological effects, as well as the different ways medical metaphors have served the philosophical, theological, pastoral, and literary discourses about the "cure of souls." We will mostly sidestep what modern research has taught us about the psychology of benefit expectation, psychosomatic responses to therapeutic attention, and so on. For modern people, the shorthand for these dynamics is "the placebo effect," while for medieval people it was, simply, "faith." Treating the psychosomatic phenomena associated with faith healing or mysticism is untenable in the present context. Historians face a nearly impossible task when it comes to judging, let alone verifying, the actual effectiveness of the therapies to which the people we study, now long dead, once submitted. To the extent that we can grasp these expectations in their concreteness and reality at all, we can deal only with collective perceptions, popular lore, the teachings of learned experts, and what can be inferred about the interfaces between them.

Speculation and Virtue

Readers of the preceding chapters will know that the therapeutic function we have posited and attempted to reconstruct for Dürer's *Melencolia* is grounded in the print's structure and its character as a speculative image. On this basis, I have argued for its place within a spectrum of early modern images marked by a certain kind of openness, a calculated indeterminacy capable of mobilizing the beholder's attention on several levels. The speculative image begins its work in the contemplation of the sensible world ("all our knowledge originates from the senses," declared Thomas Aquinas),[43] but immediately it urges the mind further, mobilizing in the process the whole hierarchy of mental faculties described by scholastic writers such as Henry of Ghent (ca. 1217–93), Neoplatonists such as Marsilio Ficino, and occultists such as Agrippa von Nettesheim, who was Dürer's contemporary. In the tripartite scheme shared by these thinkers, those faculties were "mind" (*mens*), "reason" (*ratio*), and "imagination" (*imaginatio*). Yet speculative images, in the model we are developing here, are not simply stepping stones to a higher knowledge about the world or God; to describe them this way would suggest that once they had served their purpose, once knowledge or union was achieved, their material form could be left behind. For some, maybe. As sense objects and works of creative imagination, however, their mandate is to remain concretely present, to keep intellectual experience grounded in particulars even as thought is granted its freedom. (Remembering this will also help us distinguish our subject from those ancient and modern paradigms in theology and science that historians call "speculative.") Speculative images perform their office, in other words, when they engage the beholder's natural capacities, when they make new cognitive or spiritual demands, or when they instigate a process akin to meditative exercise. The speculative image rewards in direct proportion to the attention paid to it; its therapeutic benefits are vouchsafed by the performance it enables and sustains. In theory, any image, any object available to the senses, can set the stage for this kind of natural activity—the peculiarity of the speculative image is its capacity to reflect that activity back to the beholder. Speculative labor is reflexive; it finds itself as an object of contemplation amidst the contemplation of externals.[44] Mirror imagery and mirror metaphors are, for this reason, never far from its operations.[45]

To better appreciate these operations, we turn to an ingenious colored woodcut that survives today in Munich. Dated 1488, it bears the title *Spiegel der Vernunft*, "Mirror of Understanding" or "Mirror of Reason" (figure 3.13).[46] Widely cited as a popular counterpart to Hieronymus Bosch's *Seven Deadly Sins* panel in the Prado, where the central roundel represents the sinful world as reflected on the convex surface of the eye of God, the Munich *Spiegel* is both more didactic and more interactive. As a vehicle for speculation, it can be situated historically between the systematic diagrams used to illustrate medieval treatises—in which doctrinal, devotional, or moral matters could be condensed and arranged for contemplation within a circular field—and the so-called *Vexierbilder* of the sixteenth century, perplexing allegorical tableaus such as Giorgio Ghisi's "Allegory of Life" engraving (1561)[47] and, of course, Dürer's *Melencolia*.

The transitional character of the *Spiegel* woodcut stems not only from its date, but from its commodity status. Published as a single-leaf woodcut, with its designer left uncredited, it may be compared with a roughly contemporary sheet that likewise presents itself as a "mirror" for speculative activity, the so-called *Hand as the Mirror of Salvation*, dated 1466 (figure 3.14).[48] Both woodcuts combine word and image to address carnal man for the sake of his eternal soul, promising to ease distress and banish the fear of death; both offered their purchasers a form of progressive interactive exercise in a single, simultaneously visible image, as opposed to sequenced pictures in a book. Once engaged, both stimulated memory and enlisted a higher reason in order to overcome the blockages and blindnesses arising from the lower passions—the "perturbations" (*perturbationes*) of the soul. For these reasons, both sheets count as exemplary late medieval *Lehrbilder* and *Spiegelbilder*. But only the Munich sheet moves decisively toward the conditions of the speculative image. Seeing that the mirror motifs it puts into play are no mere metaphors for self-reflection, but phenomenological prompts and affordances within the meditative environment it establishes, will help illustrate this point. The mirroring processes that speculative images set in motion allow them to function as instruments for self-observation, self-recognition, and self-reform.

Prints such as this might be held in hand, moved and rotated to bring their elements into visual range, or could be hung on the wall. Standing back fosters the illusion of a polished medallion at the

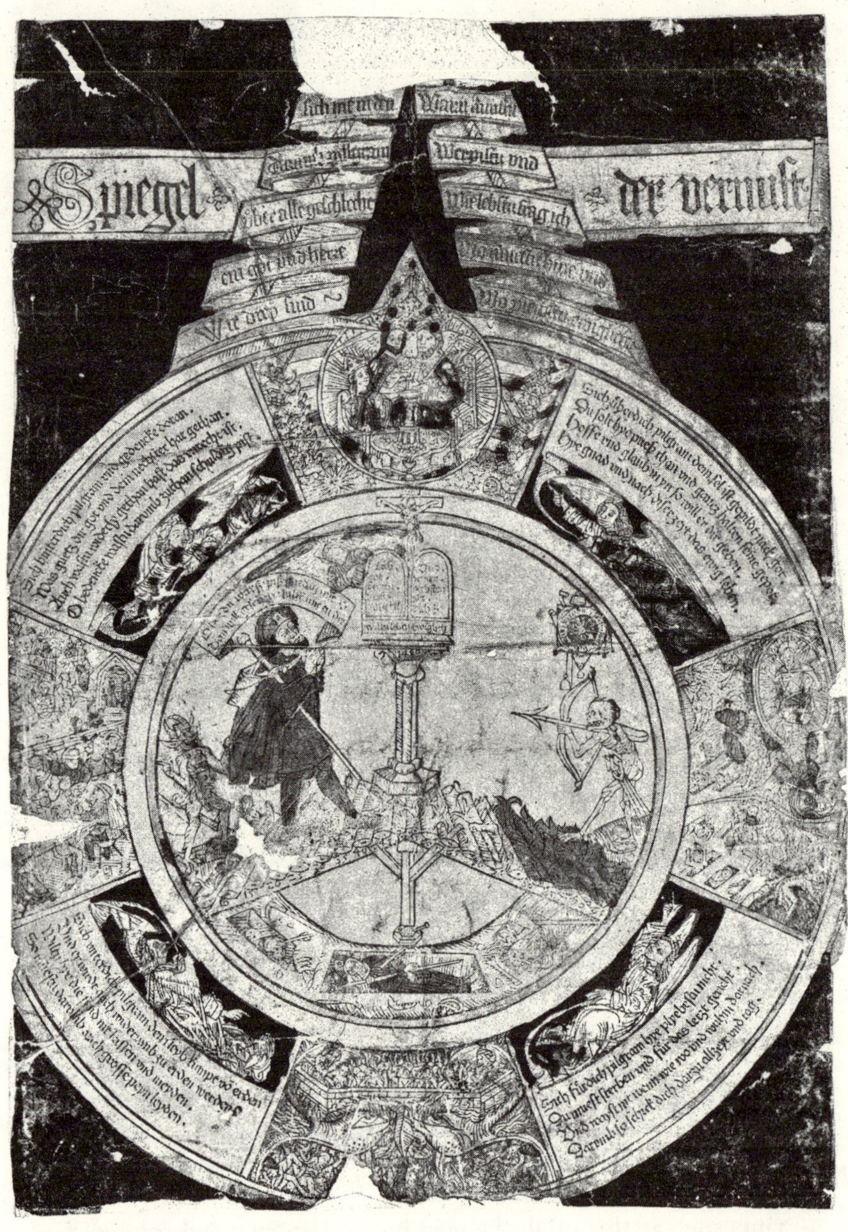

Figure 3.13. South German, *Mirror of Understanding* ("Spiegel der Vernunft"), ca. 1488, colored woodcut, 40.4 x 29.1 cm (Munich, Staatliche Graphische Sammlung).

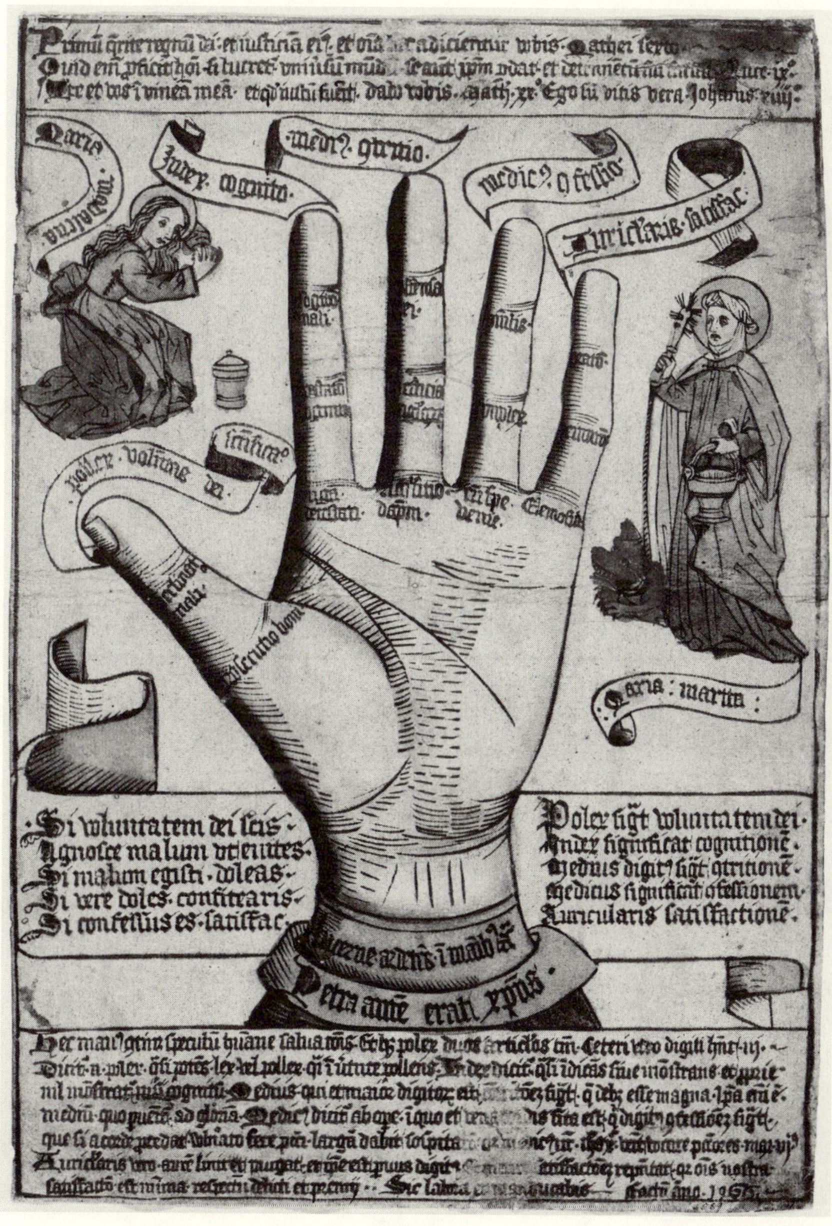

Figure 3.14. Netherlandish, *The Hand as the Mirror of Salvation*, ca. 1466, hand-colored woodcut, 38.5 x 26.5 cm (image) (Washington, D.C., National Gallery of Art, Rosenwald Collection).

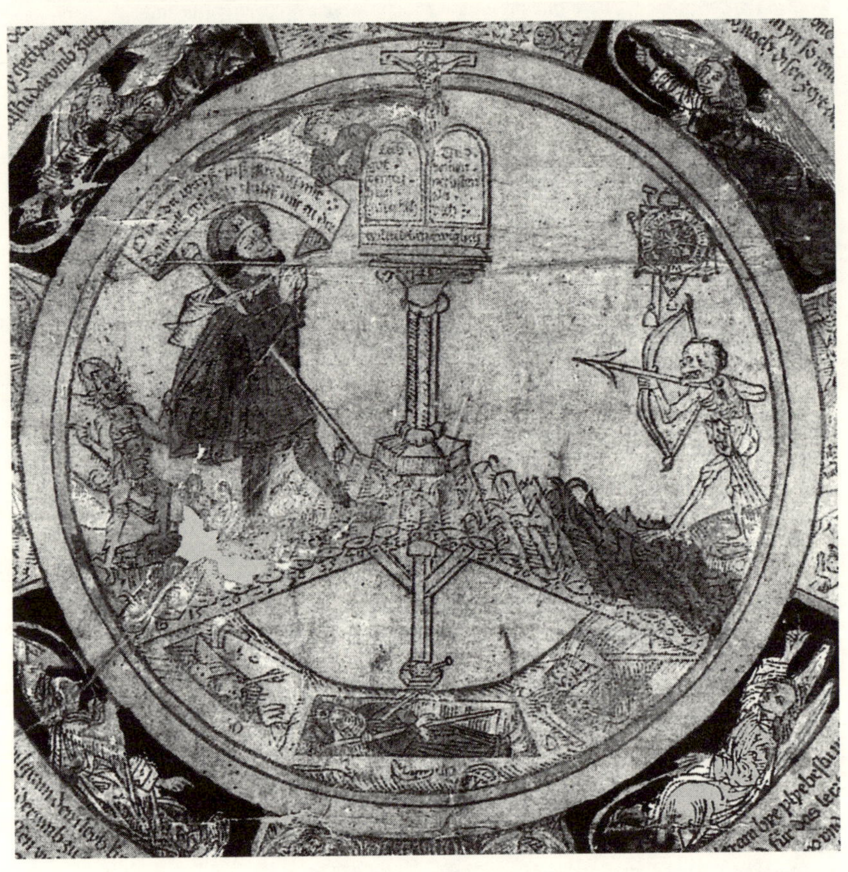

Figure 3.15. Detail from *Mirror of Understanding*: The Wayfarer. (See figure 3.13.)

center, bulging outward toward the eye like the fashionable convex silvered mirrors that decorated bourgeois homes. Inside this looking glass (figure 3.15), we see an improbable monument, the Mosaic tablets of the Law crowned by a crucifix and displayed atop a stone column. This column rises just as improbably from the apex of a rickety boardwalk, stretched across an open ravine strewn with bones. Over this precarious pathway comes striding a pilgrim, recognizable by his hat, knapsack, and traveler's stave. Hands clasped, he utters the prayer inscribed above him on a scroll: "O her du wayß piß gnedig mir / Dein will gescheh, hilff mir zu dir" (O Lord, you know the way to grace for me / Thy will be done, help me to [come to] you). He is *homo viator*, man the wayfarer in this world, an Everyman who is also the beholder's surrogate in the image. Urged on by an angel and threatened by a devil who tugs at his mantle from behind—symbolizing the temptations of the world—he is confronted on the opposite side of the footbridge by Death the Archer.

Arrayed around the mirror's fictive frame are four scenes indicated by angels, each one with his own speech scroll featuring a rhymed quatrain. With word and gesture, the angels urge the pilgrim, and by implication the beholder, to "look!" (Since the mirror's frame has the appearance of an independently turning outer wheel, one can in theory begin anywhere, though the pointing arms indicate a counterclockwise rotation.) One angel says to the pilgrim-beholder, "look behind you" (into the past), to examine how well you've returned your neighbor's charity; the next implores, "look before you" (to the imminence of death), to consider the unatoned sin you carry, to be paid for in purgatory; then we're told, "look before you" (into the future) to anticipate God's judgment; and finally, "look above you" (toward eternity), to glimpse the heavenly reward awaiting those who do proper penance. At the frame's apex, a roundel shows the "unbounded heaven" (*coleum empyreum*), replete with angels and an enthroned Trinity and Virgin Queen reposing before the Fountain of Life.

If we take seriously the claim of the woodcut to be a kind of virtual mirror, a mutable glass for picturing the self in time, then the direction one must face in order to heed the angels' injunction to "look" immediately becomes a function of one's place in the life cycle and one's own biography. Here, the *Spiegel* woodcut draws nourishment from the so-called Ages of Man theme, a diagrammatic image tradition that found one of its most brilliant applications in the Psalter made between

1310 and 1340 for the English nobleman Robert de Lisle (figure 3.16).[49] Ten roundels set against a patterned ground carry emblematic figures spanning the cycle of life, from infancy and youth to adulthood and old age, decrepitude, and death. Virtual clockwise rotation is implied, so the diagram begins to resemble Fortune's wheel. In such a mutable world, the only anchor is God's will, a notion trumpeted from the hub of the spoked wheel, where the Holy Face appears, surrounded by an inscription: *Cuncta simul cerno: totum racione guberno* (I perceive all at once: I govern the whole with reason). In the *Spiegel* woodcut, there is of course no omnivoyant gaze to center the composition, nor does the "mirror" resemble God's eye, as it does in Bosch's *Seven Sins* panel in Madrid. Instead, God watches mankind from a great hierarchical remove, leaving the cross-topped Decalogue, the unity of new and old covenants, as the hub and certification point of the Christian's earthly life. Everything else in creation is in flux: a world tossed by fortune, corrupted by sin, and prey to the devil.

Another metaphorical association of the mirror that the Munich sheet thematizes is theological and anthropological: the conception of the human soul as the "living mirror" of God's perfection, the *imago Dei* (derived from Genesis 1:26–27, the idea was given authoritative shape by Thomas Aquinas in the *Summa Theologica*).[50] The *Spiegel* woodcut refers to this idea explicitly in the banderole held by the angel pointing toward the Trinity: "dein sel ist gepildt nach got" (your soul is fashioned after God). Soiled by the Fall and by an enduring perversity, every soul's inner mirror is compromised in its reflective purity. Yet, Aquinas argued, by virtue of reason, which imparts to humans a special dignity, the possibility of renewing this image is ever-present. Participation in the church's sacraments and rituals was one fully orthodox way the *imago Dei* could be cleansed and restored.[51] Devout practices such as pilgrimage, charity, prayers for the dead, the earning of indulgences, and meditation on Last Things could also further the process. Spiritual exercises of the type fostered by the *Spiegel* woodcut or the *Hand as the Mirror of Salvation*—exercises geared toward to the self-recognition of the sorrowing sinner as a being "tested" by God, a pilgrim in mournful exile, but hopeful of return—likewise worked to brighten the inner image of God in the soul.

Earlier, we spoke about perceptions of an inherent or natural efficacy accessed by the body and its extended apparatus of sensory perception (including vision alone, wherein it acts as a form of touch).

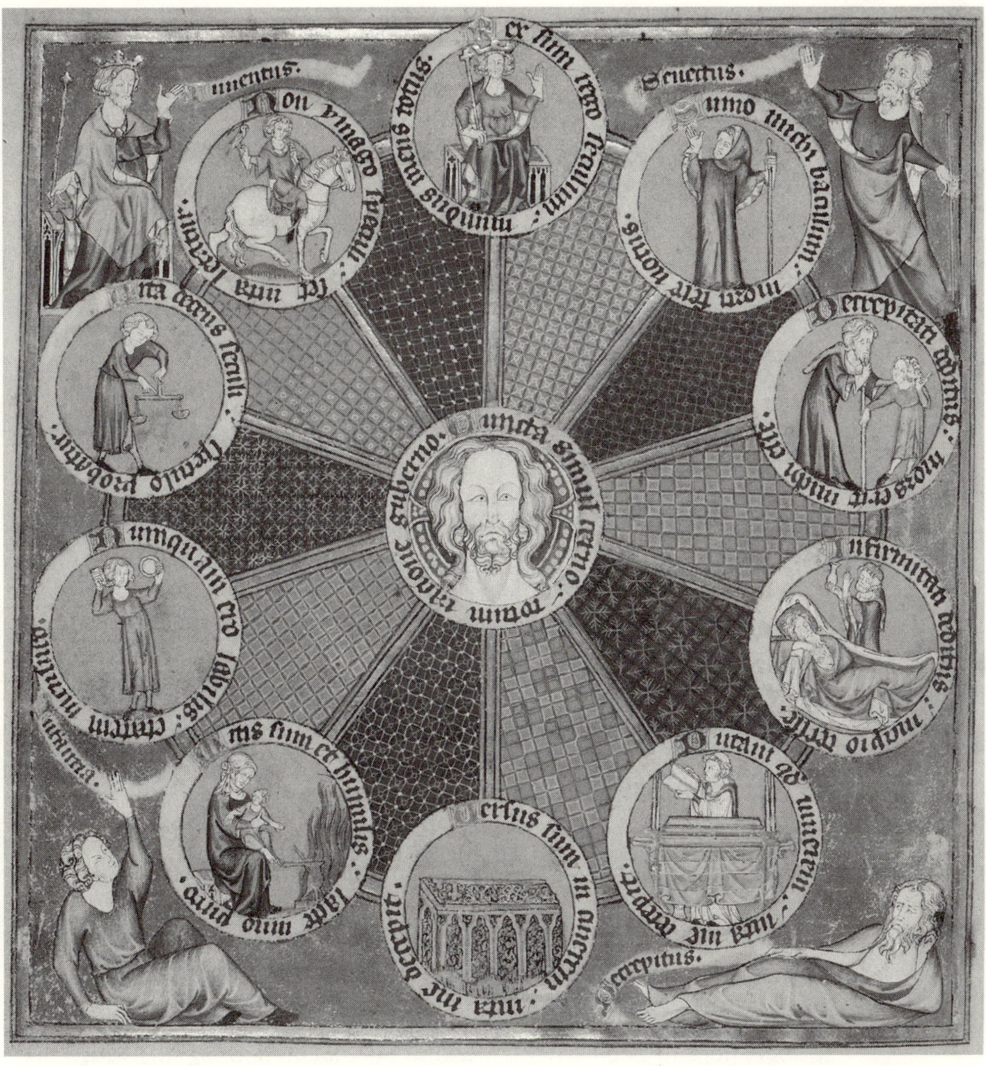

Figure 3.16. Madonna Master (English), *Wheel with the Ten Ages of Man*, illustration from the *Psalter of Robert de Lisle*, ca. 1310 and 1330–40 (London, The British Library, Ms. Arundel 83, II, fol. 126v).

With speculative images, we have entered upon a wholly different category of medicinal art, this one centered upon the collaboration of the eyes and the mind—the interface, as it were, of perception, cognition, and emotion. To recall Reindert Falkenburg's point (see Chapter 2) about the woodcut illustrations to Petrarch's *De remediis* (1532): "Their true subject is not the point of view represented in the image, but the insight and self-knowledge that the viewer forges in his speculation on the image."[52] Because efficacy is a product of the subject's self-activity, rather than being something transposed from an outside cause, I am calling this therapeutic mechanism *efficacy by proxy*. To put it another way: it is not the sense object acting upon the soul—the visible sign or image, the word materialized in writing or speech—that moves "the patient" from illness to health. Rather, action and effect arise from a praxis involving these objects.

To dramatize the contrast, we might borrow from modern pharmacology the distinction between drugs that have direct therapeutic effects, such as the antimicrobials that target specific pathogens in the blood or tissue, and those that stimulate immune responses, enabling the body to do the work of combatting disease (in general, this is called immunotherapy). Both types of drugs act upon the natural body, but the latter produces therapeutic effects by mobilizing the body's own resources, its own healing powers. Lasting health, of course, requires the restoration of the whole immune system; maintenance requires vigilant attention to the movements of the "lower" part of the soul, from which springs the desire for worldly attachments and emotions that bring distress. Battles won against pathogens in the here and now must be consolidated and fortified by regular tempering of the creaturely passions and by the inclination of the will toward humility. Just as the metaphorical function of the late medieval *Spiegelbild* as a mirror of self-recognition does not end with the sinner's acceptance of the need for penance, the therapy it offers does not end with some kind of "inoculation" against sin, vanity, or pride, contrary to what recent commentators have suggested.[53] Neither did it measure spiritual progress according to an ecclesiastical checklist of penance, as in its contemporary *Hand as the Mirror of Salvation*. Rather, the speculative image offered resources for a meditative performance that merges self-examination with the recognition of sin, self-observation with vigilance against the "perturbances" of the soul, consolation with conversion to reason.

Even with this finer-grained definition, however, we still face a serious methodological quandary. Is every kind of image that lends itself to meditation or speculation potentially a vehicle of rhetorical therapy? Is every image that facilitates the examination of conscience, the self-recognition of the Christian subject, the need for penance or conversion to God by definition therapeutic? How can we give greater clarity to the concept of the therapeutic image or therapeutic genres in the visual arts, where the proliferation of examples threatens to exceed our control? Therapy by proxy, I have argued, occurs when images, objects, and the material word are enlisted as instruments of a healing practice whose efficacy lies beyond them. The healing practices we discover behind such proxies will tend to be either psychosomatic or somatopsychic, and in any case, entirely ephemeral, impossible to document in straightforward empirical terms, thus triply beyond the reach of historical reconstruction. And yet, as the foregoing has tried to show, they can be recovered from a close analysis of particular artifacts and the structural emotions they were designed to mobilize, their capacity to propel thought and perception along multiple possible routes.

Attention to Self

Images that structure a therapeutic meditative practice, moving the beholder to heightened states of inwardness and reflective attentiveness, represent another form of what we have been calling efficacy by proxy. An example with important implications for our analysis of *Melencolia* comes from a print series Dürer completed just a few years earlier: the nineteen-woodcut cycle devoted to the life of the Virgin Mary (*Marienleben*), which was furnished with Latin verses by Dürer's occasional collaborator, Benedict Schwalbe (aka Chelidonius; d. 1521), a scholar, poet, rhetorician, theologian, historian, and astronomer who was abbot of the Stift St. Aegidius in Nuremberg (only a few streets away from Dürer's house) and a member of the humanist circle that gathered at the home of Willibald Pirckheimer. The project, one of Dürer's three "large books," was published in 1511 and dedicated to Willibald's sister, Caritas Pirckheimer (1467–1532), then abbess of the Sankt Klara Convent, a community of Franciscan nuns in Nuremberg.[54] As a self-consciously artful program for stimulating visual meditation, the entire cycle of images merits our attention; however, I want to focus on one block that has already received more than its fair share: the fourteenth in the series, the *Holy Family in Egypt* (figure 3.17), which Dürer completed in 1502.[55] And although our woodcut has several interesting focal points and features—the audacious perspective view, the fantasy farmhouse stage setting, the alignment of Holy Family and Holy Trinity—it is important for our purposes to zoom in on Joseph as a pivotal figure (figure 3.18). With axe in hand and his gaze directed toward the beholder outside the frame, Joseph the carpenter labors over a wooden beam, hollowing it out into a gutter or trough (or something of the sort) while industrious putti gather up the splinters and shavings around him. Casting him as a prototype for the Christian artist and craftsman, Chelidonius in the accompanying verses calls Joseph a "second Daedalus" and extols his skills in carving, casting, polishing, and molding.[56] But whether Dürer had the Daedalus prototype in mind when he conceived the image (nearly a decade before Chelidonius supplied the poetry) still remains an open question. In the interpretation put forward by Cynthia Hahn, Joseph emerges as a different kind of *homo faber* figure, a metaphorical "artisan of the soul [who] trims off our vices all around, takes the axe to the unfruitful trees, cuts off that which is worthless, saving the well-shaped shoots, and softening the rigidity of souls in the fire of the spirit." These are the words of Ambrose of Milan, whose commentary on the Gospel of Luke, according to Hahn, Dürer used as the source text for his distinctive interpretation of the scene.[57]

To make sense of the connection and its meaning, Hahn proposed that the figure and his overt appeal to the beholder function in the picture as a call to penance, betokening the promise of salvation through Christ's sacrifice, given to those who would properly flee from sin. This interpretation is more or less satisfying in light of late medieval piety's penitential emphasis, but something more is required, I think, if we are to take the picture seriously—and likewise the folio sequence as a whole—as an instrument of spiritual exercise. To do this means understanding the image not simply as a delivery module for an idea that, once apprehended and decoded, rewards pious reflection and brings the interpretive process to an end. Our therapeutic model must also take into account the active process the work instigates and then sustains in the real time of devotional praxis. This, in turn, requires some careful thinking about pious meditation and the role visualization plays in it.

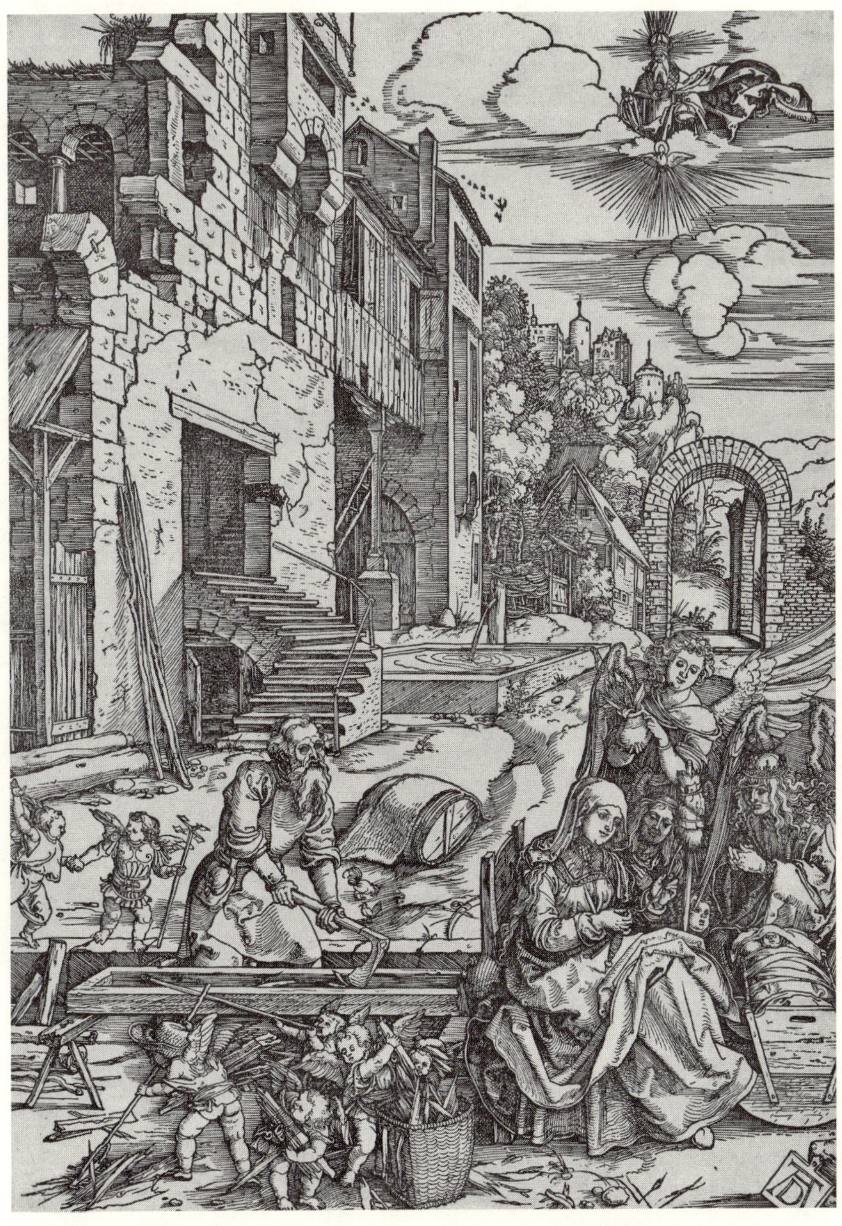

Figure 3.17. Albrecht Dürer, *Holy Family in Egypt*, 1502, woodcut, 29.5 x 20.8 cm, from the *Marienleben* series (Washington, D.C., National Gallery of Art, Rosenwald Collection).

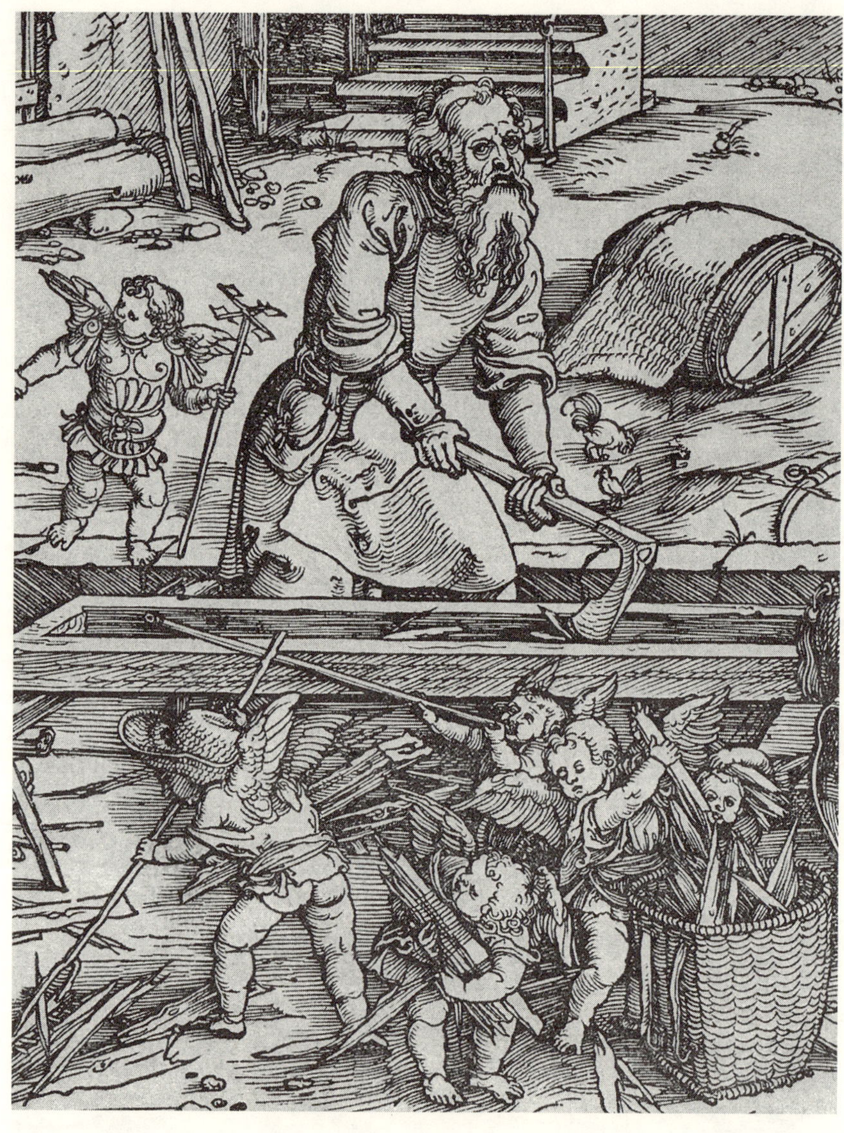

Figure 3.18. Detail from Dürer, *Holy Family in Egypt*: Joseph the Artisan. (See figure 3.17.)

To make oneself "present" at the events of sacred history; to bear witness to the suffering of Jesus and Mary with deep sympathy and awe; to start from the simplest description of an action and spin it into an elaborately wrought, quasi-visionary experience, captivating in its detail and familiarity—these were the methodological building blocks of Catholic meditation in premodern Europe. Among the insights generated by recent research is that this kind of pious meditation, undertaken with or without images, was conceived as a "mode of [internal] picturing,"[58] one that, in the process of its unfolding, entailed a kind of running reflection on the vividness and emotional power of the "internal imitation" each person produced. Later advocates for this pious practice would draw an explicit analogy with the way a painter examines the rightness of his pictorial imitation, the success of his illusion, in the process of fabricating it. In the same way, they argued, the meditating subject should engage in constant self-correction of the internal image, this as a way of measuring one's closeness to or distance from the holy models of charity, humility, and ardor being summoned.[59] Ethical and emotional conformity to Christ or the Virgin was one measure; the progressive purification of the *imago Dei*, present but latent in every soul (discussed above), was another. As the diligent "artisan of the soul" (*faber animae*), Dürer's St. Joseph offers the beholder a running course in spiritual self-observation from within its fictive space; he is, in this sense, what Andrea Catellani has called a "delegate" figure.[60] Not exactly a surrogate or double for the beholder, a delegate can assist and enjoin the beholder to do many different things with and within the image. Dürer cements Joseph's delegate role through the direction of his gaze outward from the picture, so it transgresses the strict separation of virtual and real spaces and places the beholder himself or herself under observation.

What we must not fail to appreciate is how this very same pictorial device, as it forges a connection with the beholder, also calls attention to the artifice of the picture, its status as an image, a graphic trigger for subjective perception as a creative process. Internal picturing allies itself with rhetorical healing to produce a heightened "attention to oneself" as the soul crafts its own right relation with God. Thus does the meditative image, in Walter Melion's words, mobilize and heighten "the soul's awareness of its own image-making powers"[61] and harness that awareness to a therapeutic goal.

That Dürer's *Marienleben* was designed as an instrument of meditative practice is clear enough; Junhyoung Michael Shin has argued persuasively for its conformity with the methods of pious visualization espoused by authors such as John of Caulibus and Ludolph of Saxony.[62] What must be emphasized here is that, as a point of departure for healing praxis, ambitious images such as Dürer's do not exhaust their potentiality in semiosis, in the signifying operations (betokening, promising, pointing, projecting, and so on) that animate pious desire. Rather, the meditative-therapeutic image fulfills its charge most forcefully when it is *engaged*, when it serves as an open-ended resource in a practical technique for affecting the state of the soul. This returns us to what I have been saying concerning the speculative image and allows us to differentiate several types among those discussed in this chapter.

One type, descended from medieval theological diagrams, we discovered in the Psalter of Robert de Lisle and the *Spiegel der Vernunft* woodcut in Munich; a second, informed by the tradition of visual meditation and the crafting of sacred tableaux in the "mind's eye," is manifest in the *Marienleben*; a third, coming somewhat later and exemplified by the woodcut illustrations prepared for the German edition of Petrarch's *De remediis* (Chapter 2), exploits visual ambiguity, inversion, and perplexity in order to target and reform the beholder's ethical judgment. Finally, a fourth type, taking on the appearance of an allegorical tableau and engaging the viewer as a rebuslike puzzle with no easy solution, is what we find in *Melencolia I*. In all four types, the speculative process is preprogrammed, as it were, to remain open-ended, albeit through different visual means. Whatever separates them thematically, theologically, or sacramentally, their common therapeutic identity lies in the way each sustains a real-time process of inner and outer reflection. A progressive clarification of the passions permits a form of self-recognition and an understanding of soul's true orientation.

Self-recognition is therefore more than a movement of the soul from a state of sinfulness to one of repentance; it is also a shift from the passive perception of externals to an active observation of self. Stoic philosophy dubbed this contemplative ideal *prosochē* (προσοχή), best translated as "attention to oneself." Fundamental to the ancient philosophical imperative toward self-examination and vigilance against destructive passions, *prosochē*, according to Pierre Hadot, forms a crucial bridge between ancient philosophy's therapy of the passions and Christianity's foundational self-understanding as *philosophia*, the search for wisdom concretized in the practice of virtue. Traces of this ancient ideal appear again and again in the theory and practice of Christian meditation, from the Desert Fathers to the Modern Devotion.[63] And it resurfaces in the sophisticated tools late medieval devotional culture developed for rebalancing the mind and, along with the mind, the entire personality.

Charged Matter

Vigilant attention paid to the movements of the lower part of the soul, the tempering of the creaturely passions, and the inclination of the will toward virtue formed the ethical-spiritual imperatives behind images that I have been calling speculative. In the course of treating the latter separately from images and objects possessed of an inherent efficacy, this chapter has also exposed some of the stress points in any such distinction. That distinction, in fact, breaks down in fascinating ways when we turn to the final class of therapeutic images I wish to consider. Like the late antique amulet made of heliotrope, discussed above, these are images whose very matrix, whose presence as material things, incorporates the healing properties of natural substances, substances familiar to artist and pharmacologist alike; and yet it is still by proxy that they affect the soul. Art historian Karin Leonhard's recent investigations into *sottobosco* painting in the Netherlands—the genre that dwells on the exotic flora and fungi, fluttering insects and slithering fauna, of the forest floor—offers a most compelling example. According to Leonhard, artists working in this genre, for example Otto Marseus van Schrieck (1619–78) (figure 3.19), conceived the picture plane as a point of convergence for both the representation of natural life forms and the presentation of charged matter: that is, the coloring agents right there on the painter's palette, some derived from minerals, others from plant and animal extracts, many of them toxic. Through their use, the painted image approaches the conditions of a visual *pharmakon*, a colorful cauldron of poisons and poultices, expressive of but also embodying the "antagonistic forces in nature's great realm of matter and form."[64]

For centuries, medieval artists displayed varying degrees of awareness of the medicinal properties of the natural derivatives they used as coloring agents; this knowledge was readily available in lapidaries and botanicals. The attitude displayed by an early modern painter such as Marseus, by contrast, carries with it a sophisticated understanding of the implications for art. In Leonhard's account, the practitioner of *sottobosco* lodged a novel claim about the vivifying powers of his own representational practice and did so on the basis of a strong "analogy between pharmaceutical and aesthetic values."[65] Marseus uses his art to battle pathogens symbolically, in other words, drawing on "the principles of sympathy and antipathy, contrasting cold with warm, wet and dry and the identical with the different, like a physician curing a poisonous attack or threatening disease."[66] This turns the pictorial surface into a field where "meaning effects" and "presence effects"—to use Hans Ulrich Gumbrecht's terms—converge and condition each other.[67] Speculation on the hidden sympathies behind nature's pharmacopeia, productive of a therapeutic knowledge, goes hand in hand with a felt efficacy in the presence of substances known to be apotropaic or antidotal.

Early modern artists seem also to have been more aware than earlier generations of the close association of imaginative power and moral peril in the tradition of optical naturalism. Combining this ambivalence with the homeopathic principles of toxicology, Marseus innovated a new kind of pharmacological art, according to Leonhard, in which poisonous substances are transmuted into rapturous color ("danger is transformed into attraction"). Pleasurable appearances, if not recognized for what they are and what they conceal, can kill.[68] *Sottobosco* painting aspires to be a visual "book of secrets" in which poisons and medicines are shown to derive from the same natural substances. Thus does painting become a source of therapeutic knowledge as well. Even more, it becomes a means for transposing that knowledge into an aesthetic experience that could claim to be a counterpart to natural efficacy.

Painters such as Marseus might even lay claim to being a kind of secular "god-doctor-pharmacist-magician" in the sense suggested by Jacques Derrida in his analysis of the terms *pharmakon* and *pharmakeus* in Plato's *Phaedrus*.[69] Or perhaps this is taking things too far? What is certain is that Marseus's paintings represent a hitherto unrecognized way in which early modern artists could participate in the "vernacular science of matter," as Pamela Smith has called it.[70] And they return us to that fascinating transitional moment in the long history of visual therapeutics—when a Dr. Mancini could

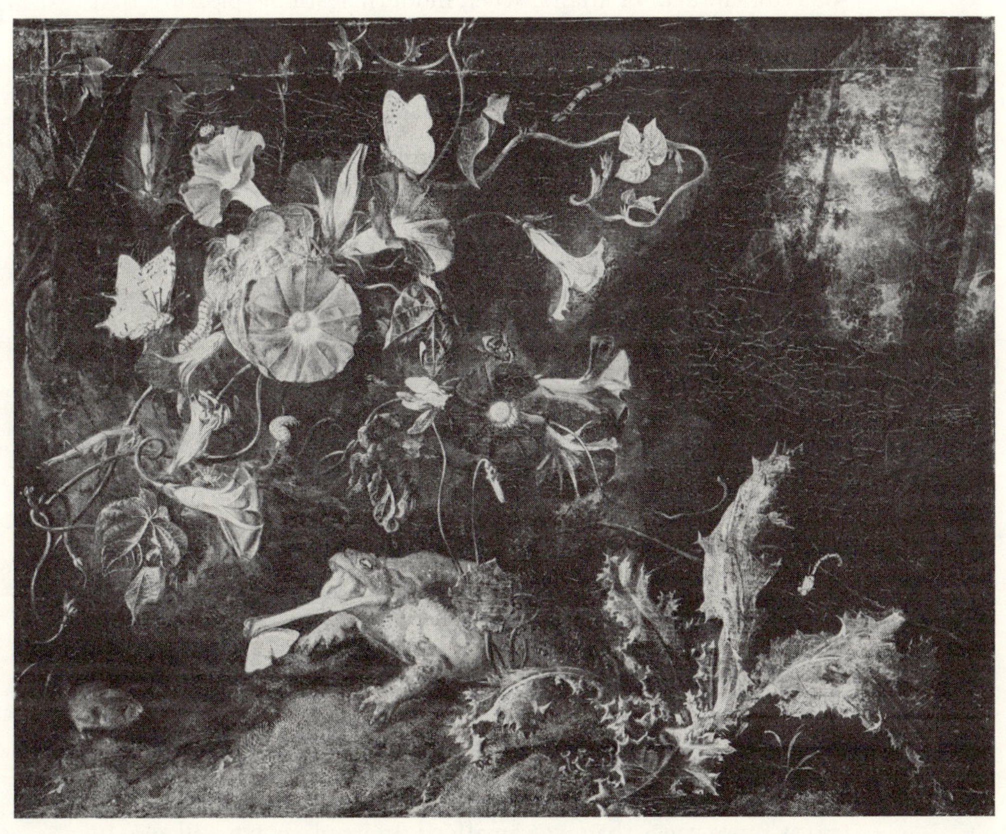

Figure 3.19. Otto Marseus van Schrieck, *Toad, Insects, and Morning Glory*, 1660, oil on canvas, 54 x 68 cm (Staatliches Museum Schwerin, Schwerin) (photo: bpk Bildagentur/Elke Walford/Art Resource, NY).

prescribe an invigorating dose of landscape imagery for the dragged-out Roman man of affairs, when modern aesthetic pleasure first became a distinct resource for the restoration of health.

With this chapter I have tried to show something of the variety of material means for activating the therapeutic expectations of beholders, expectations that were deeply etched in collective perceptions about the interplay of natural and supernatural forces, learned and folk attitudes about the processes governing body and mind, and the sacramental value of substances both under and outside clerical control. With our last example we have touched upon a highly complex mode of efficacy by proxy, one in which the artist's claims to agency in the therapeutic process, now cast in art-theoretical terms, take center stage. When, in the next chapter, we turn back to Dürer and *Melencolia*, we will find him operating within and across these intersecting traditions and anticipating some of what was to come in sixteenth-century art and science.

All of this, we should remember, took place against the backdrop of a long-standing and many-sided alliance between art and medicine that included the illustration of medical treatises, the collaborative study of anatomy, and a fluid commerce between art and pharmacology that, we have just seen, brought artists into a "common specialist culture" based on a practical-scientific knowledge of natural substances.[71] To encompass that entire history and the vast interdisciplinary literature that has grown up around it would require many more pages than we can afford. In its place, we will zero in upon an issue that scholarship on both sides of the art/science divide has still not sufficiently considered, though it is already implied by the metaphorical and actual alliance of the two professions, painter and healer. I mean the degree to which the Christian artist, under certain circumstances, might see himself as a *medicus* of the soul and of the mind—an artisanal counterpart to the rhetorical healer charged with the consolation of souls through reason and wisdom. Unearthing that possibility will be our task in Chapters 5 and 6, where a broader swath of Dürer's work will be considered in light of the unique therapeutic claims we are discovering in the *Melencolia*.

Before that happens, though, the therapeutic challenges proclaimed by the engraving's subject, the singularly distressing syndrome of melancholia itself, must pass review. Our next chapter will look at the affinity and rapport Dürer establishes between the engraving's theme and its metatheme, so to speak, its interrelated levels of "diagnosis" and "cure." That alignment, I hope to show, reveals Dürer's familiarity with a number of long-standing conceptions of psychosomatic imbalance that had filtered down through the medical, philosophical, and occult discourses of the preceding centuries, conceptions that found new meanings among the Northern humanists who were the artist's closest advisors and friends. If all the present study sought to do was deepen or refine our understanding of the picture's allegorical contents (Chapter 1), a review of melancholia's special status in the history of mental illness would be wasted labor. An abundant literature resides elsewhere.[72] Yet because the self-aware Dürer addressed his work to an implied beholder or community of beholders, a notional sufferer or solidarity of sufferers in need of assistance, the picture's address to the individual, the beholder who consciously steps into the therapeutic relationship, demands our attention. There is, embedded in Dürer's masterwork, a dianoetic logic that transforms the beholder's real or vicarious experience of melancholic disturbance into a kind of tragic knowledge that his own destiny, and his own prospects for well-being, are also at stake.

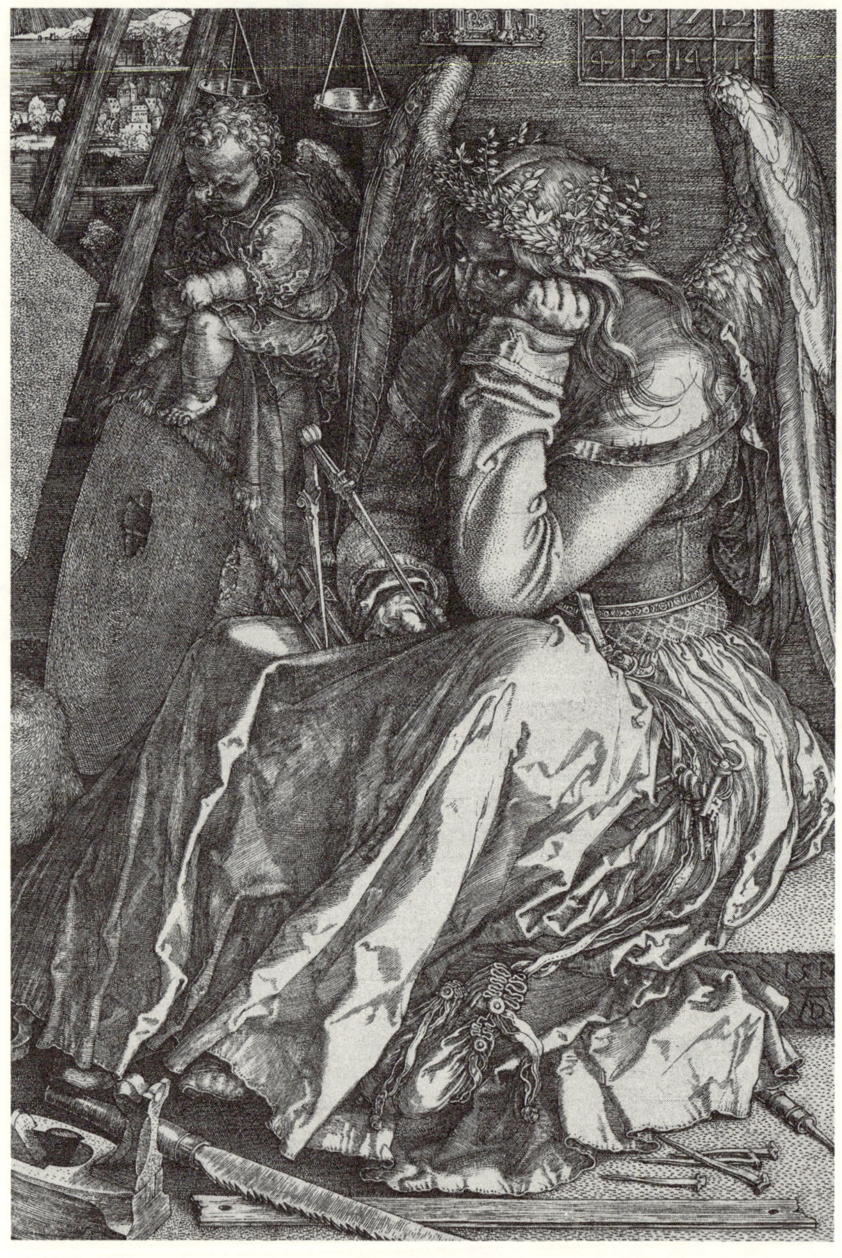

Figure 4.1. Detail from Dürer, *Melencolia I*: seated genius figure. (See figure 1.1.)

The Narrative Quality
of Melancholia

One who is living does not have it in his power to stop time, to find rest outside time in the perfect conclusion, in a conclusion of joy as if there were no tomorrow, in a conclusion of sorrow as if it could not be a drop more bitter, in a conclusion of the contemplation as if meaning were entirely finished and the contemplation were not in turn a part of the meaning.
—Søren Kierkegaard, "At a Graveside"

Five centuries of zealous commentary has raised before our perception of Dürer's engraving such a dense screen of projections concerning the identity of the winged personification, it is hard to remember that her iconographic origins were rather humble, and the expressive idea behind her pose rather straightforward (figure 4.1). There she sits at the base of a mysterious large structure, half squatting, it seems, her bent knees pushing upward through thick robes splashed with light, those knees forming a mighty mass that anchors her muscular arm, crooked and rising up to meet her cheek—and then there is that majestic head, noble features saturated in darkness, sinking into the clenched fist that supports it. Every limb contributes to the total effect, every part of Melancholy's body, even her wings, unite in this single gesture. It is a masterful study of dejection, a human state at once immobile and powerfully intense. Neither exertion nor relaxation, vitality nor passivity prevail. Setting aside the many other attributes Dürer has attached to his allegorical figure—from the keys dangling below her belt and the purse crumpled into the folds of her gown to the disheveled hair, the head wreathed with watercress, the tools on the ground, half concealed near her feet—aside from all this, we readily grasp the defining characteristic of the seated figure, the *Gestalt* on which all else depends: her *inaction*. Panofsky observed this

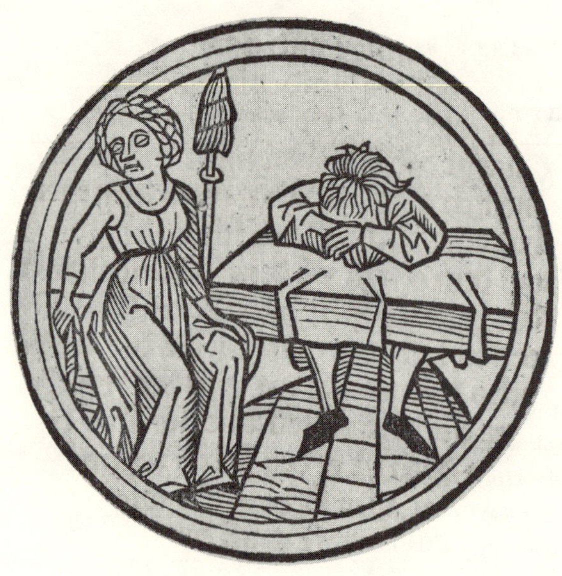

Figure 4.2. Augsburg, *Figure of the Melancholic*, woodcut from cycle of the Four Temperaments, in *Kalendar* (Augsburg: Hans Schönsperger the Elder, 1484), 19.7 x 13.6 cm (New York, Metropolitan Museum of Art, Harris Brisbane Dick Fund, 1926) (photo courtesy of the Metropolitan Museum of Art, www.metmuseum.org).

early on. From that intense stillness arises the whole mood of the scene. And the perfect counterpoint of that impotent immobility: the busy concentration of the putto atop his grindstone, scribbling or etching a *cartellino* of the kind Dürer often used to embed his signature and date within a scene.[1] Few observers have missed the opposition of the two figures.[2]

To convey "the general idea of gloomy inertia," Panofsky showed, Dürer drew from medieval representations of sloth (*acedia*), one of the Seven Deadly Sins, long considered inimical to all spiritual advancement and often associated with the dryness and numbness of melancholia.[3] Genrelike realisms pepper this tradition; the image of a woman falling asleep with her distaff, used to illustrate the melancholic complexion in the Augsburg Calendar's cycle of four temperaments (ca. 1480), is typical (figure 4.2).[4] But in contrast to a figure such as hers, the *Hausfrau* who has "gone to sleep out of sheer laziness," Melancholy's frozen pose is suffused with a kind of passionate energy held in abeyance, a vigilant repose that betokens inner processes.[5] Those bright, intense eyes that pierce the gloom tell the same story. Her visible lethargy, lifted out of time, is belied by movements that are unseeable, beating to a rhythm as sure as any natural process. But what does she see, what does she think, what does her condition permit? Because Melancholy's creative energy "is paralyzed not by sleep but by thought," she seems to exist in a precariously heightened mental state, one so striking that Panofsky had to coin a term for it: "super-awake." We have, in short, the opposite of the sinfully sluggish housewife: we are face to face with a "superior being"—"superior not only by virtue of her wings but also by virtue of her intelligence and imagination." At the same time, she is a being whose capacity and vocation have been compromised, as it were, by something unseen, perhaps by excessive reflection . . . who knows? Panofsky, attuned to medical opinions in Dürer's time about the morbidity imposed on thought by the "coldness" of melancholy, considered the magnificent seated figure, hindered in her natural activity, as the very image of a "thinking being in perplexity."[6] Cognition loses its fluidity and "warmth" under Saturn's influence; it circles back on itself and becomes self-obsessed, ungenerous, and ungenerative. Melancholy's creative praxis, whatever we might take it to be, melts into the air of unrealized purpose. Without the prospect of revealing or advancing knowledge, the danger of delusion draws close.

Given his commitment to hidden concepts and the diagnosis of symptoms—psychological as well as cultural—it is not surprising how keenly Panofsky perceived the manner in which Dürer's immobile genius, slumped in the shadows and outwardly impotent, could illuminate the mind's silent and invisible machinery, the intensive mental and even emotional activity going on behind the stilled surfaces of the body. Attributing that deep cognition to the dramatis personae of Dürer's allegorical print—and by inference to the artist for whom the image served as a spiritual-vocational mirror—Panofsky nevertheless stopped short of asking how the sixteenth-century beholder might have been coaxed beyond a strictly "exegetical" response, to see something of his own situation in the struggle against creative turpitude and spiritual sadness. Although Panofsky, in other words, was fully ready to pronounce the engraving a "spiritual self-portrait of Albrecht Dürer,"[7] he did not draw the implication that the artist may have intended Melancholy's "super-awake" state to mirror the heightened attentiveness the print demands from its viewer. That is the very possibility we should now explore.

To get at this, let me suggest that the signs of Melancholy's hidden cognition betoken the print's phenomenological relationship to the viewer. Taking her place in a long line of seated-thinker portraits, not least of all the late medieval "devotional" figures of Christ in repose, which Dürer himself first interpreted while a journeyman in Strasbourg, presumably for a humanist patron (figure 4.3),[8] Dürer's melancholic genius models and mirrors in her active stillness our own cognitive activity with the print.

Where do we look for confirmation of this idea? Earlier, we described the beholder's interaction with the print in terms of the cognitive free play of *speculatio*; this analysis, however, relegated to the background another dimension of experience, one to which we must now begin attending: narrative. I want to suggest that when the beholder consents to active engagement with the print, he or she invariably enters upon a dynamic form of narrative identification, one in which the "fiction" of the image is assimilated to the "truth" of the beholder's own life and vice versa. Imitation, always carrying with it an element of transference, begets ethical knowledge as well as spiritual insight. Through it, both the notional sufferer and his or her proxy within the image pass from a stopped-up "thinking in perplexity" to a clarification of imagination, reason, and memory, a restoration of function, a renewal of creative thought and action.

Whether the inherent instability of melancholia as an "assemblage" of causes, effects, and interpretations lies at the heart of this kind of transference remains unclear.[9] What does seem clear is that this passage from perplexity to clarification already betokens therapy. That is the premise of this chapter, and we will go on to explain why the genial melancholic, as a special kind of psychosomatic sufferer, benefits from precisely this kind of movement of the soul. At the starting point of this analysis, however, we need to say more about identification. For it is hardly obvious why the generic viewer of Dürer's print should feel drawn into a reflexive relationship with a dejected, androgynous winged figure, why the picture might engender a mimetic contemplation of her plight, and why she insistently relates to the beholder's lived situation, rather than standing still as a timeless allegory of creativity in crisis.

Reflecting the Self in Time

Consider first the fundamental respect in which Dürer's portrayal of pensive inaction in *Melencolia I* resembles the moralizing image of the slothful housewife: both play upon our implicit understanding, our awareness, that theirs is not a permanent state, but one into which

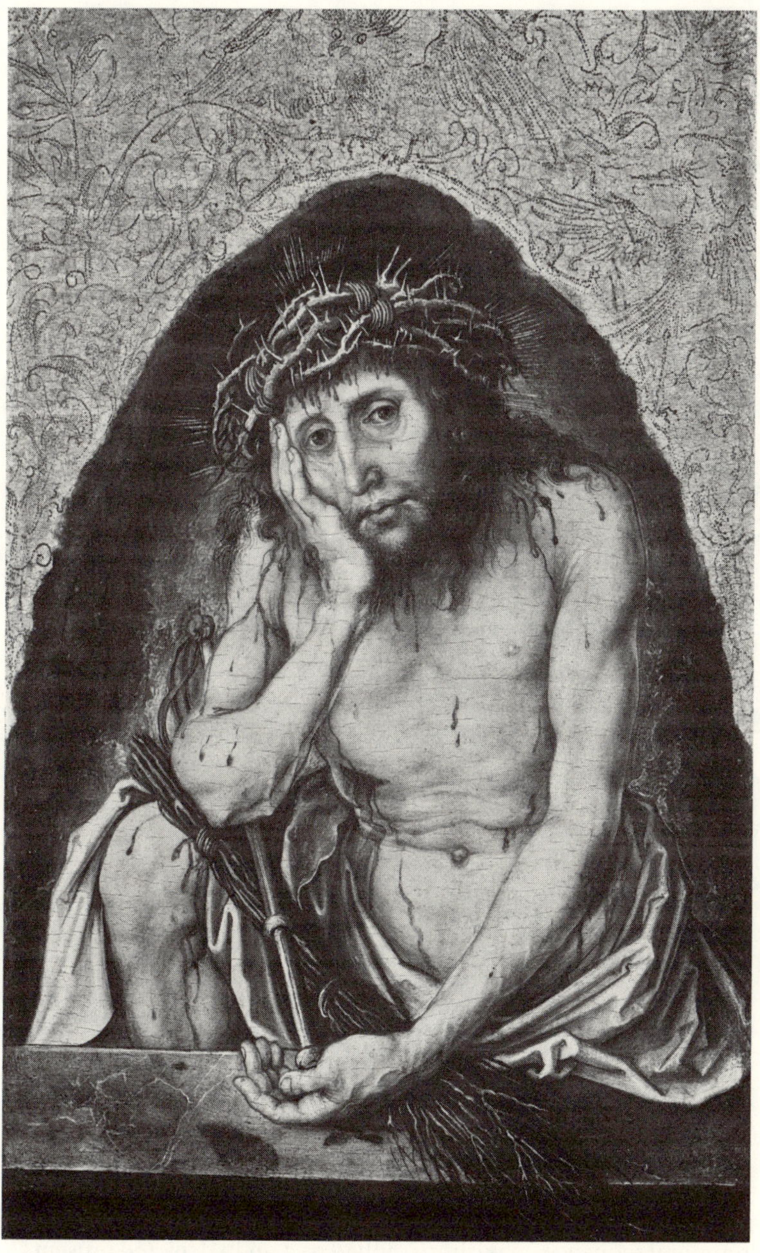

Figure 4.3. Albrecht Dürer, *Man of Sorrows in Repose*, ca. 1493, oil on fir panel, 30.1 x 18.8 cm (Karlsruhe, Staatliche Kunsthalle) (photo: bpk Bildagentur / Annette Fischer / Heike Kohler / Art Resource, NY).

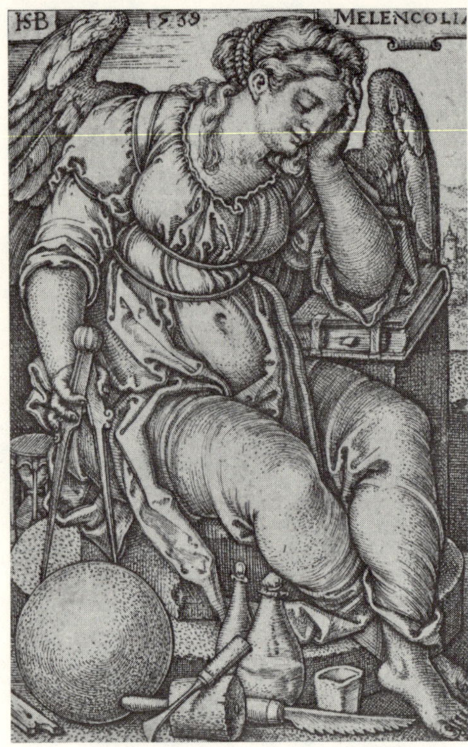

Figure 4.4. Sebald Beham, *Melencolia*, ca. 1539, engraving, 7.8 x 5.1 cm (Washington, D.C., National Gallery of Art, Rosenwald Collection).

they've passed from some other. (Even those of melancholic disposition, complexion, or constitution were not, in the view of most ancient and medieval authorities, crippled by an unchanging morbidity; as we will see later in this chapter, the worst symptoms were known to come and go.) Sleep follows wakefulness and wakefulness, in turn, follows sleep; similarly, Melancholy's creative paralysis has evidently followed upon its opposite, "a past state of activity." This can be judged by the ostentatious sprawl of tools and implements lying at her feet, objects cast away before their use has accomplished anything lasting.[10] Among modern commentators, it has been Philip Sohm who has most thoroughly explored the indications of temporality and narrative in the print, arguing that the scene demands to be "read as a temporal sequence . . . with an implied past and a depicted present."[11] Sohm points first of all to the measurable correspondence between Melancholy's compass—its angle of extension—and the radius of the sphere at her feet. With it, Dürer seems to be encouraging his learned

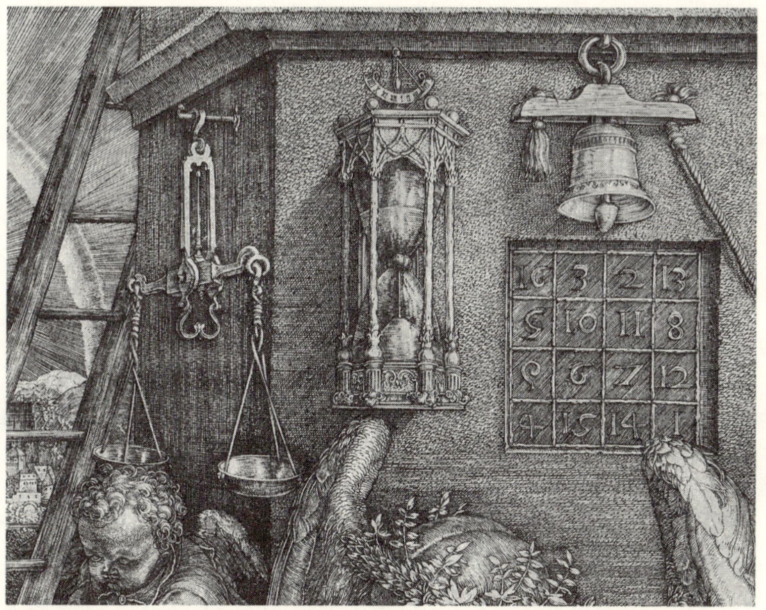

Figure 4.5. Detail from Dürer, *Melencolia I*: scales, sundial, and bell. (See figure 1.1.)

audience "to reconstruct the prior act ... of gauging the radius," something his fellow Nuremberger Sebald Beham (1500–1550), who may have worked in Dürer's shop for a time, captures more or less explicitly in his pared down version of the theme, produced around 1539 (figure 4.4).[12] Here the relationship of the geometrician's instrument to its object, disconnected in Dürer's version, is restored in the gesture of Beham's wistful and sensuous genius figure. The idea behind this modification, however, which hints at a subversive intention found elsewhere in the artist's oeuvre, remains unclear.[13]

Augmenting the little drama of the compass in Dürer's image, we find other objects arrayed around Melancholy alluding to the passage and measurement of time: the instruments attached to the wall of the tower, in particular, the hourglass crowned by a sundial, but also the bell (figure 4.5). The scales close by the putto's head may refer to the Last Judgment, the null point of the *saeculum* and the eternal beyond time's reach.[14] To these symbolic evocations of temporality we may add the bat-dragon fluttering through the sky, the cosmic burst over the horizon, and the sense of deepening twilight, lengthening shadows, flames flickering down, and so on, all richly allusive of the slow approach of death, the negation of the self in time. Heightened consciousness of mortality is set within a cosmic time marked by the planetary movements and conjunctions—astral influences that come into being with mathematical precision and pass away just as surely. Melancholy's bright eyes are not the "the only true sign of life in the . . . lifeless world of *Melencolia*," as one recent commentator put it.[15] Saturn's radiance touches everything in the scene, while something in the atmosphere, something we can not quite pinpoint, a glint of hope that renders the shadows evanescent, keeps terror at bay.

Credit is due to Sohm's superb analysis, which as we have seen focuses on the implied narrative movement from a past moment of inspiration into the present state of dejection, from activity to inactivity. Yet what these mood-generating motifs also suggest, perhaps even more powerfully, is a countervailing movement: time's flow forward, the anticipation of future events about to unfold. By restricting his reading of the allegory's temporal frame to past and present, Sohm joins hands with those other interpreters who have understood Dürer's engraving fundamentally as a diagnosis of the malaise and misfortune associated with the saturnine temperament:[16] *melancholy is like this, and this is how it comes about.* But diagnosis and warning, we suggested in earlier chapters, are only part of what made the print an effective resource for the suffering soul. How do we account for the fact that every evocation of temporality in the scene's saturnine glow, every narrative motif alluding to a past state out of which the present has emerged, provides equally for the postulation of an opposing movement—a resumption of practical activity, a clarification of confusion and disorientation, an alleviation of symptoms? To the picture's acknowledged status as a visual diagnosis, even a pathology, Dürer, I suggest, has added the claim to be an etiology, as well: *melancholy takes this course; it comes on and recedes like this.* Saturn's influence is not unchanging and unyielding; Dame Melancholia is not the helpless victim of tragic action, irreversibly caught in a web of destiny and suffering she can't escape.

This suggests that among the responses Dürer's engraving is capable of arousing is an ingrained awareness that every beholder's own experience has an ineluctable temporality, trajectory, and purpose (*telos*), a beginning and a progression toward an end. Furthermore, it asks whether it might not be the creative melancholic, above all other exemplars of the self in time, who finds consolation, relief, and renewal in contemplating this ebb and flow. In another context, the literary scholar Stephen Crites has written of the "narrative quality of experience,"[17] and it is with his model that I would like to test some aspects of the premodern experience of melancholy, aspects that play a role in the therapeutic conception of Dürer's print as I have construed it.

By encouraging the beholder to anticipate Melancholy's passage back into inventive activity, Dürer's tableau taps into a fundamental demand that informs both our experience of narrative, broadly speaking (that is, across genres), and the narrative quality of spectatorship historically (that is, prior to the rise of "disinterested" aesthetic experience in modernity): I refer here to the idea of an imaginative merging of tragic situations fictional and real, "inside" and "outside" the space of representation. According to Aristotle's scheme, representations of tragic suffering—whether poetic, dramatic, or even pictorial—always aim toward a "clarification" (κάθαρσις, *katharsis*) of the very same emotions stoked by the represented action. In the *Poetics*, those canonical emotions are "pity" (ἔλεος, *eleos*) and "fear" (φόβος, *phobos*). The end result is the sweeping away of ignorance, sorrow, confusion, and the affective states accompanying them. "Recognition" (ἀναγνώρισις, *anagnōrisis*) and "reversal" (περιπέτεια, *peripeteia*) set this movement toward clarification on its course. By enlisting the viewer's compassion, by connecting the demand for resolution and self-knowledge internal to Melancholy's "story" to the situation of the beholder, the print not only mobilizes the viewer's human sympathies as a witness to a form of suffering. Crucially, the demand also styles the spectator as an *agent* of this passage toward clarification, a collaborator in the return to creative functioning.

This point must be emphasized, but also explained before proceeding. Let us distinguish two concentric circles each with a different mode of agency at its center. One mode arises from the kind of speculative engagement with the print I described in Chapter 2. Giving the work of art its due as a philosophical pastime, as an ethical and spiritual workout capable of alleviating the symptoms that block the free flow of imagination, helped us understand this mode of agency as a technique of self-cultivation, a therapeutic inwardness that mobilizes the soul's higher resources. The second circle of agency is more intersubjective. It arises from an engagement with the germinal narrative or "plot" into which the beholder imaginatively projects—a paradigmatic problem of human life, one shared with other persons. One might even call it a "tragic situation" that works on the emotions of the beholder much as the spectacle of undeserved suffering works on the audience in Attic tragedy. Vicarious experience means that the represented action is imagined as a possibility in the life of the spectator, a predicament toward which his own fate could easily carry him.

In the case of the peculiar distress produced by melancholia, and in particular the variant linked pathogenetically to the "combustion" of bile (*melancholia adusta*), said to be brought about by everything from immoderate passions to red meat or heavy wine, the therapeutic challenge is greater. At its extremes, the overheating of blood and bile, whatever its causes, threatened the patient with a violent delirium, just as excessive cooling led to the worst form of torpor, depression accompanied by suicidal thoughts.[18] Inciting the beholder to see an open-ended "story" of suffering reflected in Melancholy's chaos amounts to an invitation to enter time's rhythms and anticipate a relaxation of symptoms, a restoration of potencies (cognitive, spiritual, emotional, creative). This points to a mode of therapeutic rebalancing that is, strictly speaking, neither a spiritual consolation nor a magical neutralization of debilitating astral influences. By appealing to Aristotle's well-known theory of *katharsis*, I am suggesting that this therapeutic effect is akin, rather, to a therapy of the passions, a form of purgation aimed at restoring "pleasure" to the organic system, a rebalancing at once psychological and somatic, a remedy both moral and medicinal. Addressing itself to a broad audience of melancholic aspirants "born under Saturn," from fellow creative geniuses and great men of action to overworked art students stuck in the mud, Dürer's portrayal of melancholia poses as both diagnosis and remedy— not a cure, but an alleviation of symptoms sufficient for getting on with things.

Combustive, Delusive, Demonic

Shimmering with astral radiance and pulsing with unseen affinities among the scatter of things, the "intense atmosphere" of Melancholy's thought space, described by Frances Yates as a projection of the occultist's visionary stance (Chapter 1), borders on the hallucinatory. Had Dürer left to posterity only this one document of his life and art, we would place him alongside Bosch as one of the great surrealists *avant la lettre*. *Melancholy is like this*, we intuitively hear the artist saying, and in the crowded tableau we imagine we have the mirror of an inner state. But whose inner state? Is Dürer's notional sufferer a "melancholic by nature," or an example of the *melancholia artificialis* that Panofsky saw personified in the winged genius?[19] Is he or she an unfortunate victim of Saturn's influence, or one who suffers from a devastating alteration in the humoral or thermal balance, that is, a form of morbid melancholia? Given the dazzling spectrum of moods and disorders associated with black bile since antiquity—in categories ranging from "illness," to "condition" to "disposition"—the situation faced by our surrogate in Dürer's picture is far from clear. Perhaps it is not as dire as the penumbral mood of the scene suggests. A fuller diagnosis is in order.

Consider the worst-case scenario first—the deeply pathological. Medical writers since antiquity described the most extreme clinical manifestations of morbid melancholia as a disoriented state akin to mania—a "madness" marked by delusions of the kind otherwise associated with demonic possession (at the very end of the nineteenth century, the term "manic-depressive insanity" was coined by German psychiatrists to distinguish this form of delirium from other depressive states).[20] How would a sixteenth-century artist picture this condition from the inside, as it were? Ready with one answer to this question is Dürer's contemporary, Lucas Cranach the Elder (ca. 1472–1553), who produced at least four painted "Melancholia" allegories between 1528 and 1533. The earliest of this group, now in Edinburgh, is illustrated in figure 4.6.[21] Sitting close to the floor in an open-air mess hall of sorts, a lynx-eyed enchantress is seen sharpening the end of a wooden stick while watching several naked, wingless *spiritelli* mount and harass a bony hound. Annoyed by their rough play, the dog is close cousin to Dürer's slumbering hunting dog in *Melencolia*, one of several obvious borrowings Cranach made from the engraving. (Others include the orb, the compass, and the carpentry tools scattered on the floor.) Just beyond the fictional parapet that separates the room from the deep landscape, hovering opposite an apple tree that likewise marks the threshold between the goddess's strange domain and the earthly *mundus*, we see naked women riding a menagerie

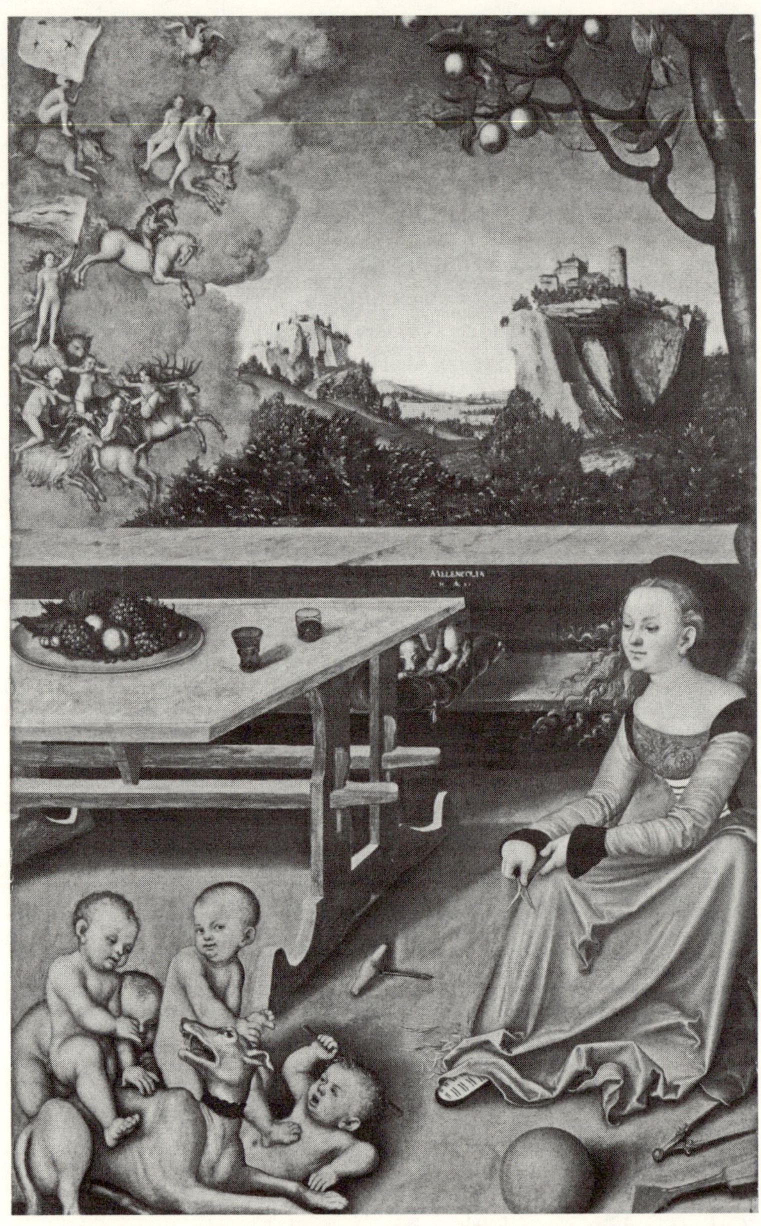

Figure 4.6. Lucas Cranach the Elder, *Allegory of Melancholia*, dated 1528, oil and tempera on wood, 112.5 x 71 cm (Edinburgh, National Galleries of Scotland) (photo: National Galleries of Scotland. Long loan in 1993).

of animals in orgiastic abandon through bursts of charcoal fumes (figure 4.7). Unseen by the room's inhabitants, the clamorous cavalcade takes on the character of an apparition visible only to the beholder. Surging forward from the picture space into ours, this image within the image doubles as a glimpse inside the mind deranged by melancholic distemper.

Yet the imagery of rampaging demonic beings was hardly Cranach's invention. Popular tales of a "furious horde" of wild, satanic riders (*Wütisches Heer*) were an established feature of witchcraft beliefs and iconography, at least from the later fifteenth century, and appear elsewhere in South German, Alsatian, and Swiss art before the Reformation (figure 4.8).[22] When reported, their terrifying appearance was understood by learned commentators as a delusion induced by sorcery, not an actual klatsch of satanic beings. In the witchcraft imagery produced for sophisticated audiences by Dürer's German contemporaries, notably Hans Baldung (ca. 1484–1545), whose witch imagery predates Cranach's by a decade, the lines separating eyewitness observation, medical diagnosis, and anal-erotic fantasy are mischievously erased (figure 4.9).[23] In parallel fashion, it seems, Cranach's purpose was to link melancholy to "the delusions of witchcraft," as Charles Zika has argued. Conversely, by relying on "the key visual codes for the representation of witchcraft" and the identification of the wild riders as Saturn's children, Cranach levels a powerful indictment of melancholy as a delusional state that "spawns violent and destructive forces that endanger right order, similar to the destructive forces of witchcraft."[24] Here we are halfway between the Renaissance era's persistent fear of demons—a persistence that fascinated Aby Warburg, among others—and the Aristotelian-Galenic observation of natural causes, an "enlightened" view of witchcraft that scholars have detected, for example, in Goya's *The Spell* of 1798.[25] Without fully displacing demonological thinking, psychomedical explanations of witch sightings and accusations of this kind were already gaining ground in the early sixteenth century.

With his Edinburgh panel, Cranach needles us to decide whether it is the satanic riders who induce, through black magic, terrifying visions akin to melancholic mania, or whether a "delusional melancholic mind" has conjured them into being in the first place. As we will see in more detail shortly, ancient and medieval medical writers held that atrabilious imbalance lent itself to such visions, for it made

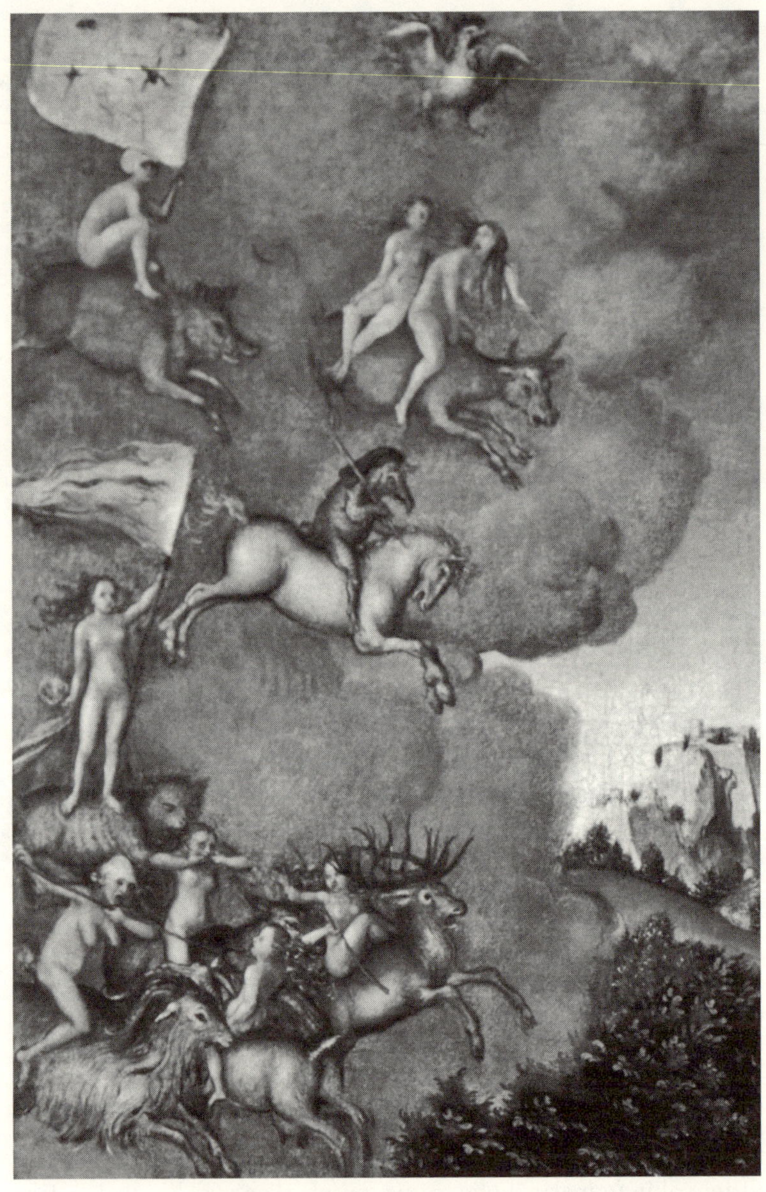

Figure 4.7. Detail from Cranach, *Melancholia*: vaporous cloud with wild riders. (See figure 4.6.)

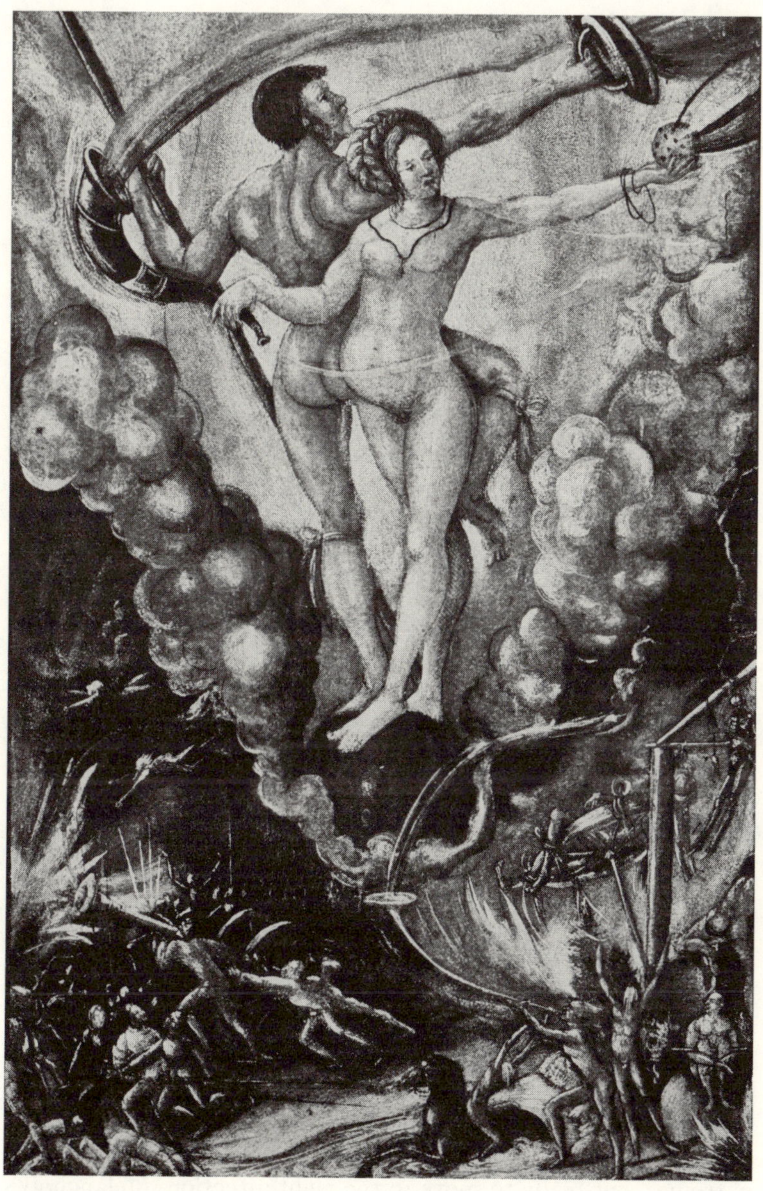

Figure 4.8. Urs Graf, *The Furious Horde*, ca. 1513–15, tempera on paper on limewood panel, 27.3 x 17.2 cm (Kunstmuseum Basel, Amerbach-Kabinett 1662) (photo: Kunstmuseum Basel, Martin P. Bühler).

the mind both vulnerable to outside attack and productive of fearsome apparitions from within.

It is all the more striking, then, that no such demonic forces break to the surface in the luminous atmosphere of Dürer's *Baustelle*. The uniform space secured by geometry is not interrupted by visionary cloudbursts of the kind Cranach pictured. Only the bat, a demonic figure Dürer directly associates with the soul's sickness by virtue of the words scrawled upon it, hints at such a threat. (At any rate, the winged messenger, as Konrad Hoffman has argued, appears to be leaving the scene.)[26] Yet the battle to banish melancholy's demons is far from over. Signs of a resolution to the crisis of despondency and gloom are indeed all around; time is poised to flow toward the future, toward a restoration of function, but the darkened mood of the engraving, which has impressed so many of its admirers, can not be denied. Dürer knew from experience that the "hot" melancholic genius could easily overheat, bringing frenzy, or it could run cold and descend into despondency and madness. For centuries, medical writers pointed out that melancholic distress had no single etiology, and what causes could be identified manifest differently in different types of persons. As a somatopsychic syndrome, melancholia had, in short, an unstable identity. Its resistance to straightforward diagnosis, we will see, derived from a kind of relational hydraulics of humoral substance, heat, and moisture. Each organic factor affected the other and was affected in turn, producing a kaleidoscopic range of conflicting clinical symptoms.

My argument will be that as an emblematic feature of the narrative, the "intense atmosphere" of Dürer's engraving thematizes melancholy's unique power to suspend the sufferer between contradictory states—between overheated frenzy, the stuff of ecstatic visions, and frozen torpor, a despondency that despairs of health and tragically searches for its own annihilation. Warning the beholder about this dangerous borderline is not, however, the engraving's only answer to this crisis. Laying out the ground for the mind's resistance and suggesting possible itineraries, it also proffers a kind of consolation, as well as a way clear of the predicament. Poised between extremes, but ready to move in the right direction, Melancholy's narrative "situation" invites and instigates a tempered response in the beholder, a moderate and modulated speculation with the power not only to model, but to restore the mind's creative functioning.

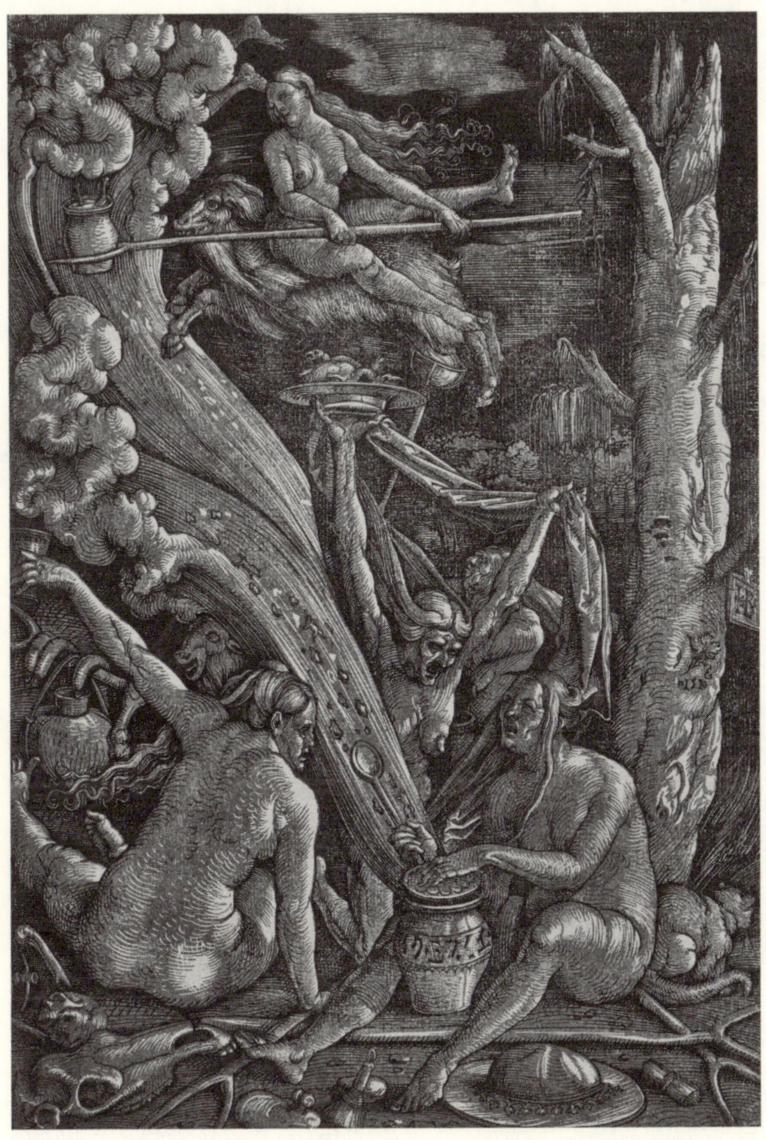

Figure 4.9. Hans Baldung Grien, *Witches' Sabbath*, 1510, chiaroscuro woodcut on gray paper, 37.9 x 26 cm (Berlin, Staatliche Museen, Kupferstichkabinett) (photo: bpk Bildagentur/ Jörg P. Anders/Art Resource, NY).

Melancholia—A Mutable Affliction

From the earliest identification of melancholia as a distinct illness in the Hippocratic corpus (fourth to fifth centuries BCE), Greek medical writers placed it on the line separating clinical syndrome from functional psychosis and defined it variably as an acute or chronic condition.[27] Generally recognized was the fact that normal persons were susceptible to an everyday form of depression marked by "aversion to food, despondency, sleeplessness, irritability, and restlessness"; to blame were those various disturbances in the balance (δυσκρασία, *duskrasia*) among the four humors (blood, phlegm, black bile, and yellow bile), organic substances whose optimal blend (εὐκρασία, *eucrasia*) signaled health.[28] Persons with higher concentrations of black bile, the humor thought to be in the ascendancy in autumn and associated with coldness and dryness, were always at a higher risk of feeling "thoroughly penetrated" by these symptoms; when left untreated, the ill effects of this *duskrasia* could intensify. Canonical for ancient symptomology was the equation put forth in the Hippocratic *Aphorisms* (4.23): "fear and despondency persevering for a long time means melancholy."[29]

Meanwhile, a special minority of patients shared in what the author of the Aristotelian *Problemata physica* described as a distinctive melancholic "mixture" (κρᾶσις, *krasis*)—a unique blend of humors, elements, and temperatures that would later be called the individual's "complexion" (*complexio*) or "temperament" (*temperamentum*).[30] Of the four canonical temperaments (figure 4.10), the melancholic was especially idiosyncratic: disposed toward paralyzing gloom, but also endowed with an extraordinary potential for creative accomplishment, "susceptible to particular diseases, but also particular modes of perception."[31] "Why is it that all those who have become eminent in philosophy or politics or poetry or the arts are clearly of an atrabilious temperament?" is the question with which Pseudo-Aristotle begins his influential investigation.[32] Along with these special gifts, he explains, came special burdens. Solitude, despair, sadness, and greed were the melancholic's birthright; to overcome them, and return to optimal functioning, his ever-renewing challenge.

We have already registered the outsized role this notion played in the Renaissance construction of an "inspired melancholy" (*melancholia generosa*) that was a key attribute of the Saturnine mind (as well as in the modern construction of melancholia as a subjective mood).[33] But let us return to Greek medicine prior to the systematization of the four cardinal temperaments by the Roman physician Galen (131–210) and his followers. It is important to see how the contradictory symptoms of this particular humoral excess were thought to stem directly from the strange properties of black bile itself. We have just noted that the author of the *Problemata* (number 30, section 1) describes the humor as a "mixture [*krasis*] of heat and cold," an unstable infusion that tilts the body toward extremes: chilling the system beyond measure in one case, overheating it in another. Bile is naturally cold, Pseudo-Aristotle explains, and "if it abounds in the body, produces apoplexy or torpor or despondency or fear." Alternately "it produces cheerfulness accompanied by song, and frenzy, and the breaking forth of sores, and the like," especially when "this heat approaches the region of the intellect." It is in this way that some become "affected by diseases of frenzy and possession; and this is the origin of Sibyls and soothsayers and all inspired persons, when they are affected not by disease but by natural temperament."[34]

Here Aristotelian naturalism and the medical notions derived from it betray the influence of Plato's theory of divine madness. Their convergence was prepared, as Klibansky, Panofsky, and Saxl realized, by the correspondence dreams and prophecies—the "gifts" of a pathological melancholy—already had with the Platonic equation of "mantic" and "mania."[35] Even from a strictly humoral basis, however, black bile was judged to have a "heightened pathogenic potential."[36] In working out the various processes by which this thick, earthy humor was formed, how it moved and separated, how it was transmuted, filtered, and absorbed in the body's organs, Galen also recognized its distinctive qualities.[37] As the accumulated medical wisdom of the Greeks filtered down through later Hellenistic, Roman, Arabic, and Scholastic accounts of melancholia and the cardinal temperaments, this notion of melancholia's singularity, rehabilitated and reinterpreted in the Renaissance by Neoplatonists such as Marsilio Ficino, faithfully followed. Across centuries of medical discourse, black bile anchored the paradoxical idea of an "eucrasia within an anomaly"; thus the enduring perception of melancholia's uniqueness among the somatopsychic illnesses.[38]

That melancholia's special contradictory character fascinated medical authorities well before the mystical dualism of Ficino is attested in the most important handbook dedicated to the syndrome

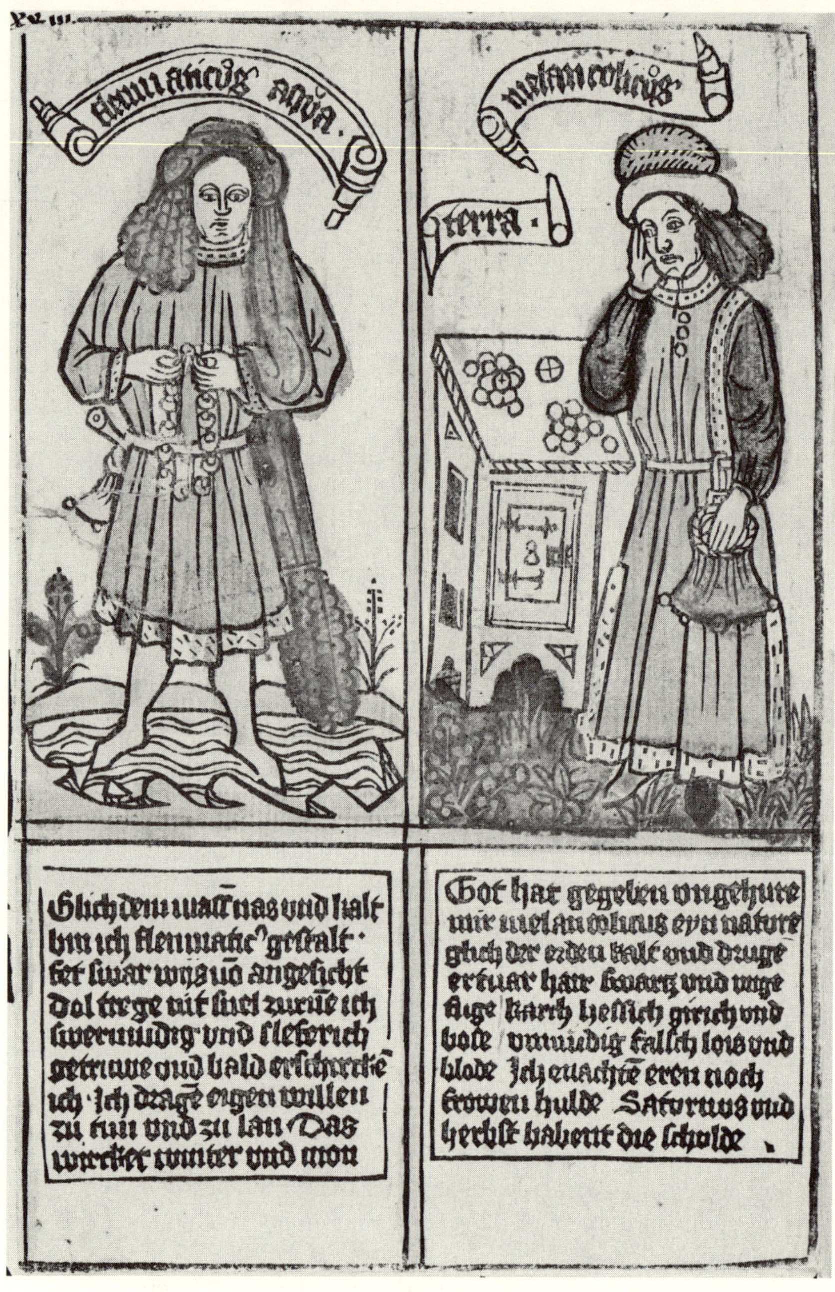

Figure 4.10. *The Four Temperaments*, hand-colored woodcuts in manuscript of Gall Kemli (d. 1481), *Diversarius multarum materiarum*, assembled in the fifteenth century; each page approximately 21.2 x 14.5 cm (Zurich, Zentralbibliothek, Ms. C 101, fols. 25v [Phlegmatic and Melancholic] and 26r [Sanguine and Choleric]) (photos: courtesy of Zentralbibliothek Zurich).

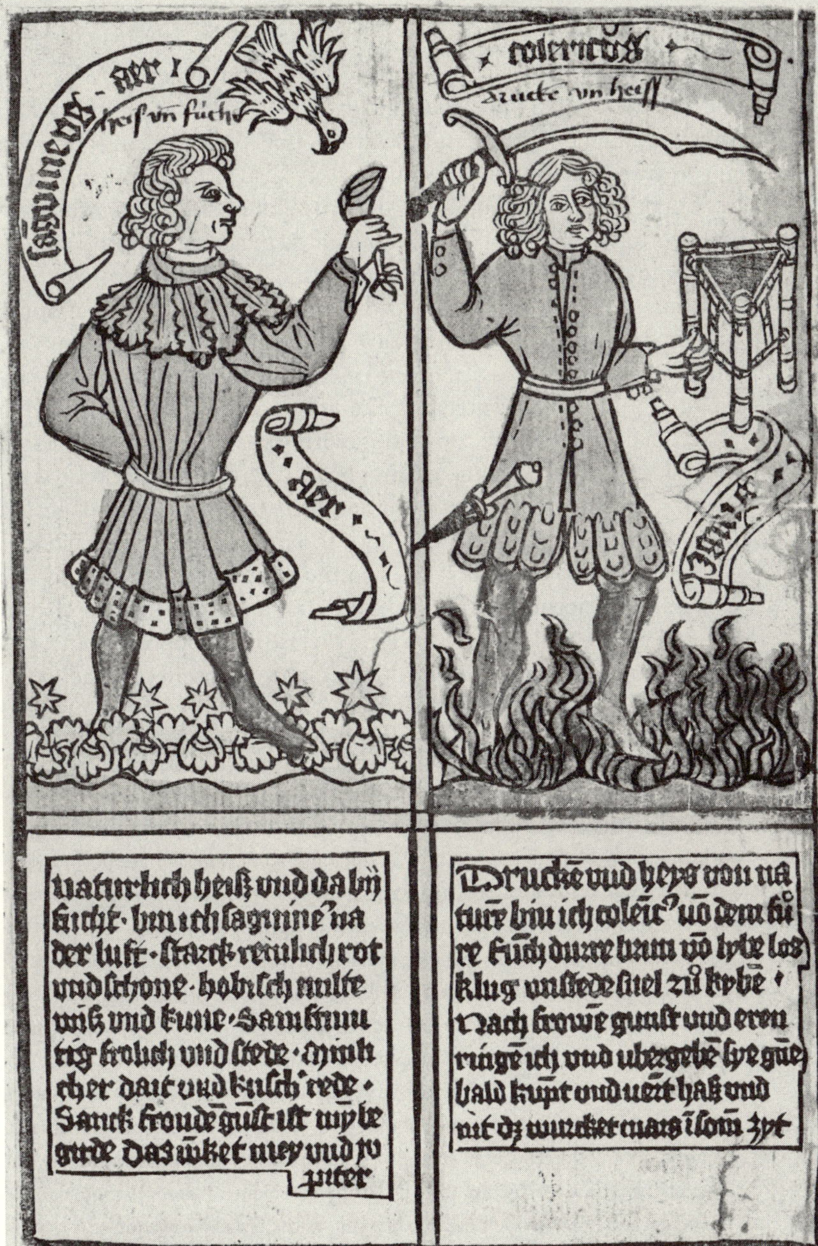

natürlich heiß vnd da bij
sicht · bin ich sanguineus na
der luft · starck reinlich rot
vnd schone · hob ich mitte
witz vnd kune · Sam bruu
tig frolich vnd stete · Minh
eher dait vnd kusch rede ·
Sanck froude gnst ist witie
gnde das ubket nuy vnd ju
piter

Drucke vnd heis von na
ture bin ich coleir· vn dem fi
re fuch durre bram vo hite los
klug vnstede snel zu krbe ·
Nach frowe gunst vnd eren
ringe ich vnd ubergebe ire gue
bald kupt vnd uert hass vnd
nit dz wunket mars in sein zyt

in the medieval West. Composed by Constantinus the African, a Benedictine monk (and convert) who ended his days at Montecassino Abbey around 1090, the handbook reproduced the writings of Ishâq ben 'Amrân (d. early tenth century) while also synthesizing material from Galen and, via Galen, the doctrines of Rufus of Ephesus (late first century), who had likewise connected melancholy with intellectual genius.[39] Variety and contradiction must have run through Constantinus's case files like red threads, for as he tells his readers: "Some [patients] love solitude and the dark and living apart from mankind, others love spaciousness, light, and meadowy surroundings, and gardens rich in fruits and streams. Some love riding, listening to different sorts of music, or conversing with wise or amiable people.... Some sleep too much, some weep, some laugh."[40] It was likewise with regard to etiology. Constantinus found so heterogeneous a collection of causes—climatic conditions both too dry and too moist, lack of exercise but also overexertion, too much voluptuousness and too severe an asceticism—he confessed to find it "astonishing...that in our experience melancholy can always arise from opposite causes."[41] In a pointed warning to those who specialize in intellectual achievement, Constantinus even identified "the activities of the rational soul" as potentially harmful—especially where one is prone to overdoing it. His list includes:

> strenuous thinking, remembering, studying, investigating, imagining, seeking the meaning of things, and fantasies and judgments, whether apt [founded on fact] or mere suspicions. And all these conditions—which are partly permanent forces [mental faculties], partly accidental symptoms [passions]—can turn the soul within a short time to melancholy if it immerses itself too deeply in them.... And all those will fall into melancholy who overexert themselves in reading philosophical books, or books on medicine and logic, or books which permit a view [theory] of all things; as well as books on the origin of numbers, on the sciences which the Greeks call arithmetic; on the origins of the heavenly spheres and the stars, that is, the science of the stars, which the Greeks call astronomy; on geometry, which bears the name of 'science of lines' among the Arabians, but which the Greeks call geometry; and finally the science of composition, namely of songs and notes, which means the same as the Greek word 'music.'... Such men...assimilate melancholy...in the consciousness of their intellectual weakness, and in their distress thereat they fall into melancholy. The reason why their soul falls sick lies in fatigue and overexertion, as Hippocrates says.[42]

To the historian of medicine, this sounds like the standard warning that Greek and Roman physicians issued against immoderation in any area of life: when it comes to movement and rest, ingestion and elimination, sleeping and waking, copulation and continence, you just have to take it easy. Much the same advice was offered by Rufus of Ephesus, who attributed the descent into melancholic gloom to an excess of mental effort. "People of excellent nature are predisposed to melancholy," he writes as if in answer to the Pseudo-Aristotle's lead question, "since excellent natures move more quickly and think a lot."[43] In weighing melancholy's multiple causes and identifying "overexertion" as a key risk factor, medical writers such as Constantinus were paying special attention to the interaction of bile with the body's animal heat. All bodies possess an "innate heat" (*calor innatus*), according to Galen, on which depends not only circulation, digestion, the absorption of nutrients, healthy elimination, and fertility, but sound cognitive function as well. Regulation of the body's thermal balance thus was critical, and fever was indicative of a wide range of ailments. Just as immoderate coldness or dryness could cause "thickened superfluities,"[44] excessive combustion, especially in the gut, could scorch the body's juices, spelling danger. Yellow bile, in particular, was prone to being dangerously transformed in this way; once blackened, it became an unstable humoral compound the great Persian scientist Avicenna (Ibn-Sīnā; ca. 980–1037) called *melancholia adusta*, "burnt" bile.

Eventually, medical authorities accepted that, in addition to yellow bile, blood and black bile itself, if not properly eliminated, could also be transmuted by inner combustion into darkened excesses. (According to Galen, after the spleen had absorbed all the bile it needed for its own nutrition, or transformed it back into blood, the rest was deposited in the stomach to aid in digestion.) In synthesizing this principle fully with the doctrine of the four humors, Avicenna opened the door to a more differentiated set of atrabilious conditions. "From now on," Klibansky, Panofsky, and Saxl explain, "melancholy illness could have a sanguine, choleric, phlegmatic, or 'natural melancholic' basis," a system that "had the advantage of coupling the variety of symptoms with a variety of causes."[45] Physicians in Dürer's time knew the special dangers of atrabilious blood and the combustions that produced it. The Netherlandish physician and poet Jason Pratensis (1486–1559), for instance, attributed the *affectus melancholicus* primarily to the admixture of bile with corrupted blood, stinking and black."[46] This transmutation of the humors multiplied the already countless variety of symptoms—more euphoric, more depressive, more frenetic, more listless—exhibited by those suffering from melancholia. Ultimately, according to Klibansky, Panofsky, and Saxl, the medical recognition of this dyscrasic cross traffic in the organic body, mutable and unstable, "disrupted the cogency of the scheme of the four humours."[47]

Most harmful were the toxic vapors produced by this pathology of combustible substances. By virtue of the distinctive effects these fumelike byproducts had on the brain—on perception, thought, and imagination—*melancholia adusta* was considered the basis for one of three canonical "types" of melancholia. Black bile was central to each of these types and, again, Galen's account was the authoritative one. Accumulation of the cold, dry, and toxic substance could occur, according to Galen, in the head, the whole body, or the hypochondrium—but the part most crucially affected in all three cases is the brain. For it is here, as Angus Gowland explains, "where the psychic pneuma (or spirit) mediates the functions of the rational (or hegemonic) soul, such as thought, memory, knowledge, imagination, understanding, and sensation."[48]

Consider what happens to the brain when bile is localized pathogenically in the upper abdomen. As Galen notes in *De locis affectis* (On the affected parts), this "hypochondriacal" variety of melancholia is marked by severe flatulence and other digestive disturbances; inflammation of the stomach thickens the blood there so it becomes atrabilious, and "an atrabilious evaporation produces melancholic symptoms of the mind by ascending to the brain like a sooty substance or a smoky vapor."[49] Because the internal divisions of the body were deemed permeable, in other words, smoke produced when blood and bile were "cooked" in the upper abdomen could rise through the thorax and into the head. Patients suffering from an affection of the spleen risked having even more of this "noxious serum" flowing into the stomach for combustion, the end result being fumigation of the brain. Hopelessness, sadness, the loss of mental clarity, even a delirium bordering on hallucination, were the results, according to Galen. Purgatives that opened the bowels and moved excess bile and atrabilious blood down and out of the stomach were an important means of combating these pathogenic humors.

Ancient and medieval medical authorities routinely noted the manic, fear-struck delusions their patients experienced in the grip of bilious excesses. Noting the extraordinary diversity of the "abnormal sensory images" that presented themselves, Galen describes how

> one patient believes that he has been turned into a kind of snail and therefore runs away from everyone he meets lest [his shell] should get crushed; or when another patient sees some crowing cocks flapping their wings to their song, he beats his own arms against his ribs and imitates the sound of the animals. Again, another patient is afraid that Atlas who supports the world will become tired and throw it away and he and all of us will be crushed and pushed together. And there are a thousand other imaginary ideas.[50]

Theological commentators in the Middle Ages, though offering different explanations of causes, would likewise come to diagnose melancholia in terms of its deleterious effects on cognition, imagination, and sense perception, especially vision. Hildegard of Bingen (d. 1179), for instance, associated a dulling of vision with the *humor melancholicus*, the origin of which she related to the infirmities wrought by the Fall. Only a demonic assault upon the passions, she reasoned, could stir up comparable images. But, as we have seen, the medical understanding of a runaway combustion, and the takeover of the senses and intellect by toxic fumes permeating the body and rising up into the head, had already rendered Hildegard's demons terrifyingly concrete. In premodern medical culture, the congestion of the brain's permeable chambers by sulphurous gases coming from the abdomen was no mere metaphor: built-up pressures demanded release. Unchecked and unevacuated, sooty vapors would begin to mix with the invisible "animal spirits" flowing into the brain, impeding the essential functions—imagination, memory, reason—that depend on them.[51]

When Cranach borrowed from the established schema for depicting visions and explicitly showed those infernal rampages of blasphemous beings, ringed by black smoke, as attributes of his melancholic enchantress and the spells she cast, he was certainly drawing upon the doctrine of "burnt" bile and its delusion-inducing byproducts current among the medical naturalists of his day. That his multiple renditions of the melancholia theme coincided closely with his involvement in the creation of a reformed "Law and Gospel" iconography, in collaboration with Luther, has not escaped the notice of scholars. Does the crossing of medical and demonological discourses in the sulphurous vignettes carry specifically Lutheran ideas about melancholia?[52] Almost certainly the answer is yes. Michael Stolberg has, in this connection, detected strong resonances of Philip Melanchthon's medical thought as it would soon be worked out in his treatise on Aristotle, the *Commentarius de anima* (1540), a work that took up Luther's notion of "the whole man" as the true object of salvation from the perspective of Christian naturalism.[53] Galenic anatomy is here joined to natural philosophy to argue that medical knowledge of the body, God's creation, must join with a spiritual knowledge of the soul to address fully and holistically the incapacities of man in his fallen state. Cranach refers to that postlapsarian infirmity—blamed by Hildegard for the beclouding of natural perception—in his image of the Tree of Knowledge with its dangling apples, shown growing at the threshold of Melancholy's portico, opposite the satanic night riders. Absent the therapy of the Word, thought and affect, grounded in the body, fall prey to demonic forces, compounding spiritual blindness with the noxious byproducts of a humoral *duskrasia*. For all their visual allure, then, Cranach's melancholia pictures would seem to narrow, rather than widen, the range for speculative free association as they demystify the syndrome along Lutheran lines. They become, in short, a colorful, dreadful, even entertaining species of *Lehrbild*—certainly not an arena for meeting the melancholic sufferer halfway.

A parallel, but wholly different effort to "demystify" the syndrome and its uncanny power to becloud perception, thought, and affect are at work Dürer's portrayal of the "inner atmosphere" of the melancholic mind. Standing immediately prior to the concerns that informed Cranach's renditions, the disorienting spell Dürer casts in *Melencolia* is broken as a function of its therapeutic mode. The restorative, "passive exercise" of speculation enabled by the print is what brings this about. To further this insight, we must spend a little more time with the doctors, and set the cognitive work instigated by Dürer's engraving (see Chapter 2) within the total spectrum of treatments and therapies recommended for the various types of melancholia. Like the account of melancholia's etiology sketched above, our discussion of medical opinion on its treatments will have to remain selective. Nevertheless, it will be crucial for better appreciating how the unique ethical and spiritual exercise *Melencolia* facilitates relates to the inherent "changeableness"[54] of the illness itself. And it will further our understanding of how the engraving's narrative elements, once activated, could serve as the pathway toward clarification—the *katharsis* of the passions that restores equilibrium and alleviates the suffering of the soul.

Return to Pleasure

Treatment options for a syndrome with such a multiplicity of causes and so many contradictory symptoms as melancholia were, to risk understatement, extremely varied. Practitioners, it seems, tried everything. The therapeutic challenge was compounded all the more since, in the case of melancholia, etiological factors could also be psychological.[55] A few representative views must suffice.

On the conservative side of things, Soranus of Ephesus (early second century) has left us a detailed description of the two-tiered treatment regimen he favored.[56] Beginning when the illness was acute, his patients would undergo—in various sequences and combinations—fasting, bloodletting (though here he advised against using hellebore, due to its toxicity), various fomentations and annointings, all in combination with a light diet; also cupping with scarification, clysters (enemas), and poultices could enter the picture. Soothing remedies might be applied locally, "particularly to the region over the cardia and between the shoulder blades." To offset wakefulness, he prescribed "passive exercise, first in a hammock and then in a sedan chair"; anticipating New Age relaxation techniques, the sound of dripping water he considered helpful in calming the nerves before sleep. Once the acute phase had passed, Soranus introduced a carefully regulated diet, the application of plasters, oils, and ointments, massages and baths, more passive exercise, some walking, modest entertainments, and various kinds of mental exercise. Sitting in on philosophical discussions could qualify among the latter, he explains (with Cicero apparently in mind), "for by their words philosophers help to banish fear, sorrow, and wrath, and in so doing make no small contribution to the health of the body." Soranus was not alone in acknowledging the benefits of "treating" pathological melancholia through reasoned reflection and exhortation; this long tradition of philosophical remedy was taken over by Christian moral and pastoral theology, where the cure of melancholia was closely bound up with the treatment of *acedia*, a spiritual inertia, boredom, and "carelessness" that left the mind vulnerable to delusion.[57]

In the view of Rufus of Ephesus, whom Galen would join in recognizing three types of melancholia, treatment should begin with bloodletting, especially "where the whole body is full of melancholy blood." But, he adds, "when only the brain has been invaded, the patient does not need to be bled." (Galen would express this opinion too.)[58] In the latter type of case, and likewise with the hypochondriacal type, therapy had to focus on relaxing the stomach and opening the bowels. Among the purgatives, cathartics, and diuretics Rufus trusted for expelling bilious humors were those composed of "dodder of thyme and aloe," wormwood, colocynth, and black hellebore. Anything that improved digestion, reduced flatulence, and soothed internal pains—from simple walking to the application of mustard plasters to the area of the stomach—should also be tried. Melancholia drove premodern doctors to inspired heights of pharmacological creativity, exemplified in the "sacred remedy of Rufus," a cathartic formula containing colocynth, yellow bugle, germander, cassia, agaris, asafetida, wild parsley, aristolochia, white pepper, spikenard, cinnamon, saffron, and myrrh; the mixture was to be combined with honey and administered in four small doses with hydromel (a fermented honey beverage similar to mead) and water. Specialty compounds like those of Rufus and Galen acquired legendary status in later medical traditions as "holy bitters" (*hiera picra*), formulas whose ancient variants allegedly dated back to Asclepian temple medicines.[59]

Especially prized were therapies that helped expel humoral excesses and simultaneously dispel negative ideas from the soul. Galen advised "exercise, massage, and all kinds of active motion,"[60] while Rufus, with the same goals in mind, recommended coitus. His opinion was taken up by several Byzantine compilers, for example Oribasius of Pergamon (325–403), personal physician to Julian the Apostate. Sexual intercourse calmed the passions and "dissipated fixed ideas from the soul," according to Oribasius.[61] Paul of Aegina (625–90) transmitted this idea with complete assurance: "the best possible remedy for melancholia is coition."[62] Constantinus the African likewise repeated Rufus's advice: "Sexual intercourse pacifies, turns pridefulness into austerity, and aids those who suffer melancholy."[63] All of these authors naturally took it for granted that to avoid thermal overcompensation, intercourse should never be too strenuous.[64]

Effective as these treatments might be, ancient and medieval medical writers knew that the system's rebalancing through cathartics, purgatives, palliatives, stimulants, and strengthening agents rarely ended in cure. Symptoms could be brought under control for a time, and the disease might subside, but recurrence was an ever-present possibility. Aretaeus of Cappadocia (ca. 150), a contemporary of Galen, emphasized the inherent "changeableness" of the illness in the chapter he devoted to melancholia in his *On the Causes and Symptoms of Chronic Diseases*: "It is impossible, indeed, to make all the sick well, for a physician would thus be superior to a god; but the physician can produce respite from pain, intervals in diseases, and render them latent."[65] Every disease follows a clinical course, and the course recognized for melancholia in ancient and medieval medicine was one of ebb and flow, onset and remission, urgency and latency. Likewise did Renaissance medical writers recognize, as Noel Brann has shown, "that the goal of the physician should be not so much to *eradicate* as to *regulate* melancholy so that it can better fulfill its God-given role as a material aid for the enhancement of human genius."[66]

If we return to Dürer's engraving with these considerations in mind, the therapeutic imperative behind the germinal narrative (described earlier in this chapter) and its potential role in a course of a treatment becomes clearer. The diagnosis has been made; every square inch of the picture communicates it. Now, how will the disorientation arising from the picture's calculated chaos be overcome? How will the confusion wrought by the contradictoriness invading every object, every symbol, be clarified? How will the hallucinatory unease stemming from the picture's "structural obscurity" be relieved?

A work of art printed on paper is neither a poultice nor a purgative, of course. But as our foray into the therapeutics of melancholia in naturalistic medicine has already suggested, we *can* speak, recognizing the limits of the analogy, of a relief that comes from "passive exercise": a form of mental flexing and free play that consciously avoids overexertion, a gentle "warming" of what has grown too cold, a metaphorical "moistening" of what has become dry.[67] This, I have argued, is precisely the opportunity that Dürer's print, understood as a speculative image, offers: a moderate mental workout that calms rather than excites the passions, a stimulation of the soul's higher powers, an evacuative that dispels the vapors beclouding the mind (in Galenic terms, a freeing of the psychic pneuma, or *spiritus anima-lis*, in the brain from the corrupting effects of bile). This, in a word, is a form of *katharsis*—not in the medicinal or religious sense of a "purgation" of negative emotions, but a "clarification" of the passions with both ethical and spiritual consequences.[68] Ethical *and* spiritual, we must insist, because the beholder's natural activity has been reinstated through a virtue-forming attention to oneself (*prosochē*), a return to reason over against the debilitating effects of a "cold" and "dry" mental state.

Astral Forces and the Thinking Being

Before we rest with this conclusion concerning *Melencolia*'s therapeutic mode, a key Renaissance alternative to traditional humoral medicine must be accounted for. Medical astrology, or "iatromathematics," answers the question of melancholia's proper remedy very differently—replacing the naturalistic conception of the body as a microcosm in need of humoral, thermal, and hydraulic engineering with the idea of unseen forces penetrating the body and determining its rhythms. Planetary "influences" do just that, and for this reason astrology teaches that they must be propitiated and harnessed or fought and counteracted before any real flourishing can be possible. For centuries, this conceptual framework informed naturalistic medicine. Doctors, for example, relied on an established set of correspondences between zodiacal signs and specific regions or organs of the body when planning therapeutic interventions such as bloodletting and surgery; these diagrams became standard in illustrated medical books (figure 4.11). A similar conceptual link between macrocosm and microcosm motivated the occultists' use of talismans and magic images to propitiate planetary influences, as we will see. Dürer's relation to contemporary astrological and magical thinking about Saturn's negative inspiration has been such a foundational issue in modern research on *Melencolia* since Karl Giehlow's pioneering—and unfinished—studies of 1903–1904,[69] and it has occasioned so much discussion since then (see Chapter 1), that we can hardly avoid the issue here.

We can address it in a relatively short space, however, because occult science is only part of the engraving's intellectual background, not, in my view, its sole inspiration. It is no longer tenable to assume that iatromathematics constituted, for Dürer and his intellectual circle, the same total worldview that it did for those philosophers who

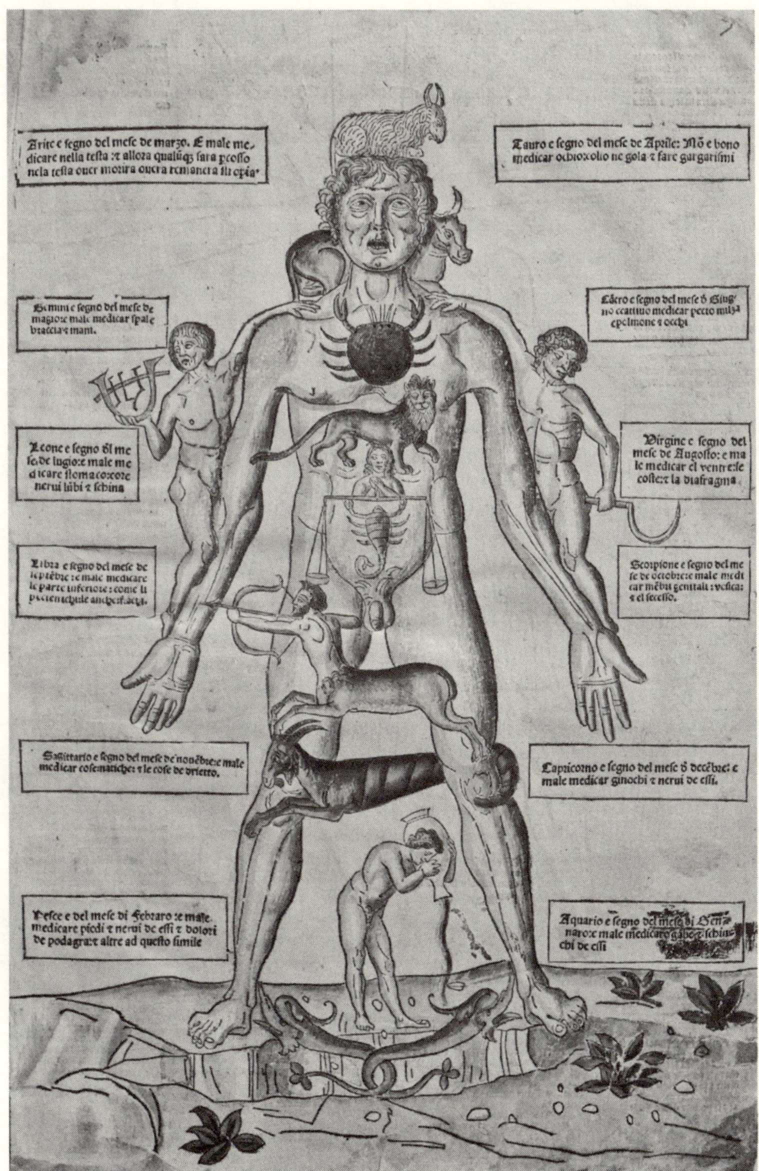

Figure 4.11. Italian, *Phlebotomy Man with Planetary Symbols*, colored woodcut from Johannes de Ketham, *Fasciculus Medicinae* (Venice: Johannes and Gregorius de Gregoriis, 5 February 1493–94), fol. bii recto (New Haven, Cushing/Whitney Medical Library, Incunabula + K-17 [Goff]) (photo: by the author).

have been claimed as sources for the *Melencolia:* the copyist(s) of the Arabic handbook of astrology and divination known as the *Picatrix* (a thirteenth-century Spanish translation of an eleventh-century compendium), the leader of the Florentine Neoplatonists Marsilio Ficino, or the occultist Cornelius Agrippa von Nettisheim.[70] The permeation of medical thinking by astrology, divination, and magic in the fifteenth and sixteenth centuries was, without a doubt, a "revolution of fundamental significance," as the authors of *Saturn and Melancholy* tell it.[71] And a new, metaphysical approach to therapeutics, with its reliance on horoscopes and talismanic images, reflects that shift. "In Ficino and his successors," Klibansky, Panofsky, and Saxl continue, "the notions based on astral influences grew to encompass so comprehensive a picture of the world that the whole art of healing was considered as nothing but a particular method of employing the general cosmic forces, and like the other sciences, it merged in the last resort with magic, which in turn was a kind of 'applied cosmology.'"[72] Central to this occult science and decisive in the Ficinian doctrine of *melancholia generosa* was the notion of Saturn and Jupiter as countervailing cosmic forces: one producing malignant, the second "jovial" effects upon sublunary bodies and minds.

By the time he began work on *Melencolia I,* Dürer had had ample opportunity to become acquainted with the new metaphysical doctrines of melancholia in Ficino and the astrologically centered approach to therapeutics: in 1497, the Florentine philosopher's letters were published in Nuremberg by Anton Koberger, and by 1505, the first two books of *De triplici vita,* a work already known in Germany by the time of Dürer's birth, had found their German translator in Adolph Muelich.[73] These facts alone would have justified Aby Warburg's confident description of Dürer's engraving, in the context of his famous study of Reformation-era prophecy and astral magic, as "that ripest and most mysterious fruit of the cosmological culture of the age of Maximilian I."[74]

But the new metaphysical conceptions hardly displaced traditional explanations of the melancholic temperament overnight. Renaissance medicine remained in thrall to the "materialist determinism" of Galen's theory of melancholy and to Galenic pathology in general until the late seventeenth century.[75] As Klibansky, Panofsky, and Saxl are quick to point out, despite the vogue of Ficino's doctrines, the influence of the *Picatrix,* and the fascination exerted by Agrippa's occult science, *the* preeminent German humanist, Konrad Celtis, still "identified himself completely with the customary views of school [that is, Scholastic] medicine, and Saturn was for him nothing but a mischief-maker who produced sad, labouring, and 'monkish' men."[76]

It is more than noteworthy, then, that Dürer's earliest documented engagement with the classical theory of the temperaments was, in fact, in direct collaboration with Celtis. I refer to the title page woodcut he designed, after a sketch provided by Celtis himself, for the *Quatuor libri amorum* (Four books of love), which the poet laureate dedicated to his patron Maximilian and had published in Nuremberg in 1502 (figure 4.12).[77] Heralded in the superscript by her own praise of the Greeks for describing, the Romans for translating, and the Germans for amplifying her, Philosophy sits enthroned inside a great garland whose foliage receives the breath of the four winds, each associated with a cosmic element and a bodily humor. Modeled in part on the prisoner's vision in Boethius's *Consolation of Philosophy*, the goddess is the first of several female personifications Dürer would devise during his career, the most famous being Melancholy. In the lower left, Boreas, the melancholic wind, cold and damp, coming from the north and associated with the earth, is depicted as a bitter old man puffing out frigid air. Icicles hang from the frozen arbor above him. Portrait roundels commemorating the great sages of Egypt (Ptolemy), Greece (Plato), Rome (Cicero, with Virgil also named), and Germany (Albertus Magnus) and a caption with verses extolling all that the goddess encompasses complete the composition.[78] By virtue of its prominent placement, Dürer's monogram—set between the roundel displaying the *Latinorum poetae et rhetores* and the obelisk furnished with the "scala artium," seven Greek letters signifying the liberal arts—proclaims the capacity of his art to mediate philosophical wisdom.[79]

That was in 1502, and it is not unreasonable to suppose that Dürer had occasion to expand and develop his views on the causes and treatments of a "saturnine" melancholy in the ensuing decade, a period that also brought the death of Celtis (in 1508). Drawing closer to Maximilian and his intellectual circles following his return from Italy, Dürer would also have grown aware of the emperor's deepening preoccupation with the dangers wrought by Saturn's influence. This preoccupation was driven in part by Maximilian's personal

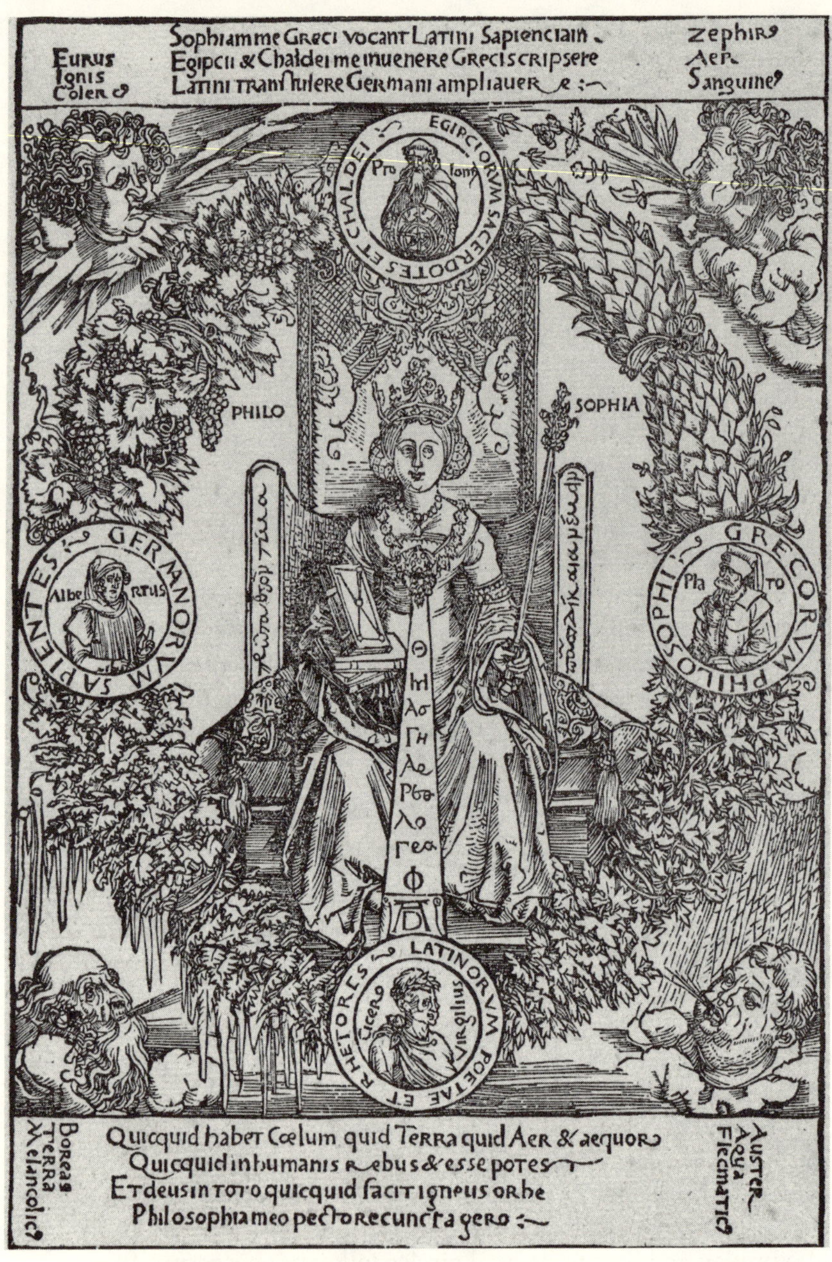

Figure 4.12. Albrecht Dürer, *Philosophia*, illustration for Konrad Celtis, *Quatuor libri amorum*, woodcut, 21.9 x 14.8 cm (Nuremberg: Sodalitas Celtica, 5 April 1502) (Washington, D.C., National Gallery of Art, Rosenwald Collection).

fascination with his mythical ancestor, Hercules Aegypticus, and that hero's tragic "frenzy"—a fascination nourished by a memorandum penned by the emperor's advisor, the Augsburg humanist Konrad Peutinger (1465–1547), who linked the melancholy of Hercules to the *Problemata*'s account of heated black bile; that linkage spoke as well to Maximilian's own sequence of medical crises.[80] Meanwhile, health worries of his own seem to have gripped Dürer at the time commissioned projects from the imperial court in Vienna were ramping up; the "diagnostic" pen-and-ink self-portrait in the Bremen Kunsthalle, to be discussed in Chapter 5, in which the artist points to his spleen, the site of black bile's production in the body (see figure 5.7), is only the most overt evidence of this. We may fairly conclude that the new position given to Boreas in the *Philosophia* woodcut and the pagan wind deity's equation with earth, night, winter, old age, and melancholy represents the "first evidence of Dürer's notion of the melancholy state." Certainly it is prophetic, not only for Dürer's identification of his art with humanist erudition and cosmology, but for the painter's personal struggle with illness, mortality, and fate later in life.[81]

From this array of evidence it also seems clear that Dürer would have known that state-of-the-art treatments for melancholia encompassed medical, magical, and psychological therapies. Ficino himself had already endorsed a multipronged approach to countering Saturn's baleful effects. Stressing the need to mobilize Jupiter's influence through talismanic images (especially in cases where the "jovial" planet was absent from the patient's horoscope), he also recognized the value of medical interventions to rebalance the body's humors as well as the fundamental importance of what we have been calling "cognitive" remedies. In book 3 of *De triplici vita*, Ficino offers a total program for accommodating human health to the "harmonic plan" of the heavens, to be accomplished

> through images . . . put together harmonically, through medicines tempered with a certain proper consonance, through vapors and odors completed with similar consonance, through musical songs and sounds . . . through well-accorded concepts and motions of the imagination, through fitting discourses of reason, through tranquil contemplations of the mind [*per imaginationis conceptus motusque concinnos, per congruas rationis discursiones, per tranquillas mentis contemplationes*]. For just as we expose the body seasonably to the light and heat

of the Sun through its daily harmony, that is, through its location, posture, and shape, so also we expose our spirit in order to obtain the occult forces of the stars through a similar harmony of its own, obtained by images . . . certainly by medicines, and by odors harmonically composed. Finally, we expose our soul and our body to such occult forces through the spirit so prepared for things above (as I have often said)—yes, our soul, insofar as it is inclined by its affection to the spirit and body.[82]

Imagination, reason, and "tranquil contemplations of the mind" participate in the soul's repair precisely by virtue of their natural operations; each in its own way disposes the microcosmic soul toward those countervailing astral forces that rebalance it harmonically. Ficino's sevenfold method accorded to natural cognitive exercise, then, a key autotherapeutic function, something Warburg clearly recognized. In his view, such "mental concentration" enabled "the melancholic to transmute his sterile gloom into human genius."[83]

Why, then, has Dürer been credited with such a singular focus on the astrological? Why else but the electrifying presence of an object directly concerned with mitigating the debilitating power of the illness—the famous "Jupiter square" (*mensula Iovis*), the sixteen-celled numerical chart that Dürer has set into the wall behind Melancholy (figure 4.13). Confronting the viewer directly, it goes unseen by the seated genius, who nevertheless seems to reach absentmindedly toward it, her folded left wing just overlapping the bottom of its frame. Just as suggestively, the chart is aligned vertically with the bell, close enough for the bell pull to graze its upper right corner as it dips down, neither slack nor taut, past the picture's edge. In this subtle choreography of contacts, separations, overlaps, and infinitesimal proximities we have another example of Dürer's knack for intimating the hidden sympathies between things. The vignette anchored by the magic square is perhaps the most appealing of the engraving's zones, a pictorial metaphor for the object's cosmic power of attraction.

Melencolia's magic square has attracted more than its share of attention from mathematicians, symbol hunters, code breakers, philosophers, astrologers, and other adepts of the esoteric—and for good reason.[84] Each row of numbers counted in any direction (vertically, horizontally, diagonally) adds up to thirty-four, as do the numbers in

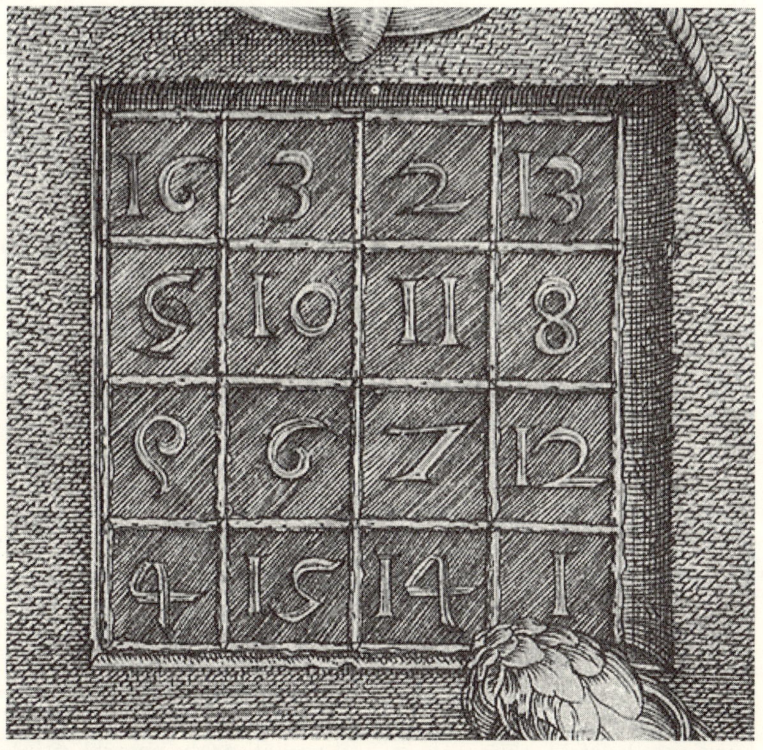

Figure 4.13. Detail from Dürer, *Melencolia I*: the Jupiter square. (See figure 1.1 above.)

the cells of the four outer corners; the four center cells; the groups of four assembled from the two inner cells of the top and bottom lines and two inner cells of the left and right column, respectively; each corner group of four; and so on.[85] Islamic mathematicians had developed this branch of number theory as early as the seventh century, and it may have entered Europe, along with other aspects of Arabic astral magic, through the court of Alfonso X of Castile (1221–84).[86] In all likelihood, the design of Dürer's sixteen-cell square derives from the occult philosophy of Agrippa von Nettisheim, for whom magic and mathematics were intimately connected. In Agrippa's conception, "formal and rational numbers" represent divine ideas, distinguishing them from the "natural numbers" used in the secular world of commerce. The former stand in the closest possible relation to truths beyond the sensible world precisely because they have no counterparts in observed nature.[87]

Some have taken the "magic constant" of thirty-four in Dürer's square to be symbolic of Christ's years on earth as a man. Others have discerned numerological meanings both far-flung and obvious: the engraving's date, for example, 1514, which is visible in the lower row. This was also the year Dürer's mother died (17 May), making the magic square, in the view of some commentators, emblematic of the whole scene's allegedly mournful mood,[88] therefore commensurate with its—again, alleged—function as a consolation in grief (see Chapter 5).

Building on the work of Giehlow, Warburg identified the Jupiter square as an astrological talisman of the kind recommended by Ficino for use by fellow scholars in warding off the ill effects of Saturn (himself a victim of dark anxiety, Ficino's horoscope showed Saturn in the ascendant position).[89] As a "magic image," its purpose is to counteract the pernicious effects of one planet by attracting the healing power of another—in this case, the deity's "joyful" nature works to dispel "all worries and fear," as Panofsky would later write, vaguely concurring with the opinion of his predecessors.[90]

Does the therapeutic potentiality of *Melencolia* come down simply to this? In the exegetical perspective common to Giehlow, Warburg, and Panofsky, the magic square symbolizes the neutralization of those rays that bring the darkness associated with melancholia and *acedia*, "lightening" those states to become the *melancholia generosa* associated with genius. As Ficino had asserted, only the right combination of the two planetary influences can produce melancholic philosophers who embrace their destiny as children of Saturn, men "whose minds are truly withdrawn from the world."[91] But only Warburg had the imagination to understand the square also in narrative terms, as the marker of a kind of astrological *peripeteia*, a triumphant reversal in the melancholic's struggle against Saturn's influence. And most significantly, he conceived this as a victory set in motion by thought itself. That account we must now quote in full:

> Dürer shows the spirit of Saturn neutralized by the individual mental efforts
> of the thinking creature against whom its rays are directed. Menaced by the
> "most ignoble complex," the Child of Saturn seeks to elude the baneful plan-
> etary influence through contemplative activity. Melancholy holds in her hand,

> not a base shovel...but the compass of genius. Magically invoked, Jupiter comes to her aid through his benign and moderating influence on Saturn. In a sense, the salvation of the human being through the countervailing influence of Jupiter *has already taken place*; the duel between the planets, as visualized by [Johannes] Lichtenberger, is over; and the magic square hangs on the wall like a votive offering of thanks to the benign and victorious planetary spirit.[92]

Magical imagery in the virtual world that Dürer's print conjures up, in other words, moves beyond symbolization to serve as an active relay for the psychic mobilization of Jupiter's aid, and then finally as a token of its efficacy. On this basis, Warburg, breaking with Giehlow, could declare the engraving a *Trostblatt*, a comforting image, since the victory of the thinking being over Saturn's dark power "has already taken place."

Yet for all his optimism, Warburg did not follow through on this founding insight into the print's therapeutic instrumentality. And he *could* not do so, I submit, as long as the "Child of Saturn" of his scenario remained a purely notional character, as long as the "medicine" offered was of a spiritualized sort, as long as the narrative passage from affliction to relief was confined within the rules of allegory.[93] Released from these constraints, however, the question and its answer become obvious. Is not the "thinking creature" Warburg invoked to be found not only in the ambivalent seated goddess of Dürer's *Meisterstiche*, but in the beholder, whose speculative exercise is mirrored by her state of vigilant repose? Whether that speculation focuses wholly on the Jupiter square or ranges freely over the entire collection of objects and bodies, the mobilization of benign planetary forces posited by Warburg can only ever be a function of the contemplative activity instigated by the print. Once set in motion by this activity, the germinal narrative that we described in this chapter's opening pages requires a beholder for its direction, its fulfillment, and the resolution of its tensions. Suspended in twilight, the passage toward a "lightened" melancholy remains to be accomplished, and the one tasked with this is the same "thinking being" who now holds the print in his or her hands. Enlisted and enabled by the incipient narrative, the natural activity of the beholder advances the cause of healing—a therapy that is neither spiritual consolation nor astrological magic, strictly speaking, but a steady, measured concentration that yields a progressive tempering of the passions, leading, finally, to their clarification. For the ailing subject, such a rebalancing appears at once psychological and somatic, moral and medicinal. That is the conceit of the image.[94]

In the foregoing discussion, I have made a double appeal to Stephen Crites's notion of the "narrative quality" of experience: I have pointed to an incipient quality of narrative in the description of melancholia itself, at least as Dürer and his contemporaries would have understood the syndrome, and I have offered it as hermeneutical pathway into the therapeutic logic of the engraving (that logic being a function of its formal structure and even its rhetorical *ductus*, the "itinerary" it sets for the beholder's speculative efforts). That the two go hand in hand is part of the brilliance of Dürer's diagnostic-therapeutic portrayal of Dame Melancholy: a figure of "thought in perplexity" who invites identification by the viewer and then enlists the aid of that same viewer in sweeping away the confusions born of chaos and obscurity, anticipating the return to creative activity.

An unstated premise in all this returns us to Kierkegaard's epigram for this chapter and the dialectical sense that experience augments itself by carrying forward what logically antedated it. German thought has long relied on the word *Erfahrung* for this dialectical image of experience as a self-enhancing journey, intimate but not identical with individual biography. In his study of the idea of historical experience, Frank Ankersmit notes that *Erfahrung*'s root verb, *fahren*, "means 'to go,' 'to sail,' [and] 'to travel through,'" and is "suggestive of the kind of encounters or . . . 'adventures' that one may have on a journey and, more specifically on the journey through one's own life and of all that may enrich and form one's personality."[95] Its opposing term is *Erlebnis*, which also means "experience," but the kind of unmediated, epiphanic experience that flashes from out of nowhere, overwhelms, and even terrifies as it exposes phenomena in their nakedness. *Erlebnis* is the stuff of revelations, recognitions, miracles, and revolutionary breakthroughs. It recedes just as swiftly as it appears, leaving experience to catch up with knowledge for which it could not possibly have prepared.

The manic delusions suffered by melancholics as a result of black bile's "combustion" in the body and the rise of vapors into the brain are one particularly unwelcome form of *Erlebnis*. With subtle descriptive skill and a strategic accumulation of signs and symbols designed to put cognition on a steady course toward renewed functioning, Dürer has effectively harnessed the natural human proclivity for *Erfahren* against the debilitating, quasi-demonic eruptions of *Erlebnis*. Rather than being a diagnosis of Ficino's *furor melancholicus* or Agrippa's "frenzy," as Panofsky had proposed, Dürer offers the viewer a therapeutic alternative—an instrument for rebalancing and restoring agency to the suffering subject as an *experiencing* subject, as an ethical self in time. No fait accompli, the work's call to virtue is heeded as a process. Surrogate and emblem for those "who have once and more than once given up," Melancholy will, in just a moment, "rise to her feet" to resume the project of perfection.[96]

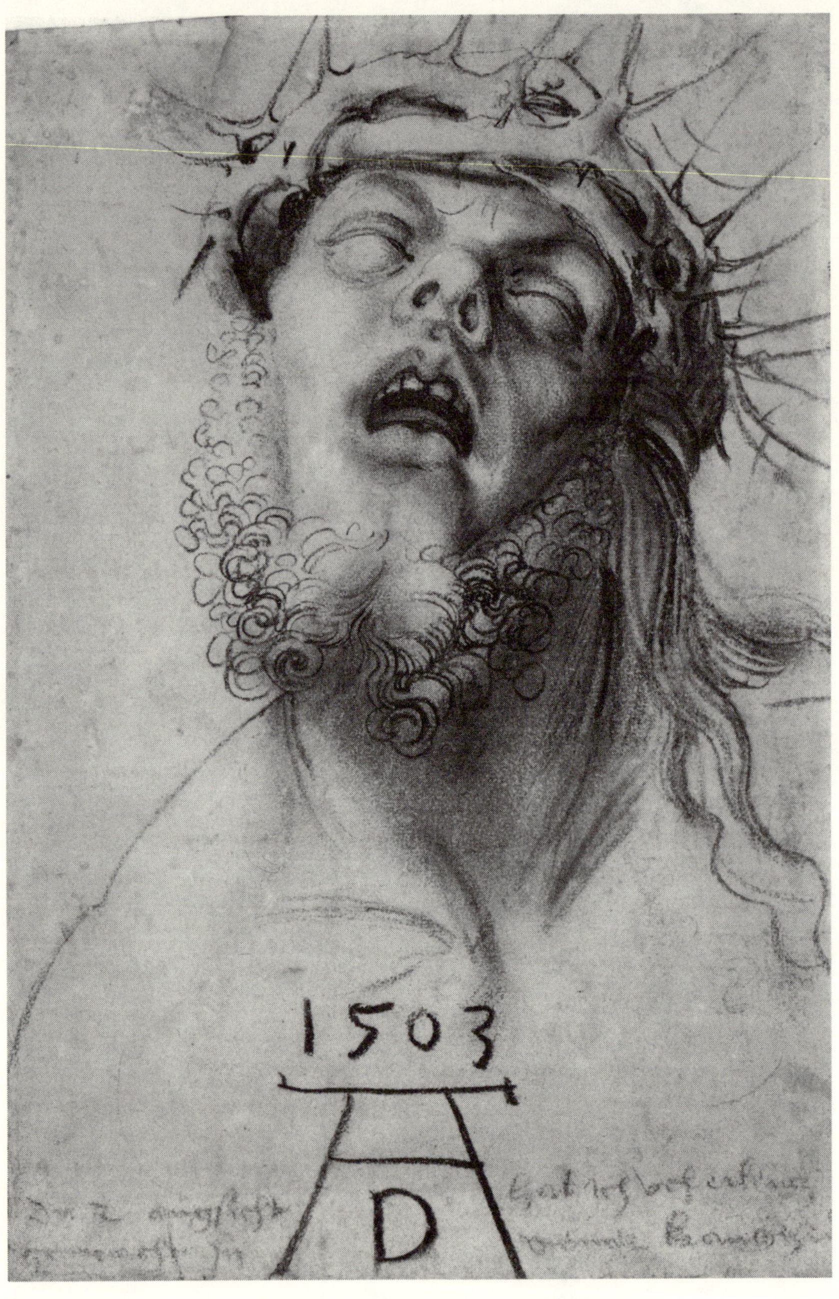

Figure P.1. Albrecht Dürer, *Head of Christ*, charcoal on paper, 31 x 22.1 cm (London, British Museum) (photo: © The Trustees of the British Museum London).

Prologue to Chapters Five and Six

The physician . . . must be able to see through his patient, as clearly as one can
see through a drop of distilled water in which not a speck of dust can remain
undetected; he has to see so clearly, as one can see, through spouting springs
the pebbles and grains of sand on the bottom—see their number, color, and
shape, etc.
—Paracelsus, *Paragranum* (1529-30)

Image and Addressee

"I produced these two countenances for you truthfully," the artist
declares below a portrait of Christ in delirious agony, "when I was
ill." Scribbled lightly at the lower edge of a sheet preserved today
in London (figure P.1), the sentence is cleaved in two by the sturdy
akimbo legs of Dürer's monogram, which is boldly crowned by the
date, 1503.[1] These same brand signs appear in the upper right corner
of the second countenance (*angsicht*) referred to in the inscription:
Dürer's charcoal portrait of exactly similar size, showing a turbaned
man with a beard of tight curls, his whole face knitted together in a
spasm of pain (figure P.2).[2] To whom has the artist addressed himself
amidst his own affliction? Gift or commission may have prompted
this exchange, though the charcoal medium suggests the former;
historical guesswork may or may not someday succeed in identifying its actual recipient. We will take up these questions further on.
Here we need only acknowledge the rhetorical force of that informal
"you" (*vch*, or "euch" in modern German). With it, Dürer stakes his
claim within a bounded community of sufferers, a claim continuous
with the powers of his art to render visible the invisible bonds of
mutual service and Christian love. Therapies betoken human relationships with active and passive roles, but these are not always fixed.

"

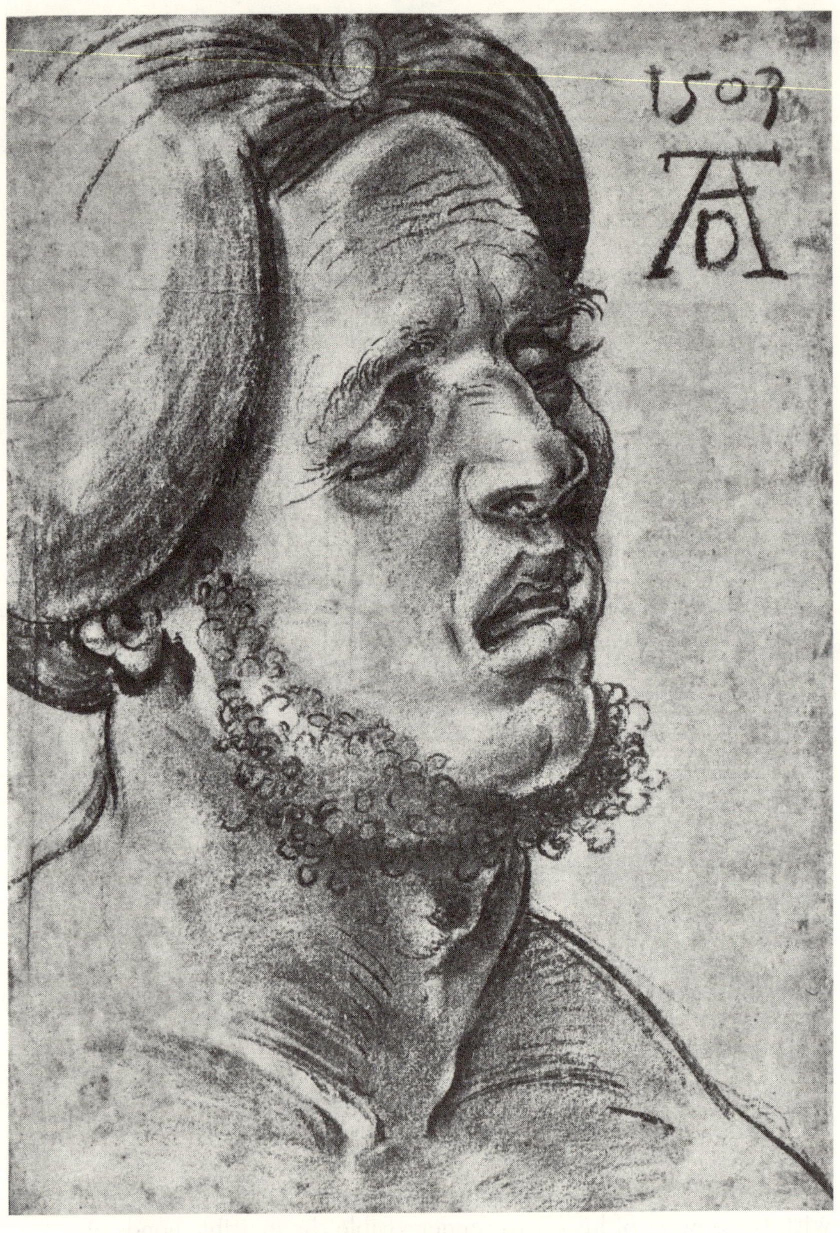

Figure P.2. Albrecht Dürer, *Head of Man in Pain*, charcoal on paper, 31 x 22.1 cm (London, British Museum) (photo: © The Trustees of the British Museum London).

Sometimes they hinge on the therapist's willingness or capacity to share in the pain he treats; other times, amidst the recognition that reciprocal aid is called for, those relationships switch, or double. This is where I would like to begin thinking about the therapeutic roles open to intensely self-aware artists such as Dürer.

Measured against the long social history of the image maker's vocation, the freedom of artists to address their works to whomever they like is a relatively recent phenomenon, characteristic, it is routinely said, of European art's modern history. North of the Alps, it was Dürer's generation of painter-printmakers who first recognized the complex demands this then-emerging freedom placed on their creative practice. Anticipating different classes of addressees meant many things. First and foremost, it meant shifting the terms by which personalized agency, the construction of an artistic persona standing behind the image, could be articulated—even, or especially, when the principal addressee of a work is oneself. More than any other of his German contemporaries, Dürer mastered the projection of self and representational agency through various modes of address and did so in all of the genres he engaged. Not surprisingly, the innovative approach he took to self-reference in his inscriptions, signatures, and monograms, not to mention his unprecedented experimentation with self-portraiture, which one recent commentator has labeled "an obsessive concern with his intellectual and social status as a painter," has occasioned much discussion and continues to be a major tributary for scholarship on the artist.[3]

But the awareness of new, or newly differentiated, audiences for the visual arts goes far beyond one artist's quest for attention, expression, and authority. Among its historic motivations, some are patently economic. Private patrons for paintings expected their particular needs to be addressed, and they paid for the privilege. Audiences for prints, by contrast, had to be cultivated in a public market where tastes ranged and where buyers of different means rubbed elbows, where vendors competed, products were positioned, inventions protected against piracy, and so on. Other causes for a differentiated awareness of audience among Renaissance artists are more intangible: the evolving character of education and training, for instance, with its demand for new forms of mobility, both physical and social; the decision to accommodate stylistic idioms that bore the prestige of an artistic center to the "local" flavors found on the periphery; or the broadening exposure to antique models and the latest trends in compositional design through prints and drawn copies. Not least of all was the growing ambition of artists, whether as members of a court or in their civic lives, to associate themselves with men of learning and what we call taste; to share in humanist pursuits, projects, and pastimes; and to cultivate friendships based on them.

Increasingly, the social circles and philosophical sodalities with which artists such as Dürer identified represented a privileged class of addressees for their art. Sharing the optimism of humanist men of letters and sympathizing with their sorrows, collaborating with the Nuremberg civic and mercantile elite in the project of spreading the fame of their city, working with the leaders of parish and cloister in the project of discerning the Christian's true identity and true vocation at a time of spiritual uncertainty and insecurity—all of these engagements brought to the fore for Dürer the problem of how best to use one's art to attend to diverse audiences. As we will see, Dürer drew especial benefit from his friendships with the scholars, theologians, poets, and scientists who made Nuremberg their home or graced it with regular visits: men such as Konrad Celtis, who, among other things, helped him compose Latin inscriptions; Benedictus Chelidonius, the abbot of Vienna's Schottenstift monastery, with whom Dürer collaborated on his devotional books; Lazarus Spengler, the city council secretary who was so instrumental in the city's march toward reform; Anton Koberger, the publisher who was also Dürer's godfather; and most of all, the wealthy patrician Willibald Pirckheimer (1470–1530)—humanist scholar, advisor to the emperor, and Dürer's closest mentor, benefactor, correspondent, and friend.

It was in the orbit of the Nuremberg humanists that Dürer would have found encouragement to explore a key question posed by classical aesthetic theory, one with several important implications for the concerns of the two chapters that follow: Could the painter enjoy the same freedom of invention as the poet? Discussion of the relative powers of painting and poetry had been robust among Italian writers since the later fourteenth century; most accepted that Horace's great dictum, *ut pictura poesis* (as is painting, so is poetry) could be applied in reverse, to the mutual ennoblement of both arts.[4] Petrarch's assertion that Homer was the "first painter in ancient memory" (*il primo pintor delle memorie antiche*) was matched repeatedly by claims that painting could aspire to the conditions of poetry, that it could and should, like poetry, find its métier between imitation (*imitatio*), invention (*inventio*), and imagination (*fantasia*) and do so within the parameters of recognized genres. This was the ground for Bartolomeo Fazio's (d. 1457) embrace of the affinity between painters and poets when he declared them equals in displaying their talent through the "invention and arrangement of their work." After all, he continues, "a painting is indeed nothing else than a wordless poem."[5] The belief that painting could model itself on the motivations, methods, and modes of poetry was widely embraced by Italian artists, some of whom even tried their hand at poetry. (For producing verses of real literary merit, however, Michelangelo represents the rare exception.)

Evidence for a parallel embrace of the equality of painting and poetry among German artists is harder to come by, in large part because of the absence of a home-grown art-theoretical discourse north of the Alps—an absence Dürer himself was determined to remedy by the time he commenced work on the *Meisterstiche*. Given this commitment, it comes as no surprise to find Dürer developing his sense of a close alliance between painting and poetry along several avenues at once: in the different collaborative projects undertaken with Celtis and with Chelidonius;[6] in the pursuit of a learned approach to classical subjects and the desire to emulate the greatest of his Italian peers; in his participation in the short-lived Nuremberg "School of Poets" (*Poetenschule*), an academy conceived by Celtis and inaugurated under Willibald Pirckheimer's father, the lawyer Johann Pirckheimer, in 1496;[7] and in the artist's proud, if partly ironic, forays into poetry (an instance of which we will examine in Chapter 6). All of these pursuits have encouraged generations of scholars to see Dürer as uniquely congenial to the theoretical alignment of painting with poetic invention and the effort to innovate pictorial equivalents for the recognized modes of poetry and drama inherited from classical thought.

To explore the possibilities of a therapeutic "office" for the painter represents a further and perhaps surprising extension of this impulse to place painting on equal footing with poetry. That Dürer undertook this within a sodality of learned men who were already engaged in various novelties and experiments in philological scholarship, ethical Christian thought, and philosophy as an indispensible guide for the conduct of life makes it less unexpected. Although the parameters for such an empowerment of the artist were nowhere

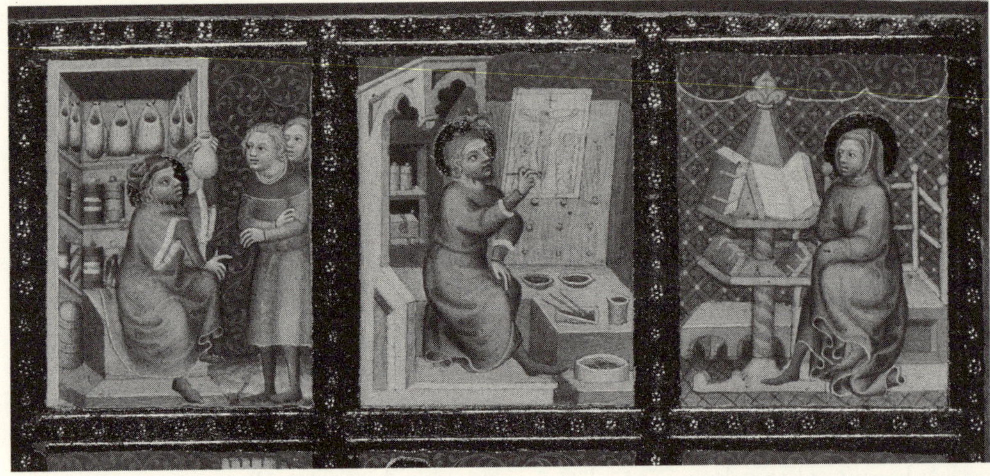

Figure P.3. Johann of Troppau, St. Luke as physician (left), painter (center), and evangelist (right), from a gospel book from Brünn, Austria, 1368 (Vienna, Österreichisches Nationalbibliothek, Cod. 1182, fol. 91v).

articulated, nowhere set down, several hallmarks of the Northern European painter's professional identity and practical training had, in a sense, already prepared the ground. In the centuries before Dürer, painters progressively nurtured the association of their profession with St. Luke, the evangelist whose legendary act of painting the Virgin and Child "from life"—a fine pious anachronism—had provided the notional archetype for miraculous Marian icons and "authentic" portraits derived from them. Painters' guilds in cities throughout Northern Europe would be named for him, especially in the Low Countries, where they grew into complex social organizations. Before he became an evangelist and a painter, of course, Luke was a doctor. That triple vocation is reviewed in a charming set of vignettes by the abbot Johann of Troppau, painted for the gospel book, now in Vienna, that he signed and dated in 1368 (figure P.3).[8] Contemporaries of Dürer might even merge the professional attributes of the painter's *studiolo* with the apothecary's shop in their depictions of St. Luke at work as a *pictor divinus* (figure P.4).[9]

Connected with these developments was the growing vocational

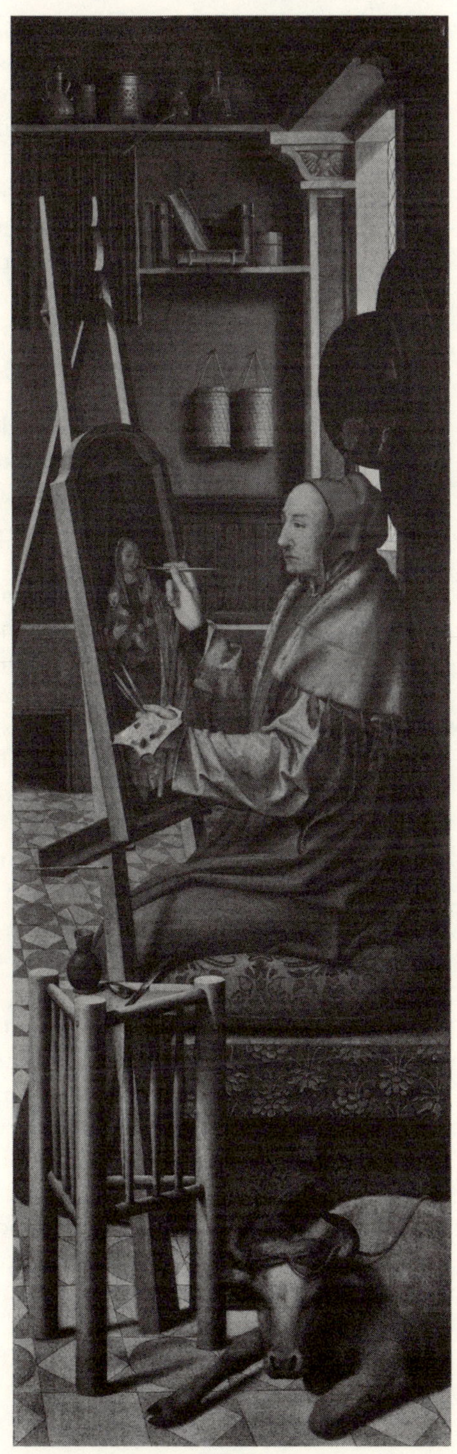

Figure P.4. Antwerp painter (workshop of Quentin Massys), *St. Luke Painting the Virgin*, ca. 1520, oil on oak panel, 114.9 × 35.4 cm, from a dismembered triptych (London, National Gallery of Art. Presented by Henry Wagner, 1924) (photo: © National Gallery, London/Art Resource, NY).

distinction conferred by the painter's knowledge of the diverse color-ing agents derived from plants, animals, and minerals—a knowledge that intersected directly with the apothecary's art. That entrepre-neurial contemporaries of Dürer, for example Lucas Cranach the Elder, could consolidate the two enterprises under one roof[10] reveals how the Renaissance artist might participate in yet another kind of "common specialist culture,"[11] a culture whose practical-empirical ethos found perfect expression in Dürer's riposte during the mock-poetic combat with Lazarus Spengler: "Something of all things I will know." Dürer's various efforts to manage and merge these cross-voca-tional associations reveal, alongside a continuing preoccupation with commercial success and reputation, a profound ethical self-awareness that, we will see in Chapter 6, realizes itself in the soul services the painter was uniquely equipped to provide his friends.

Painter, Poet, Orator, Physician

More important than their common commitment to a creative bar-gain between imitation, invention, and imagination is what painting and poetry, as mutually empowered liberal arts in the Renaissance, shared with two other disciplines that met the ancient definition of an "art" (τέχνη, *techne*): the art of oratory (rhetoric) and the art of healing (medicine). Specifically, all four of these practical crafts laid claim to the power to be able to "move" the subject from one state to another, using the materials, tools, and techniques uniquely at their disposal. A clear distillation of this doctrine appears in book 2 of *Della pittura* (1435–36), where Alberti takes it for granted that the primary purpose of the painted narrative (*istoria*) is to "move the soul of the beholder." Counseling variety in the imitation of expres-sive bodies, Alberti explains that it is visible movements (*mozione*) that reveal the invisible movements (*emozione*) of their characters' souls, for like begets like, and this in turn has the power to move the beholder: "It happens in nature that nothing more than herself is found capable of things like herself; we weep with the weeping, laugh with the laughing, and grieve with the grieving."[12] On its own, this emphasis on gesture's power to move the spectator's soul, very much at the core of Alberti's theory of painting, would be enough to show its author's indebtedness to rhetorical theory; the treatise was com-posed, after all, at a time when Cicero and Quintilian had become mainsprings for Italian humanist theories of painting and poetry—a time when, Enea Silvio Piccolomini (1405–64, later to become Pope Pius II) remarked, the arts of painting and oratory "love each other mutually."[13]

Rhetorical theory's linkage of speech, visible gesture, affect, and instruction had profound consequences for the ways painters would come to think of their addressees, cutting deeper than Alberti's practical handbook, however influential, could possibly venture. At its root, the claim that art not only pleases and instructs, but "moves" the soul of the spectator is grounded in Plato's doctrine of the communicative *logos* and its systematic transformation by Aristotle into the art of rhetoric, a familiar story in the intertwined histories of ancient philosophy, politics, and poetics.[14] The essential purpose of rhetorical persuasion, in this tradition, is to modify the beliefs lodged in the soul of the listener, to operate upon the soul in a way that rebalances the listener's "passions"—that is, the relation of those passions to higher faculties such as reason—and thus the subject's capacity for judgment. In philosophical discourse, dialectical argument can likewise move a subject from one perspective to another, but it does so only by acting on the intelligence. By contrast, rhetoric targets the emotions. Painting is bound to do likewise.

It is true that Aristotle's *Rhetoric* does not explicitly make room for a genus of rhetorical persuasion that we could call therapeutic or curative. Yet the parallel between medicine and rhetoric, already set forth by Plato in the *Phaedrus*, lends itself completely to something like a "speculative theory of verbal psychotherapy." These are the terms Spanish historian of medicine Pedro Laín-Entralgo used fifty years ago in a brilliant but overlooked book, *The Therapy of the Word in Classical Antiquity*. Laín-Entralgo argued that such a therapeutic category is demonstrably present between the pages of the *Rhetoric* and those of the *Nichomachean Ethics*, the *Politics*, and certainly also the *Poetics*,[15] a thesis that finds confirmation in more recent accounts of Hellenistic ethics, for example, in the work of Martha Nussbaum.[16] Of paramount importance in Laín-Entralgo's account is what he shows about the deep parallelism between medicine and rhetoric and what it may have suggested to Renaissance painters and poets—namely, that their enterprises, too, could move the souls of their addressees from one state to another. What's at issue is not simply a matter of persuasion, of moving the subject forensically toward a truth or a higher level of conviction, but a psychophysiological operation aimed at the emotions as well as the intellect, an operation that produces quasi-physical effects in the body, what Aristotle and his medieval commentators called "mental impressions" or "impressions in the soul."[17]

As a mode of communicative address, the psychotherapeutic operation common to rhetoric, poetry, and painting finds the subject in a starting state understood in terms of deficiency, infirmity, or a metaphorical blindness ("illness") and works to move him or her to a state of repletion, flourishing, and knowledge ("health"). Assumed in this model is the idea that three agents come together in every rhetorical encounter: the orator, the listener, and the word conveyed between them. The intended outcome (persuasion) depends on the degree to which each agent contributes its inherent capacities and powers to the interaction. Aristotle (*Rhetoric* 1.2) casts the three "agents," as I have called them, in more technical terms as the three cardinal "proofs furnished by the speech" that the skillful orator must master.[18] Those capacities and powers merit examination. For instance, in order for the listener to be properly moved, logic dictates that he or she must be movable, that is, governed by a specific configuration of passions that can be modified—in a word, persuadable. It is a defining task of the orator to ascertain this, since it will affect his or her choice of words and their arrangement. Aristotle called this thing to be ascertained the "disposition" (διάθεσις, *diathesis*) of the listener's soul, and accepted (following Plato) that it could manifest numerous possible "aspects" (εἴδη, *eidē*), depending on the passions (πάθη, *pathē*) present in the individual, in addition to other personal factors such as age, habits, virtues, and so on.[19] Realizing its central importance to political and poetical speech led Aristotle to develop a full-fledged theory of the passions—what they are, how they are provoked, and how they could be modified or stabilized, by the action of the word.

The parallel with medicine could not be more striking: in every therapeutic encounter there are, analogously, three ideal figures or agents: the physician, the patient, and the "medicine" (broadly construed as the thing introduced as efficacious, whether it's a drug or some other agent of therapeutic action). In order for the patient to be cured, he or she must be in some way disposed to cure; it is therefore central to the physician's task to discern "how and in what measure each patient is curable."[20] Taking account of the disposition toward health went hand in hand with judging the disposition toward illness. Galen, echoing Plato and Aristotle, claimed that disease arises from a "preternatural disposition" present in the sufferer (*diathesis para phusin*).[21] Conversely, an effective healing practice, under the right conditions, awakens the natural disposition toward health in the individual. The tradition of natural medicine made the body's humoral "complexion" the ultimate unifying cause of that disposition, while astrological medicine (iatromathematics) assumed it was the power of the stars (see Chapter 4), but the principle of defining the individual as a uniquely complected psychsomatic ground for therapeutic action is the same.

Another factor critical to the rhetorical encounter is the character (*ēthos*) of the orator—critical, Aristotle says, because "we have confidence in an orator who exhibits certain qualities, such as goodness, goodwill, or both."[22] Precisely the same qualities that incline the listener to the orator and cement the relationship on which persuasion must always be built—moral probity, prudence, kindness, decency, and so on—find their perfect parallels in the ancient ideal of what must happen whenever the physician makes contact with the patient. The notion recurs throughout the Hippocratic corpus. "The character of the therapist," Laín Entralgo sums up, "his natural qualities, his habits, his acquired virtues, his prestige—has considerable importance in the efficacy of his prescriptions."[23]

Renaissance advocates for a renewed "therapy of the word," undertaken within the context of the broader humanist revival of classical and patristic thought, likewise acknowledged the parallels between rhetoric and medicine and likewise set themselves the task of studying the passions. To understand the invisible synergies of mind, body, and soul in their changing states and to examine the peculiar efficacies of the many "medicines" available to treat sorrow, grief, fear, confusion, and other "perturbations of the soul"—not least of all, philosophical melancholia—this became the imperative underlying the revival of literary consolation undertaken by Italian writers as different in their philosophical orientations as Petrarch, Salutati, Conversini, Manetti, and Ficino. Summarizing their collective enterprise, George McClure explains in his masterful account, *Sorrow and Consolation in Italian Humanism*:

> Rejecting dialectic and theoretical learning, humanist writers instead cultivated a practical eloquence that spoke to human emotion, the human will, the

human psyche. Evincing a belief in the legitimacy of worldly grief, they provided a solace responsive to the vicissitudes of secular life, and they sometimes offered particular lay perspectives and solutions different from the sterner warnings and cures traditionally advanced by the confessor and pastor. Fully acknowledging the humanity of sorrow, they sought out comforts from neglected troves of Platonic, Stoic, Peripatetic, Epicurean, and Christian thought.[24]

We have already held up Petrarch as representative of the Renaissance cultural ideal of eloquence and the progenitor of humanist efforts to restore rhetorical healing to its rightful place in the empire of letters. It is his example, his project to explore and treat spiritual and secular sorrows side by side, that will structure my discussion in the two following chapters of Dürer's participation, as a visual artist, in the newly validated Renaissance ideal of philosophical medicine. Since the two men lived over a century apart and the German painter's knowledge of the Italian humanist's works can not be assumed, a few further words about the value of this comparison are needed.

Petrarch considered his calling to be that of a new—indeed, modern—type of pious intellectual. In this spirit, he innovated a distinctive practice as a rhetorical healer, a *medicus* charged with providing consolations for the soul (*anima*) and the mind (*animus*). In exploiting medical terminology in this way—elsewhere he speaks of *morbi animi*, *antidota*, and *medicamenta*—Petrarch was taking his cue from Cicero in the *Tusculan Disputations* (3.3.6), where philosophy is touted as an "art of healing the soul" (*animi medicina*).[25] Another impetus behind this language, one we can mention only in passing, was the poet's contempt for the "empty elegance of words" that medical doctors displayed at the deathbeds of their patients, part of Petrarch's public struggle with the medical profession over the relative dignity of their respective arts. "And while their patients are dying," he complains of the doctors in a letter to Pope Clement VI (1291–1352), "they knit the Hippocratic knots with the Ciceronian warp."[26]

To delineate further the proper domain of the moral philosopher and orator and their shared commitments as movers of minds, Petrarch geared his new practice toward three distinct classes of listeners/readers; in the process, he reshaped the extant genres of consolatory literature in remarkable ways. Inspired in large part by personal concerns, he began the project with himself, with his own world-weariness (*contemptus mundi*) and spiritual sickness: the major result was the three-day dialogue with his "divine" physician Augustine, the *Secretum*, composed roughly between 1347 and 1353. Meanwhile, in his many letters addressed to friends and patrons, most of them living, some dead—letters collected and edited by the poet himself in the *Epistolae familiares*—Petrarch took on the obligations of a different therapeutic office: the ancient role of the moral advisor, sage, exhorter, and comforter in times of sickness, death, bereavement, and despair; here too, in the process, he reinvented the genre.[27] Finally, Petrarch addressed himself to a third, larger class of listeners—the whole of humanity—in the massive compendium of Latin dialogues we introduced earlier in this book: *De remediis utriusque fortunae*. A project undertaken, in McClure's judgment, to "complete Petrarch's growth as a constructive Stoic healer," it holds the poet's "clearest definition of the 'philosopher' as the 'animorum medicus.'"[28]

Without pressing the analogy too far—and, again, without positing any direct inspiration from Petrarch's writings—the next two chapters will argue that the broad stream of therapeutic concerns running through Dürer's oeuvre can best be understood within a similar threefold model of Christian-humanist psychotherapy. The first of these healing offices centers on the self, another is devoted to family and friends, and a third is set in universal service to all Christians. Like Petrarch, Dürer recognized the legitimacy of worldly as well as spiritual sorrows and began his project of remedying them all by addressing his own, most intimate miseries. Like Petrarch, Dürer, I will argue, took seriously the ethic of mutual assistance, consolation, and soul service within his circle of learned friends, intellectual advisors, patrons, and family members. And like Petrarch, he accepted that his unique talents and "genius" not only qualified, but practically obligated him to enter upon the office of universal healer with the medicine at his disposal: the eloquent image. Chapter 5 therefore concentrates on Dürer's role as a self-consoler and self-healer; Chapter 6 goes on to uncover the therapeutic impulses behind the exchanges and works addressed to friends, family, and finally the greater community of believers. As we will see, wherever Dürer assumed the role of the *medicus*, he reshaped the genres appropriate to each context where misery called out for attention, just as Petrarch had done in the empire of letters. Though its resources are exhausted by none of them, *Melencolia*, perhaps uniquely in Dürer's oeuvre, holds a significant place in all three of these therapeutic contexts.

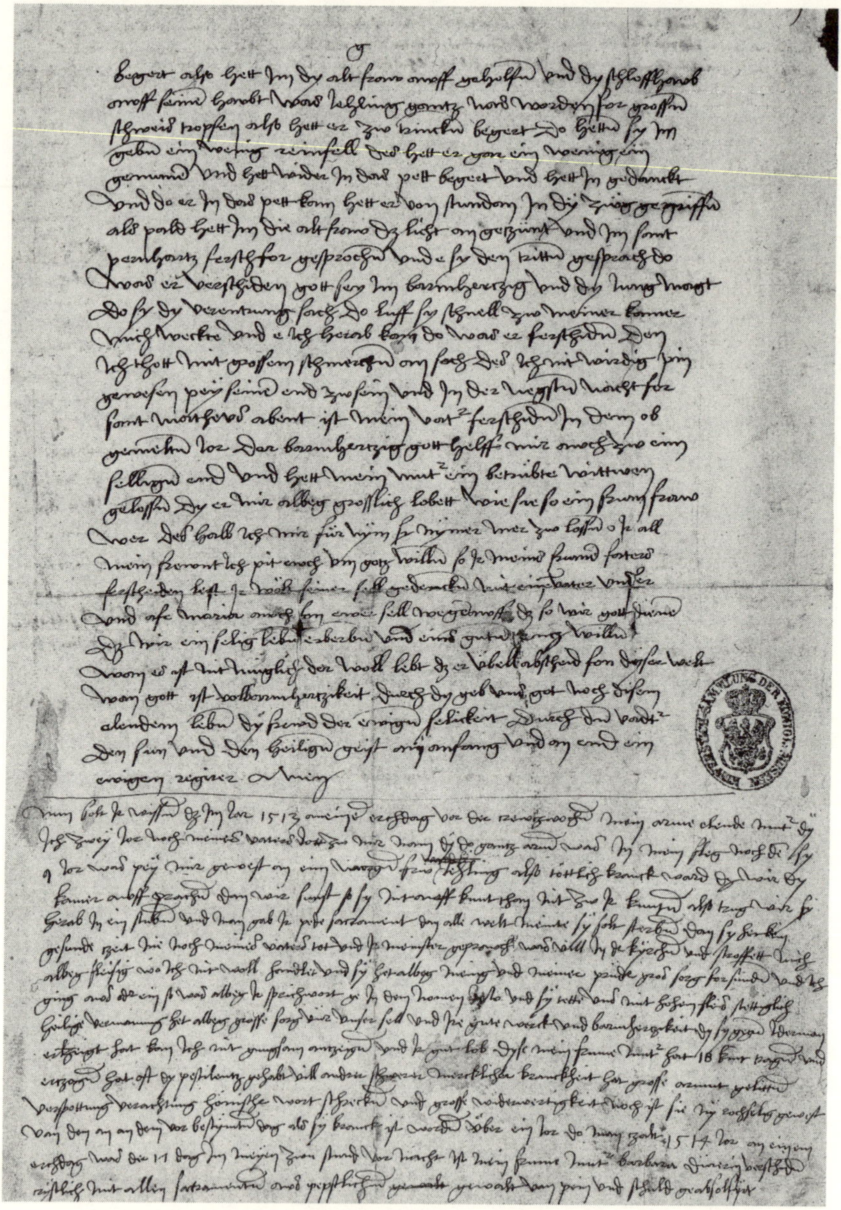

Figure 5.1. Albrecht Dürer, page from the artist's *Book of Remembrances (Gedenckbuch)*, ca. 1502–1514, pen and brown ink on paper, 31.2 x 21.5 cm (Berlin, Staatliche Museen, Kupferstich-kabinett, Sign. Clm. 32, fol. 19r) (photo: bpk Bildagentur/Jörg P. Anders/Art Resource, NY).

CHAPTER FIVE

The Artist as *Medicus*, Part One:

Practices of the Self

Our starting point is what is, to us, the only possible and lasting center, namely, that of the suffering, striving, and acting individual, of what he is, always was, and will be; in this way our observations will be, to a certain extent, pathological.
—Jacob Burckhardt

The Suffering Son

A tremulous twilight that replaces normal vision with weird apparitions, a world-weariness expressed in every sinew of the seated figure, a sense of energy and ambition ebbing as the time of earthly life ticks away, a mourning of all endeavor. With Panofsky's indelible notion of a "spiritual self-portrait" set in their minds, interpreters have often insisted that biography is the key to understanding the uncanny mood of *Melencholia I*, and perhaps also Dürer's very choice of subject. What appears to be the visualization of a depressed state of mind must also be a secret wish for solace, a release from sorrow. A particularly acute time of bereavement in the artist's life is said to be the source. That personal sorrows and intellectual worries informed Dürer's conception of the engraving and the development of its "allegorical" imagery can hardly be doubted, but such a pathway into its unique function and meaning, as we will see, is strewn with pitfalls.

In the autumn of 1513, Dürer saw the passing of two men who had figured prominently in his life and that of his family circle: first it was Anton Kress (b. 1478; called Cressus), the chief pastor of St. Lorenz in Nuremberg and a close associate of Dürer's collaborator Benedict Chelidonius, who composed the elegy for his funeral; he died on September 7.[1] Then it was the revered Nuremberg publisher

Anton Koberger (b. 1440/1445), who had been a good friend to Albrecht Dürer the Elder, then a benefactor and godfather to his son the painter, naming the boy after his good friend; Koberger died on October 3. These deaths surely rattled Dürer, then in his early forties. Koberger had lived to the ripe old age of seventy-three, but Kress, at the time of his passing, was three years younger than Dürer himself.

More grievous was the long illness of his mother, Barbara (née Holper), a devout woman who bore eighteen children—though only three reached advanced adulthood—and for whom her son had great affection. Barbara had come to live with Dürer's family two years after the death of Albrecht the Elder (in 1502) and handled the local sale of Dürer's prints while he was in Italy.[2] Little else is known about her situation in the intervening years, but it has been assumed that her health gradually deteriorated. In April of 1513, amidst a period of intensive work on the so-called *Kaiserbilder*—large pendant portraits of the emperors Charlemagne and Sigismund that Dürer was preparing under commission from the Nuremberg City Council—the elderly woman suffered an acute episode. In the ensuing confusion, according to Dürer's own account, the family was forced to break down the door to her room. Fearing the end, they carried her downstairs to have the sacraments administered, only to see the crisis pass. One year later she would be gone, and Dürer recorded his experiences in the bas-de-page of the sole surviving page of his *Gedenckbuch* (Book of remembrances)—the same page where, in 1502, he had already described the unfortunate circumstances of his father's death (figure 5.1).[3]

> From that day, on the aforementioned date when she was taken ill, more than a year later, in 1514, as they reckon it, on a Tuesday, the 17th day of May, two hours before nightfall, my mother, Barbara Dürer, died a Christian death with all the sacraments, absolved by Papal power from pain and sin. But first she gave me her blessing and wished me peace with God, and exhorted me with beautiful words to keep myself from sin. She also asked to drink St. John's blessing [consecrated wine], which she then did.
>
> She feared death very much, but she said that she was not afraid to come before God. Also she died hard, and I noticed that she saw something frightening; for she asked for the holy water and then said nothing for a long time. Then her eyes closed. I saw, too, how Death gave her two strokes to the heart, and how she closed her mouth and eyes and departed in pain. I prayed for her. I have such sorrow from this, that I cannot express it. God be merciful to her.[4]

Something of the painful fragility of advanced age, the other-worldliness of one approaching death's threshold, appears in the nearly life-sized charcoal portrait Dürer made and inscribed about two months before his mother passed away (figure 5.2).[5] Insisting that the picture, with its boldly sculpted forms, was drawn from life, and certifying it as such on the very day it was made, the artist wrote across the top: "1514 an oculy Dz ist albrecht dürers / mutter dy was alt 63 Jor" (On March 19, this is Albrecht Dürer's mother, when she was 63 years old). Returning to the sheet sometime after her death, he added the following, this time in ink: "vnd ist verschiden / Im 1514 Jor / am erchtag vor der crewtzwochen / vm zwey genacht" (and she passed away in the year 1514 on Tuesday before Cross Week [Rogation], two hours before nightfall).[6]

While there is surely something too romantic in the suggestion that the son worked directly from his mother's bedside,[7] the sheet does place the artist's determination to record visual facts on full display. Every bone and tendon of the woman's lower neck is captured by Dürer's unerring eye and hand, the temporal artery bulging from below its thin covering of waxy skin is unsparingly depicted, and the striking divergence of the sitter's right eye, noted by so many commentators, is shrewdly observed and rendered. (Claims that this represents a ophthalmological condition are probably misplaced.)[8] Here again we find Dürer exercising, in Otto Benesch's choice words, "the perception of an eye trained by physical experience and accustomed to building up a notion of reality from empirical facts."[9] For all this, however, the artist has not treated his beloved mother as a mere specimen of old age or her illness as an occasion for anatomical fact-gathering. Alongside his career-long interest in portraiture, family history was for Dürer an ongoing project. As early as 1490, possibly right before setting off on his journeyman's years (*Wanderjahre*), he had portrayed his parents in a diptych whose panels are now divided between Nuremberg and Florence.[10] Later, as an established artist-entrepreneur in Nuremberg, the good son would come to embrace the role of family chronicler (he began assembling his *Famlienchronik* in 1524). If the portrait of his ailing mother has a surplus that goes beyond recording, we have to look for its meaning in Dürer's intuitive grasp of the portrait's function as a memorial, where private solace meshes with social memory. Peerless in his experience as both subject and object of the drawn portrait, Dürer was

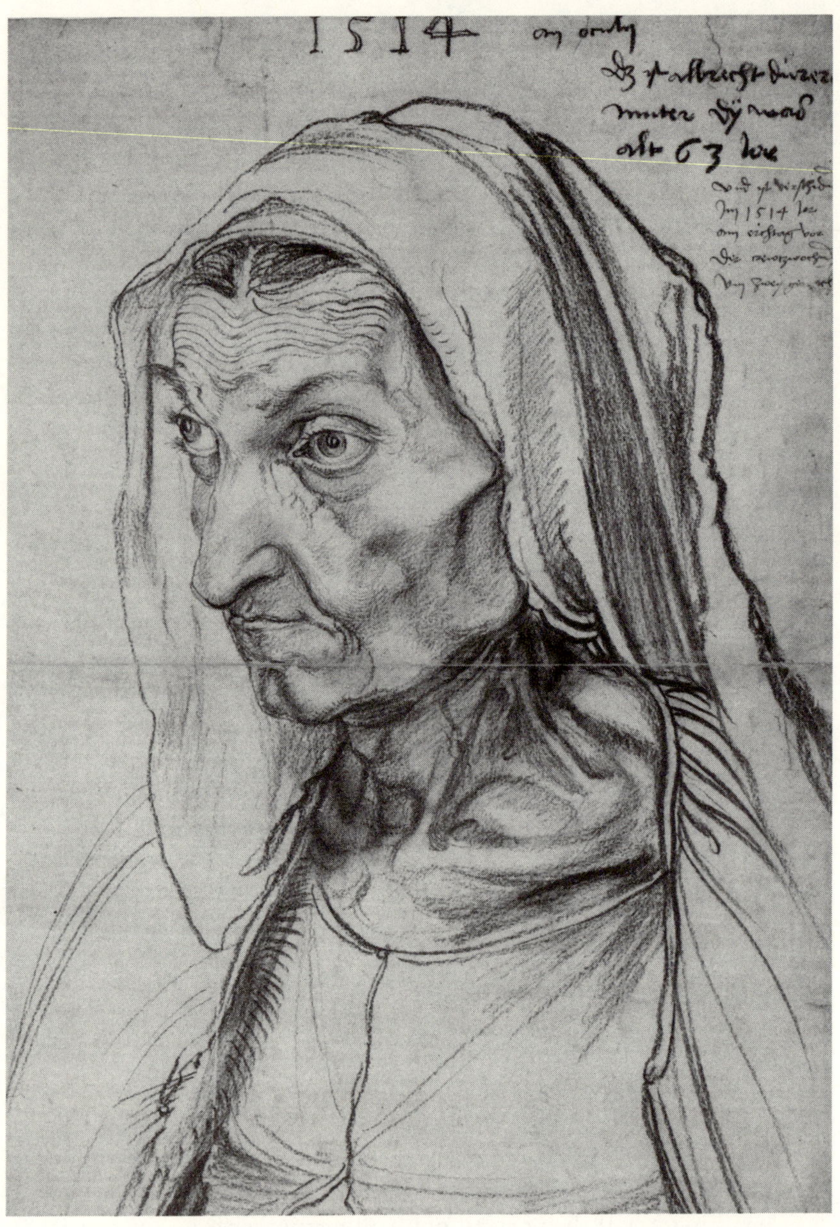

Figure 5.2. Albrecht Dürer, *Barbara Dürer at the Age of 63*, dated 1514, charcoal on paper, 422 x 306 cm (Berlin, Staatliche Museen, Kupferstichkabinett) (photo: bpk Bildagentur / Jörg P. Anders / Art Resource, NY).

uniquely equipped to adapt the genre to his emerging practice as a self-consoler.

Since antiquity, the portrait image of the deceased had provided for the preservation of *memoria* and the perpetuation of a person's "essence and standing" (*substantia et dignitas*). For the deceased, being remembered was the principal way to "live on after death" (Petronius); for the loved ones left behind, however, the perpetuation of *memoria* was just as much a form of consolation.[11] Sophisticated late medieval portraits such as Jan van Eyck's likeness of a certain "Timotheus," featuring the honorary inscription "Loyal Remembrance" (*Leal souvenir*) in simulated carved letters, functioned in this way, lending the presence-effect peculiar to images to the poetic feeling of the classical *consolatio* (figure 5.3). As therapeutic practices attending loss and sorrow, consolation and memory go hand in hand, and as therapeutic performances, each enhances the other. Reading the signs of death on the face of his mother, and casting ahead to his own grief as a survivor, anticipating memory when her absence became final, Dürer creates a bridge between private sorrows and the stoic duties of a family chronicler.[12] In life, the pious Barbara Dürer had addressed herself constantly to the "health" of her children's souls. Dürer had remarked on this concern in the *Gedenckbuch* (though not quoted above) before narrating her demise. Now that care, that attention, that need for vigilance, was passing fully to him. That Dürer relies on a draftsmanly method of "research" into visible phenomena to reveal feelings about his subject that no verbal psychotherapy could possibly reach shows him modifying the portrait as a genre and standing on both sides of the therapeutic encounter.

Is *Melencolia* something like the self-consolation of a suffering son? Is it a masterwork borne of the artist's need to drown his grief in industry, in a concentrated immersion in the fine craft of engraving, one that bordered on the obsessive?[13] Few observers have missed the fact that Dürer dated the image 1514 and that he did so twice. First, in his customary manner, he combined the date with his nested "AD" monogram, placing them in the shadowy recess under the stone bench on which Melancholy sits (figure 5.4), but then those same numbers, from their position in the bottom row of the "magic square," are seen being grazed by the wing of the seated genius (see figure 4.13). And adepts of the magic square will tell you something more: that the upper row of numbers — 16/3/2/13 — also can be read as

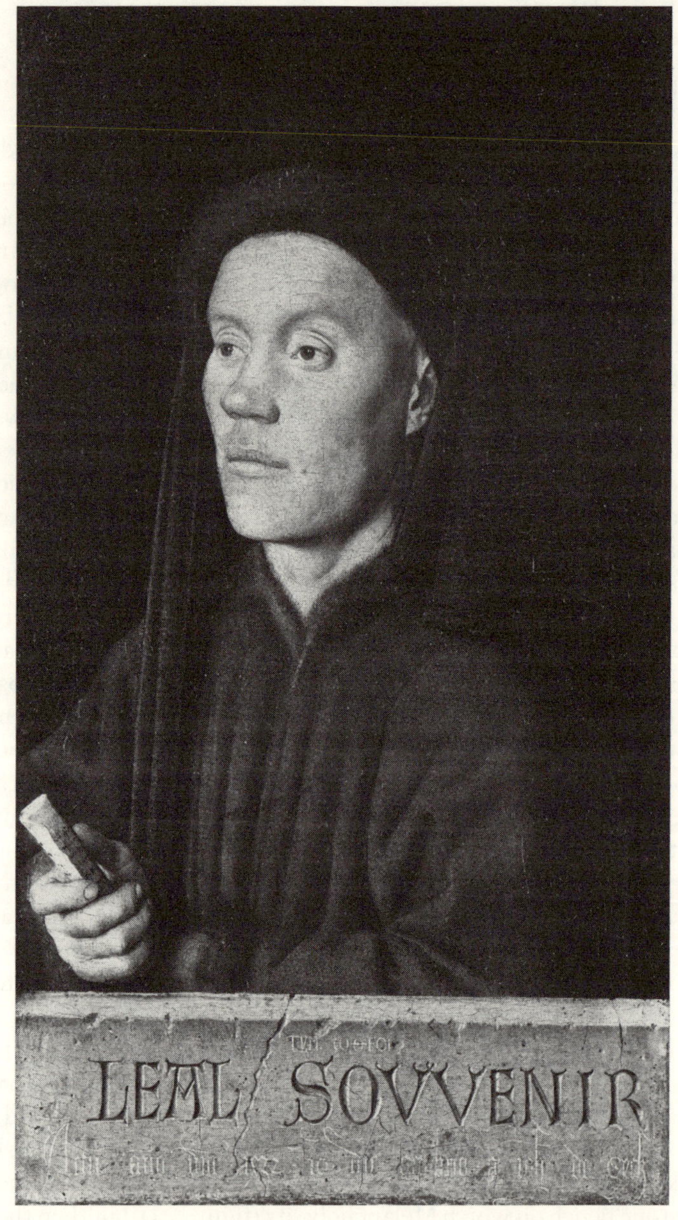

Figure 5.3. Jan van Eyck, *Timotheus/Leal Souvenir* (portrait of a young man), 1432, oil on oak panel, 33.3 x 18.9 cm (London, National Gallery of Art) (photo: © National Gallery, London/Art Resource, NY).

referring to Barbara's death date (16 indicating the day of the month; 3 added to 2 in order to stand for May, the fifth month; and when the number 13 is converted into the equation 1 + 3, it comes to stands for its product, the last digit in the death date, 1514).[14] There can be no denying that *Melencolia*'s imagery reflects a heightened consciousness of mortality, or the likelihood that its mournful mood resonates with the events of 1513–14. Interpreters have persisted in alleging a deep connection, though Panofsky had demurred, arguing that "no personal grief would have occasioned an engraving so esoteric and, at the same time, so programmatic in character."[15]

From all that has been ventured so far in these pages, it would be hard to resist that judgment. Yet for all its symbolic density and even its occult pretensions, the image is keenly psychological. Not only does it diagnose a "complex syndrome" with an accepted name (*melancholia generosa*), one Dürer would have associated with artistic genius, it also portrays a dejected state of mind. Dürer could not have missed the resemblance to his own spiritual sorrow. Perhaps the engraving, once complete, held out this kind of type of solace for him; perhaps its very making helped him refocus, carrying his mind away from cares over sickness and death. (This would be something like the "therapeutic" function of artisanal busywork as narrowly construed today.) Both propositions seem acceptable. But is all this sufficient justification for the view, flatly put forward by the Dürer expert Matthias Mende, that the engraving could just as well be called "Memorial on the Occasion of the Death of His Mother"?[16]

For all the deep interest—sympathetic and voyeuristic—that scholars have shown in the emotional life of an artist prone to confession and worry, it is surprising how consistently Dürer's commentators have missed the opportunity to connect his documentary, commemorative, and self-comforting practices with the traditions of Christian *consolatio* and its especially fertile equivalent in German religious life, *Trost*. For Aby Warburg to have characterized *Melencolia I* as a *humanistische Trostblatt*, a consoling image for humanists, required a special modification of the traditional term (*Trostblatt*, a pictorial counterpart to a *Trostbrief*) to suit his theory of opposing cultural forces in Renaissance man's psyche.[17] For ordinary Christians on the eve of the Reformation in South Germany, however, *Trost* encompassed an entire experience and psychology of pastoral care: its semantic range included notions of alleviation (*levatio*),

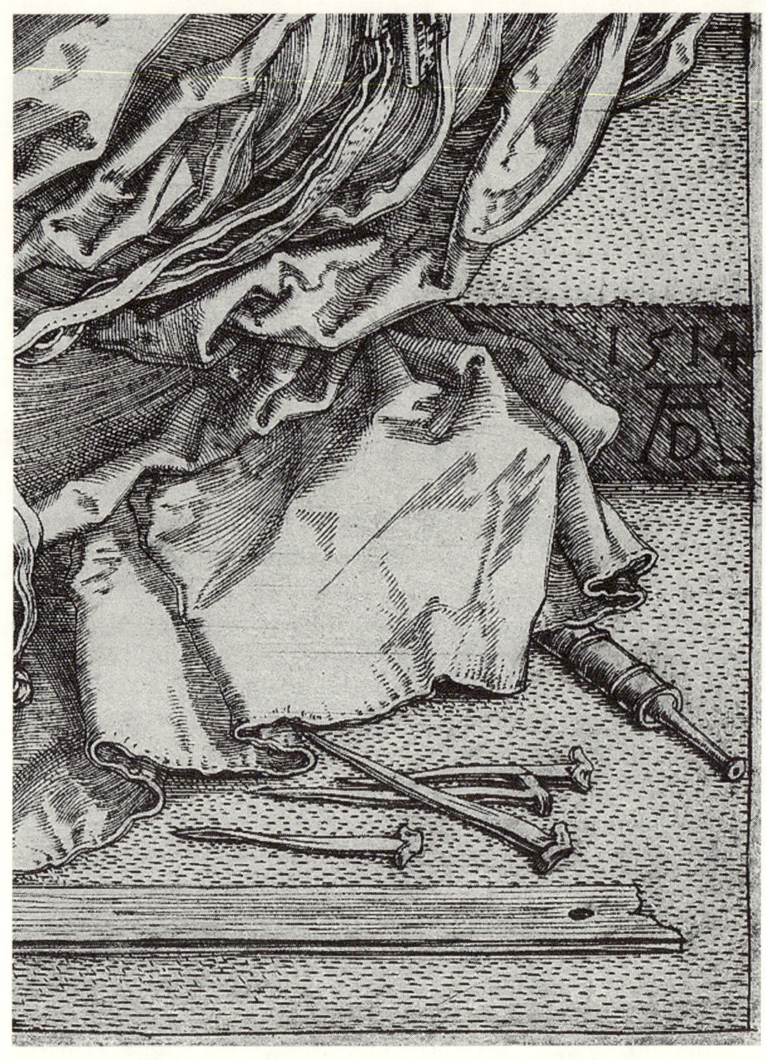

Figure 5.4. Detail from Dürer, *Melencolia I*: date and monogram in lower right corner. (See figure 1.1.)

support (*firmamentum*), assurance (*fiducia*), confidence (*confidentia*), security (*securitas*), hope (*spes*), expectation (*exspectatio*), protection (*praesidium*), and refuge (*refugium*).[18] *Trost* captured the full healing knowledge of grace in the face of worldly adversity and confusion, inner conflict, and sin—a knowledge grasped with the mind and felt with the heart. One read scripture and found solace in God's promises of salvation; one "remembered" the Passion and took refuge in the work of redemption it accomplished; one sought succor in the sacramental rituals of the church and found security and hope in God's tender compassion for his children. Each individual sought *Trost* as a balm for enduring loss and maintaining the health of the soul, but also, and perhaps more importantly, each received it as a spiritual good tendered by another, a "soul service" provided within a total gift economy grounded in God's *caritas*. Pastors and confessors charged with the sacramental care of souls were its traditional middlemen, and they, like physicians charged with the care of the body, developed their own expertise by standing on one side of the therapeutic relationship. In the first half of the sixteenth century, *Trost* emerged as a fungible good within a broader economy of mutual assistance and solace, mediated by spiritual self-help books with titles such as *Soul Medicine for the Healthy and the Sick* (Urbanus Rhegius, 1529) and *Consolation from Divine Scripture* (Caspar Huberinus, 1529),[19] a market that grew amidst the spiritual unease and uncertainties brought about by the Reformation's confessional struggles. Friendships and sodalities of like-minded, or spiritually minded, people were especially dynamic contexts for the dispensation of *Trost*. (See Chapter 6.)

Holding *Melencolia* in his own hands, Dürer could have placed himself on one or the other side of the therapeutic encounter, that of the physician or that of the patient; in all likelihood, he appreciated his own power to inhabit both roles. But if solace in grief were all that the sufferer required, the potency of the "medicine" found in this particular *Trostblatt*, a complex and contradictory allegorical image, already seems to risk overdose— a prescription for confusion, rather than clarification. From all that has been said about the engraving's *Widerspruchlichkeit* during its five-hundred-year history and all that's been ventured in these pages about its therapeutic potential, it is clear that *Trost*, however much the artist needed it in 1514, could only ever be part of the remedy available through the picture.

The Suffering Artist

"We have to pay for everything in this world," Ioan Couliano wrote in his reflections on the Renaissance melancholic, "and those with supranormal faculties must pay most dearly."[20] No stranger to the ideal of "useful suffering," Dürer nevertheless knew how to self-medicate when he had to. As a self-consoler, he actively explored ways to use his art to excavate, order, and control the battling forces within. This program extended to his much-discussed bodily afflictions, as well. In the great transhistorical confraternity of artists who fretted about their health, Dürer, prone to a kind of narcissism in both good health and ill, must be ranked high. The relevant works and documents are well known, but the peculiar way each of them blend visual fact-gathering and self-fashioning, hypochondria and self-healing, has not been fully appreciated by researchers.

It is a knotty problem into which we can afford only a glance. Consider these three exhibits from the patient's case file. Exhibit A is the lively pen drawing, now in Erlangen, that Dürer made on the verso of a sketch of the Holy Family while a young journeyman, around 1491. Judging by the bandage wrapped around his head, it appears to show the twenty-year-old in serious discomfort—possibly due to an illness, possibly from a toothache or in the aftermath of dental surgery (figure 5.5).[21] Disaffected and slightly ornery, with head slumped against an open hand, the artist stage-manages his self-regard and his self-pity at one and the same time. Exploiting self-portraiture's potential for double entendre, he also, with an almost malevolent brattiness, asks us to gauge his pain. Has the young artist turned his already well-developed knack for graphic research toward the study of a particular passion? Does he merely intend to document a health crisis? Is he showing himself—and us—how he actually copes with pain? The reality, then as now, is that the truth of pain is hard to convey to another person; all but invisible, it is ever-productive of doubt. Image makers can do no more than inscribe pain across the body's visible surfaces, capturing its indices in facial expression or gesture. Here the young Dürer shows himself—and us—that he's up to the challenge of persuading the observer that the pain behind his dejected look is real.

Calling attention to everything in the picture that is designed to persuade, however, instantly prizes open the possibility of a knowing conceit. It has two components, one graphic, the other iconographic. In the first place, we can not overlook how pain's power to

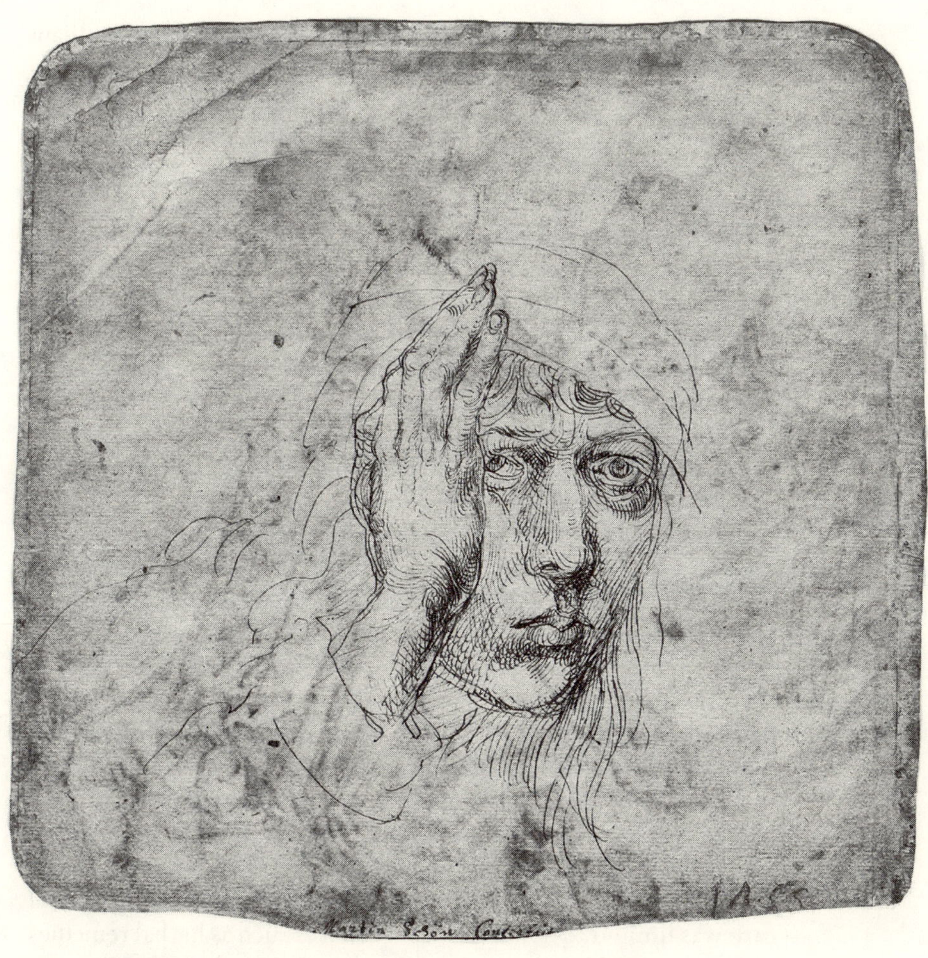

Figure 5.5. Albrecht Dürer, *Self-Portrait*, 1491–1492, pen drawing on paper, back side, 20.4 x 20.8 cm (Erlangen, Graphische Sammlung der Universitätsbibliothek).

install dark thoughts and inspire torpor has already found brilliant expression in the hurried pen strokes of the Erlangen sketch: *It hurt so much I almost couldn't bother to do this*, the sketch seems to say on behalf of its suffering subject, a subject who has nevertheless made himself appealingly visible in just this state. *You'll agree my abject state is worth seeing, however, so I did it quickly.* Keen observation and a showy mastery of line, the intimation of hot creativity and sleight of hand are never far removed. By showing the sitter's right hand, putative instrument of that line, steadying the whole head, the seat of intellect, and pressing so close to the eye, their mediator and guide, Dürer brings the "traditional centers of attention in [Renaissance] portraiture" into the closest proximity.[22] Return the convex workshop mirror to the position now occupied by the paper, however, and we realize that the head is propped up by the actual left, leaving the drawing hand invisible—and free.

The Erlangen self-portrait's cross-association of pain, visual acuity, and manual dexterity has a real-world parallel that can help us further our account of the staged quality of the scene: dental distress and its treatment in early modern Europe. Whether or not the pain of the mouth is really at issue here, Dürer was aware of the context. For many centuries before the invention of anesthesia, tooth pulling was in the hands of barber-surgeons, some local in practice, some traveling to ply their trade at fairs, where medical procedure became a form of public spectacle and, notoriously, an occasion for quackery and con schemes (figure 5.6). Moralists knew that medical fraud exploited not only the ignorant, but the special vulnerability of people in pain, or fear of pain. (For the most part, premodern dental care was limited to noninvasive procedures such as herbal remedies and analgesics, bloodletting, and amulets designed to neutralize the "caries worms" that were thought to produce painful decay—extraction was regarded as a last resort.)[23] Moralists also knew that the deceptive showmanship of the surgeon exposed the credulity of all. No wonder that the "dental martyrdom" picture, as David Kunzle dubbed it, eventually became a satirical genre in its own right. But it was, significantly, satire with serious art-theoretical overtones. Equating the illusionistic prowess of the painter with the quack doctor's sleight of hand, it poked holes in visual certitude, exposed to doubt the reality of the victim's pain, and allowed the painter a mischievous complicity in the deception.[24] Returning to the Erlangen

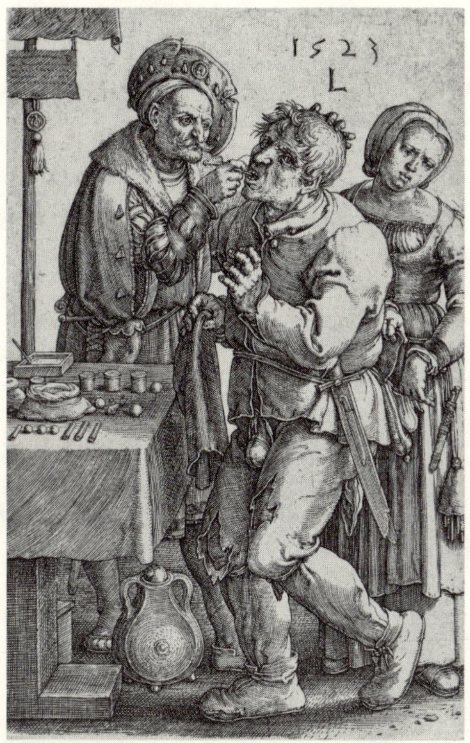

Figure 5.6. Lucas van Leyden, *The Dentist*, 1523, engraving, 11.6 x 7.5 cm, sheet (trimmed to plate mark) (Washington, D.C., National Gallery of Art, Rosenwald Collection).

sheet, one must wonder whether the dejection Dürer projects is real or feigned emotion, self-expression or self-fashioning, or whether those are false choices to begin with.[25]

To the extent that we are right in detecting a cagey, mischievous attitude behind the drawing, the iconography of its defining gesture is unmistakable: a "melancholic" head propped up by a left hand (here open, and cupping the cheek, in contrast with Dame Melancholy's tightened fist).[26] The young Dürer has appropriated a massive tradition of high religious and philosophical seriousness—the image of the plaintive, seated sufferer—that would come to inform the *Melencolia*. Its models and archetypes include Job brooding on the dung heap (see figure 6.1),[27] King David entreating God for guidance and peace, Jeremiah crying out for Israel's repentance (Lamentations 1:12), Adam grieving over the expulsion from Eden, Aeschylus writing and philosophizing in the open air, the German *Minnesänger* meditating on justice, and, not least, the wounded "Christ in misery"

(*Christus in Elend*), grieving over humanity's ingratitude as he awaits the Crucifixion from a visionary space lifted above time (see figure 4.3). Of course, only to its sufferer does a toothache feel like a crucifixion. Has the young man in the portrait already spotted the irony? Laughter, everyone knows, is cathartic and cures many ills; Paracelsus considered the medicinal stimulation of laughter a useful therapy for melancholia.[28] If Dürer is putting us on the spot and poking fun at himself, perhaps that mockery is itself medicinal. Let us not doubt the historical reality of Dürer's pain and sense of his own frailty, but at the same time, let's be careful about taking small matters too seriously. Irony can remedy pride and satisfy the secular need for consolation.

Exhibit B comes from midcareer, a period of extensive commission work for the emperor Maximilian I (1459–1519) and his court, thus surely a time of scheduling pressures, overexertion, and painful reminders of physical limits. (We know, for example, that Dürer suspended work on the painter's training manual he was planning.) Drawing himself naked but for his underpants and the sumptuous locks falling over his shoulders, and looking severely into the mirror, the middle-aged, bearded painter points to a spot on his lower abdomen, circled in pen and highlighted in yellow wash (figure 5.7).[29] Inscribing the sheet as if addressing a doctor, the patient declaims: "Where the yellow spot is, to which I point with my finger, there it hurts" (*Do der gelb fleck ist vnd mit dem / finger drawff dewt do ist mir we*). If Panofsky was right, and the painter is pointing to his spleen, the organ responsible for producing black bile, physical discomfort merges here with worry over the debilitating effects of humoral excess as well as Dürer's self-recognition as a gifted melancholic in need of repair.[30] All of this suggests an interesting linkage with the diagnostic quality and the consolatory function of *Melencolia*. Yet the fundamental question of the Bremen drawing's addressee, thus its practical purpose, remains unanswered. Dürer does what any patient is required to do in the first stages of diagnosis—answer a question about his pain—but who has asked it? For whose benefit is the deictic gesture made? I have already alluded to the long-standing assumption that this quick little pen-and-wash drawing originated as part of a consultation with a doctor, a practice well documented for later centuries.[31] Was this unconventional method of certifying the patient's pain epistolary, then, meant to close a distance neither

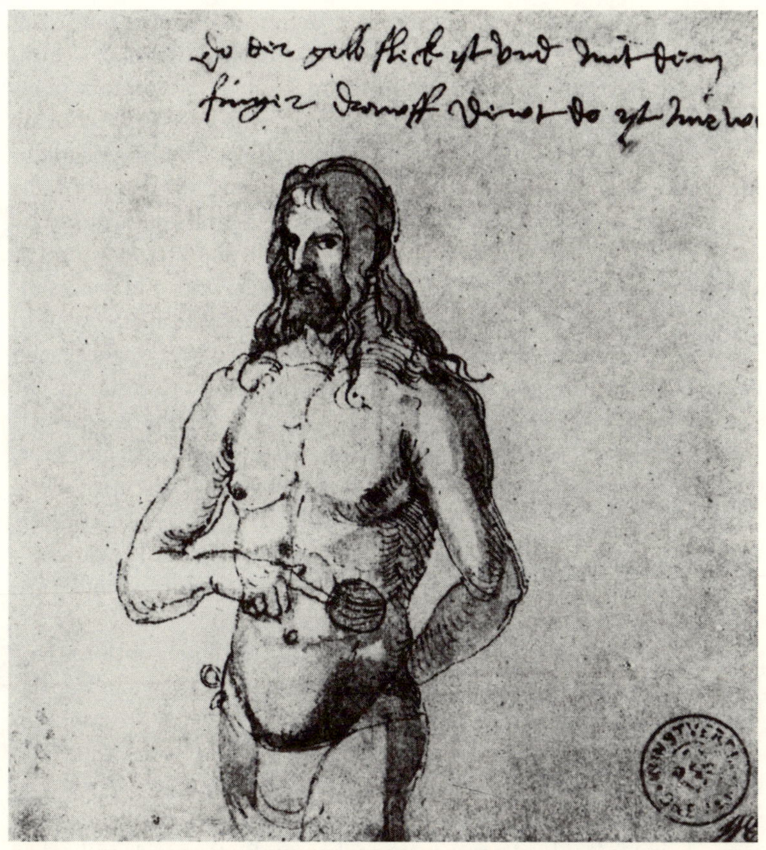

Figure 5.7. Albrecht Dürer, *The Painter Indicating His Pain*, ca. 1512–13, pen, ink, and water-color, 12 x 11 cm (Bremen, Kunsthalle) (photo: Foto Marburg/ Art Resource, NY).

patient nor clinician was able to travel?[32] Possibly it was meant to facilitate a physician's consultation with a colleague over the symptoms and possible causes of this otherwise mysterious illness. Both scenarios may be right.

Emphasizing the conventional and performative character of the drawing, Joseph Koerner has read the curious surplus of deictic gestures and references to symptoms—the pointing, the circling, the explanatory caption—as a veiled lament over the inadequacy of Dürer's art "for articulating what ails him," to wit, the shortcomings of all visual communication.[33] By contrast, we have been inquiring into the adequacy of Dürer's art for articulating what heals him. But these are really two sides of the same coin. What salutary powers would Dürer have likely ascribed to an image self-consciously made by his own hands, or to the very process of making it, or to his reflexive engagement with it? Earlier (Chapter 3) we proposed a schema for understanding the therapeutic expectations aroused by consecrated objects, holy images, votives, and so on, and hinted at the broad connection between therapeutic behaviors and representation itself. These are connections an earlier tradition of research, beginning with nineteenth-century comparative ethnographers such as Richard Andree (1835–1912) or cultural anthropologists such as Sir James Frazer (1854–1941) placed squarely in the domain of superstitious and magical thinking—sympathetic magic, homeopathic cures, iatromathematics (medical astrology), and alchemy. Built up over the course of centuries, if not millennia, collective perceptions of efficacy in the natural world are never entirely banished by the rational, modern constructs that, in the theories of Frazer, for instance, are said to supplant them—and art is no exception.[34]

Without discounting the persistence of those perceptions, this book has advanced an understanding of therapy by image in Renaissance culture that is decidedly *unmagical*, but rather grounded in Christian natural philosophy's account of the body-soul unity and classical thought's delineation of the psychotherapeutic efficacy of the word and, by analogy, the image. Earlier, in discussing the ambition of rhetorical healing as it was taken up by Petrarch and other consolers—that is, verbal psychotherapy's project to help "move" the soul from one state to another—we noted that the communicative *logos* had to operate specifically on the passions before it could properly address the intellect. Recognizing that dialectical reasoning is rarely enough to vanquish false beliefs or to bring the passions under control, rhetorical healing harnesses them, brings them out into the open, much like modern psychotherapy's investment in externalizing repressions, in "getting it all out."

Coaxing the patient into speech or image making, however integrated into an overall treatment, undoubtedly carries its own therapeutic value. Perhaps this is not so far from sympathetic magic or the use of effigies after all? These pages will skirt that question. Our immediate concern is Dürer's sense of the adequacy of the representational means at his disposal—not only line, shade, color, and light, but the written word, too—not simply to express an idea or egocentrically stake a claim to mastery, but to participate actively in the care of souls, beginning with his own. The final example of Dürer's practice as a self-consoler that I have in mind reveals the value he attached to "getting it out," even when no cure could be envisioned. Here we find the artist taking up positions on both sides of the therapeutic encounter and forging new ethical-spiritual categories for the image, a prescient testing of genres that we associate with the modern. But first some background.

Sickness and Fortune

At the center of speculations about Dürer's ill health in the final decade of his life is the "wondrous sickness" first reported in the Netherlands travel journal (*Tagebuch*) in April of 1521 and then lamented from time to time in subsequent years. Accompanied by his wife Agnes and her maid Susanna, Dürer had departed Nuremberg on 12 July 1520 and spent just under a year on the road, traversing between Cologne and Aachen, Brussels, Mechelen and Antwerp, Bruges and Ghent in Flanders, as well as making a journey north into Holland. It was business concerns that prompted the trip: following the death of his imperial patron Maximilian in January 1519, Dürer could no longer take his pension for granted and therefore sought an audience with Maximilian's successor and grandson, the young Charles V, to have it confirmed. While keeping track in his journal of every farthing spent on lodging and food, transport and tolls, doctors and trips to the spa, balancing debits against every sale of his own paintings, drawings, engravings, and books—the journal is really a ledger interlaced with observations—Dürer indulged his passion for collectibles, curiosities, exotica, and naturalia of all kinds. (The famous painter, it seems, always found time for shopping.)[35] He also showed enormous pluck in sightseeing—visiting, for example, the bones of a legendary giant in Antwerp, or viewing the treasures from Mexico then on display in Brussels.

The most elaborate of these quests for the marvelous was the ill-fated, midwinter excursion from Antwerp to Bergen op Zoom, and then onward to the islands of Zeeland, the point of which was to see a giant whale that had beached near the town of Zierikzee. Underestimating the harsh conditions of the North Sea in mid-December,

Dürer complained of being chilled, but this would prove the least of his misfortunes. While en route, the party barely escaped serious injury when their boat, docked at Arnemuiden, was accidentally rammed by a larger vessel (an incident dramatized in Ferninand Fellner's *Dürer in the Storm on the Scheldt*, among the paintings created by Nazarene devotees for the Romantic Dürer Jubilee of 1828).[36] By the time the party reached the area where the whale was been reported, however, it had already been washed back out to sea. "We wanted to see the great fish," Dürer concedes in his *Tagebuch*, "but Fortuna had carried it away again."[37]

To make matters worse, shortly after this disappointment, Dürer found himself disabled by fever and weakness. He did not describe the onset of the illness until later, however, when its recurrence clearly troubled him:

> In the third week after Easter a violent fever seized me [*stiß mich ein heiß füber*], with great weakness, nausea, and headache. And before, when I was in Zeeland, a wondrous sickness [*eine wunderliche kranckheit*] overcame me, such as I never heard of from any man, and this sickness remains with me. I paid 6 st. for cases. The monk has bound 2 books for me in return for the art wares which I gave him.[38]

Speculation about the illness had once fixed on malaria, presumably contracted by a mosquito bite; the recurrence of similar, but milder symptoms in the remaining seven years of his life, perhaps indicative of chronic anemia, would seem to reinforce this, for it is consistent with untreated malarial infection. But the bitter weather conditions Dürer reported during the journey through Zeeland very nearly rule out mosquitoes as a pathogenic cause.[39] Regardless of their origins, it's clear that the recurring symptoms became not only a strain, but a preoccupation for the traveling artist: payments to doctors and apothecaries pepper the Netherlands diary from late spring into summer 1521 and include numerous notes about medicinal herbs, for example, the East Indian myrobolens, a fruit extolled for "strengthening the heart, the liver, and the limbs," a gift from one of his Portuguese friends.[40]

Yet it is also the case that Dürer's concerns about his own physical decline and failing health antedate the wintry misadventures of 1520; the surplus of diagnostic prompts we observed in the Bremen drawing of ca. 1512–13 (figure 5.7), for example, allow us to trace this anxiety back to a period of intensifying demands and pressures. By 1520, in a letter to the secretary and chaplain of the Ernestine dukes in Wittenberg, Georg Spalatin (1484–1545)—part of which addresses the loss of his imperial pension—Dürer could remark, with noticeable self-pity, "As I am losing my sight and freedom of hand my affairs do not look well" (*Dan so mir ab get am gesicht vnd freiheit der hand, würd mein sach nit wolsten*). "I don't care to withhold this from you, kind and trusted sir."[41] Around the same time, Pirckheimer, commenting on his dear friend's situation and presumably also his health, told Thomas Venatorius (d. 1551), "Dürer's in bad shape" (*Turer male stat*).[42] For any artist, fretting about one's financial situation and worrying about physical decline justifiably go hand in hand. The active collaboration of head and hand, celebrated mischievously in the Erlangen self-portrait (figure 5.5) and seriously elsewhere in his oeuvre, formed the wellspring of Dürer's livelihood, as well as his fame. Now, for the forty-eight-year-old artist, the collaboration of incisive eye and steady hand was looking precarious from both sides. Even if the means of representation at his disposal were adequate for "articulating what ails him," would the ailing body remain up to the task? And if the body were indeed up to it, would the artist ever surrender the penitential advantages of affliction, its authenticating effects, its protean power to shape Christian identity and artistic identity at the same time—to wit, its ongoing inscription into the "Dürer myth" by the artist himself?

The Suffering Servant

No other work in Dürer's oeuvre seems to speak so profoundly to the artist's consciousness of a fragile mortality than the large-format metalpoint drawing formerly in the Bremen Kunsthalle (figure 5.8).[43] Highlighted with white chalk on green-toned paper, signed with Dürer's monogram, and dated 1522, it is the latest and in some ways the most intriguing of the Nuremberg master's surviving self-portraits. It is also the most ill-fated. Acquired for the Kunsthalle in the nineteenth century, the sheet was among the 1,715 drawings, over three hundred prints, and a small group of paintings evacuated in the spring of 1943 to the Schloß Karnzow in Brandenburg, one of the Bremen collection's four wartime depositories. Sometime between May and June 1945, amidst the castle's plundering by Soviet troops and village locals, the drawing was snatched up with a trove of other

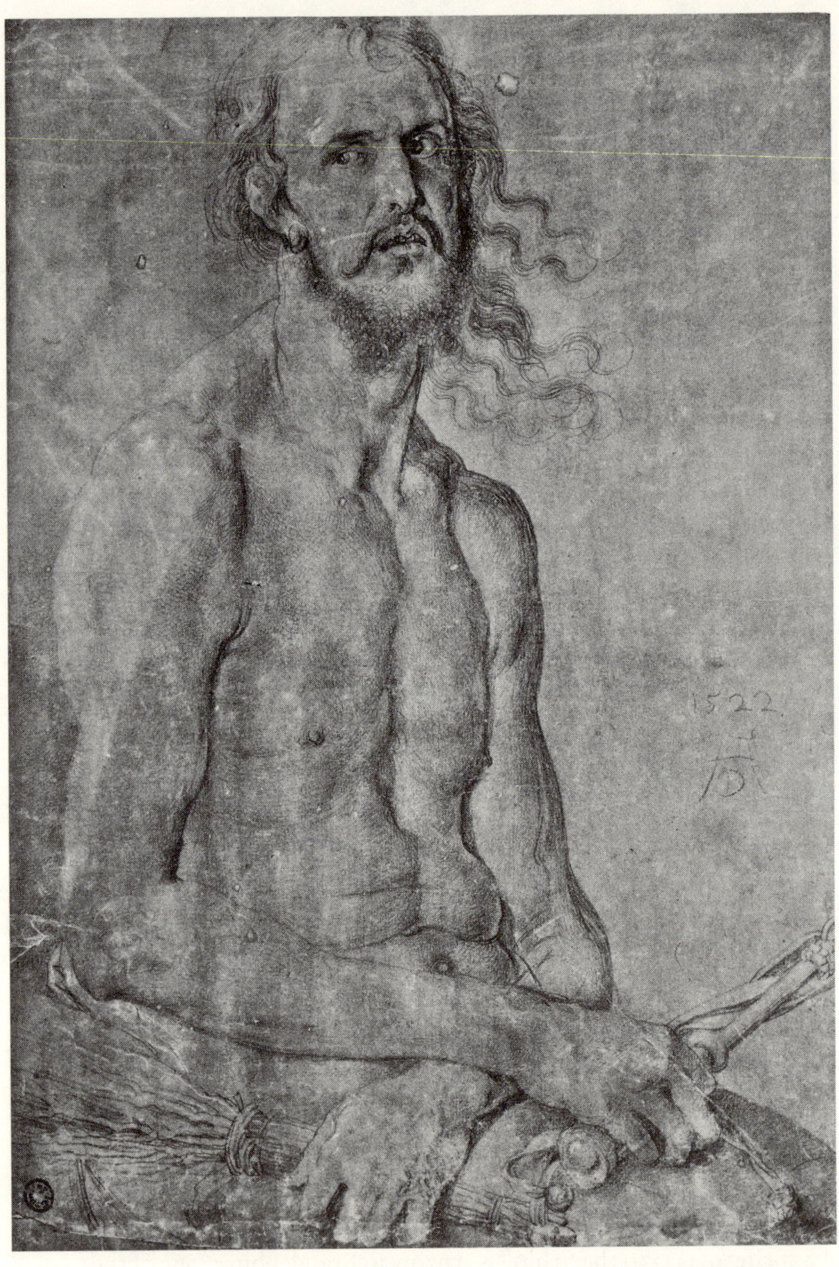

Figure 5.8. Albrecht Dürer, *Self-Portrait with Instruments of the Passion*, dated 1522, metal pen drawing heightened with white crayon on green-toned paper, 40.8 x 29.0 cm (Bremen Kunsthalle–Der Kunstverein in Bremen; presently in Moscow) (photo: Karen Blindow).

valuable works on paper (and two small paintings) by a Red Army captain named Viktor Ivanovich Baldin, who secretly transported the loot to Moscow.[44] While other displaced Dürers that were presumed lost in the war have been returned to Bremen through negotiations—*The Painter Indicating His Pain* (figure 5.7), for example, was returned in the early 1950s[45]—the self-portrait, along with most of the so-called Baldin Collection, has remained captive in Russia, its prospects for return to Germany completely uncertain.[46]

Treatment at the hands of scholars has, in truth, not been all that much kinder. Frequently invoked and remarked upon by the artist's greatest commentators, the Bremen drawing, with its unsettling fusion of Dürer's features with the attributes—notably the flagellum and birch held upon the lap—and pained attitude of Christ during the Passion, has yet to become the object of an in-depth study, even where the artist's career-long project of self-portraiture has been the focus of interest.[47] Is the dubious distinction of being both emblematic of Dürer's "late period" and yet understudied due to the drawing's post-war exile, or does the picture harbor some kind of stumbling block to interpretation, some forbidding tangle, that has yet to be recognized or confronted?

The problem of "Christomorphic self-portraiture" seems to be one such entanglement. Despite the fact that Dürer produced no other self-portrayals in the years immediately preceding or following his journey to the Netherlands (1520–21), recognizing the artist's face on the basis of authenticated self-portraits or visual documents such as the portrait medallion of ca. 1519–20 by Hans Schwarz (see figure I.1) proved easy enough for scholars early in the twentieth century.[48] Recognizing Christ in the drawing's frank and carefully observed treatment of the aging painter's body—the thinning hair, hunched shoulders, protruding clavicle, the slackening muscles of the arms and abdomen—has proven harder to reconcile. As early as 1911, Gustav Pauli, then director of the Kunsthalle in Bremen, had declared the image a seated Man of Sorrows.[49] With the general acceptance of both proposals, the figure's designation as a "self-portrait as Man of Sorrows" (*Selbstbildnis als Schmerzensmann*), or some variation on this, has gone largely unquestioned ever since. Yet Dürer's allegedly "blasphemous" gesture appears to be a matter of ongoing discomfort, even though research into the better-known case of Dürerian Christomorphy, the 1500 oil portrait in Munich, has hardly been hampered by worries over impiety—if anything, it has been energized by them.[50]

Seeking a more profound explanation for the picture's concept, scholars have rummaged around in the psychological space where the artist's health anxieties seem to have collided with a deeply felt spiritual craving for *imitatio Christi*. Panofsky, who mustered only a slender paragraph for the drawing, despite regarding it as the "epitome" of Dürer's late period, proclaimed it a kind of ascetic counterpart to the glorious Christomorphy of the Munich self-portrait. Blurring any distinction between portraiture and devotional imagery, he writes, the drawing interprets the artist's "physical pain and decay" as "a supreme symbol of the likeness of man unto God."[51] Drawing this notion of a penitential identification with the Passion closer to Freud's analysis of narcissism, Koerner set the Bremen drawing within a nexus of works that include the self-portraits Dürer produced—from about 1503 onward—in which the body's fragility is dramatized. Prominent in this group are the 1503 *Nude Self-Portrait* in Weimar and *The Painter Indicating His Pain* of ca. 1512–13 (figure 5.7); astride these are those Christ images Dürer endowed with his own likeness.[52] The synecdoche that unifies all these works, Koerner argues, is the side wound of Christ, a focal point of pre-Reformation piety rich with mystical and consolatory meanings. "By enacting the gesture of the *ostentatio*," Koerner writes of the exemplary self-pointing in *The Painter Indicating His Pain*, "Dürer can relate his own illness to the Passion, thereby assuming the pious attitude of *conformitas Christi* and invoking, for his aid, the healing power of Christ's wounds."[53] Dürer's self-therapy appears at once psychological and sacramental. Such interpretations thus attribute to the Christomorphic self-display of Dürer's late works a kind of consolatory expressionism in which pain "articulates a subjective state *and* the constitution of [the artist's] character."[54]

Despite its brevity, Koerner's remains the most complex account of the Bremen drawing to date. Shall we rest easy, then, with the notion that there is, implicit in the picture's address, a familiar claim about the conditions under which Dürer imaginatively fuses Christ's pain with his own—the same claim he inscribed below the tortured visage of Christ in the 1503 charcoal in London: "I produced these two countenances for you truthfully while I was ill"? (See figure P.1)

A different account of how the Bremen drawing can exemplify

the autotherapeutic aspect in Dürer's project of self-portraiture and at the same time stand astride its categories emerges when we scrutinize the drawing's multiple references to the "Passion portrait" tradition that Dürer knew so well and tested throughout his career.[55] Building on remarks made elsewhere,[56] I wish to demonstrate here that the guiding concept of the portrait, which I take to be the sitter's vigilant awareness of an unseen force and his ambivalent state of being "armed" for struggle, is not a direct function of Christomorphic identification. To the degree that the picture's function is therapeutic, the source of consolation is not Christ himself or conformity to his suffering. Rather, it is the reflective reason of the self in time, the *ethical self* that heeds the ancient philosophical injunction to "take care of yourself" (*epimeleisthai sautou*),[57] Christianizes it, and discovers its inner virtue in the battle against a capricious fortune. That thematic of a virtue-building inner reflection, understood as an ethical-therapeutic imperative for the new type of pious intellectual envisioned by humanism, certainly underlies the conception of *Melencolia*, whatever we may wish to say about its esoteric symbolism. To get at this thematic in a limited space, we can venture two iconographic observations, each of which, in its own way, points toward this interpretation.

The first of these details is the omission or absence of stigmata from the body. Of all the self-portraits invoked by Koerner as evidence for Dürer's special brand of Christomimetic narcissism, only the Bremen sheet emphatically avoids any reference to the wounds. Without sounding pedantic, icongraphically speaking, this means we must overrule the *Schmerzensmann* designation for good. And yet in the painting for which our drawing was made as a preparatory study, the panel preserved at Schloß Weissenstein (near Pommersfelden in Upper Franconia) (figure 5.9), the *Schmerzensmann's* attributes of death are all in place. (The panel is generally accepted as the work of a Dürer-Renaissance copyist, possibly Hans Hoffman, reproducing a painting purchased from Dürer by Albrecht of Brandenburg.)[58] The black background suggests a visionary space removed from time and narrative. Saturnine and world-weary, the muscular figure directs his dark gaze slightly off-camera, toward our left. His pose inclines him toward the *Christus in Elend* tradition, though *arma Christi* grasped upon the lap were never features of that type. The Pommersfelden panel's closest iconographic counterpart in Dürer's oeuvre, in fact, is

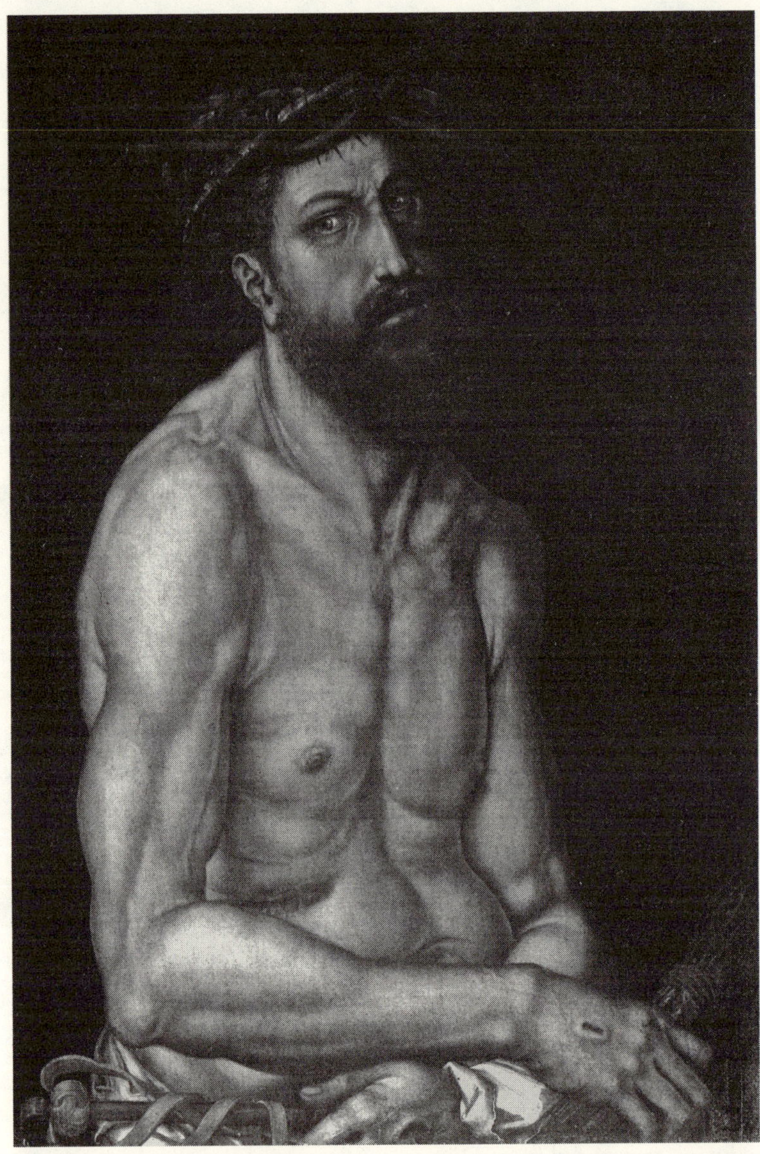

Figure 5.9. Anonymous copyist (probably Hans Hoffman), *Man of Sorrows Seated*, ca. 1600, oil on limewood panel, 86 x 59 cm (Pommersfelden, Schloß Weißenstein, Kunstsammlung Graf Schönborn-Weisentheid) (photo: Hermann Maué and Sonja Brink [eds.], *Die Grafen von Schönborn: Kirchenfürsten, Sammler, Mäzene*, exhibition catalogue, [Nuremberg: Germanisches Nationalmuseum, 1989], no. 275).

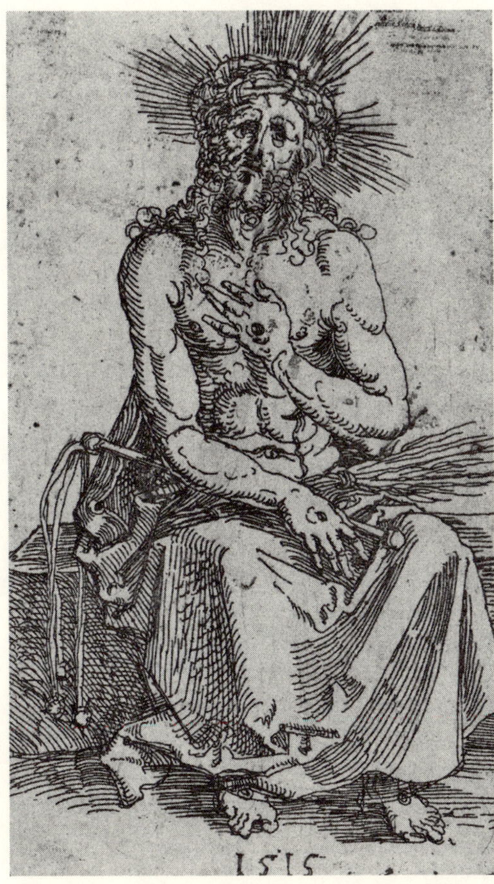

Figure 5.10. Albrecht Dürer, *Man of Sorrows Seated*, dated 1515, etching, 11.1 x 6.5 cm (Washington, D.C., National Gallery of Art, Rosenwald Collection).

found in the small *Man of Sorrows* etching of 1515, which features similar attributes (figure 5.10).[59] All of this suggests that after using himself as a model for the drawing, Dürer added all the specific attributes of the Passion—flail and birch, the crown of thorns, stigmata—to complete his concept for a painted *Schmerzensmann*, but kept the latter two out of the drawing, allowing it to remain an autonomous self-portrait.[60] The result is not a potentially "blasphemous" Christomorphy, but an image that expresses something of his own situation as a Christian man, afflicted by sorrow and tested by fortune. The self-portrait's Christomorphic overtures arose from the artist's practical decision to use himself as a model. Having done this very thing earlier in his career, Dürer knew the spiritual and psychological possibilities before him. They are rich, and they are actively evoked here, but we

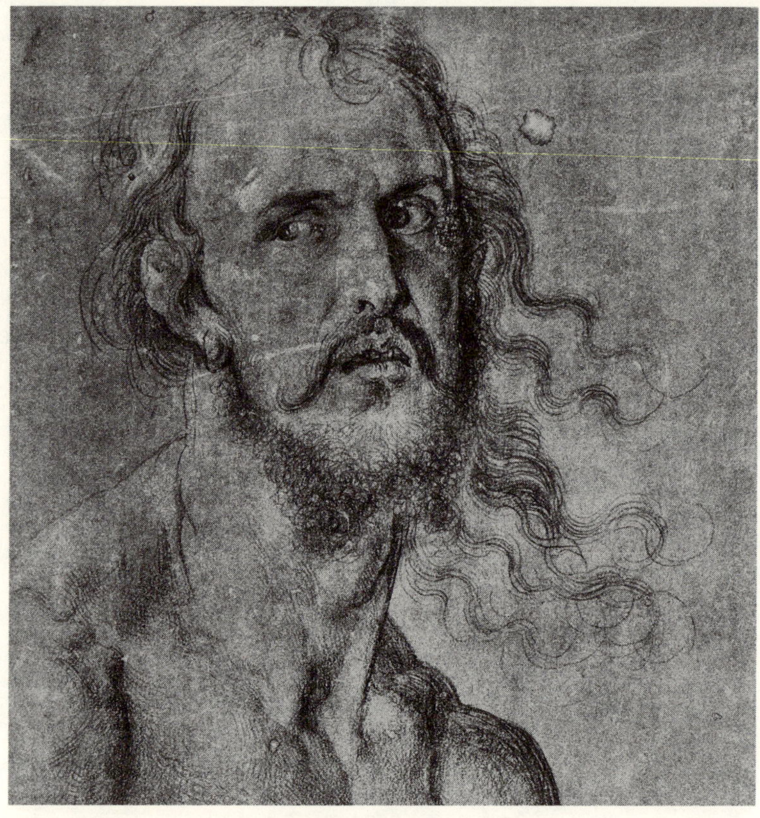

Figure 5.11. Detail of Dürer, *Self-Portrait with Instruments of the Passion*: head and billowing hair. (See figure 5.8 above.)

have not yet penetrated to the spiritual and psychological core of the picture or its true therapeutic function.

The key to getting there will be found in a motif Dürer did *not* transfer from the "study" to the painted version: the billowing of the sitter's thinning hair away from his head, as if tossed by a wind coming from the left, the same direction from which the figure is lit (figure 5.11). A seemingly naturalistic effect of atmosphere, a note of transitory movement in an otherwise stilled tableau, the motif has elicited no significant comment from writers.[61] Yet it quickly gains in symbolic intent when Dürer's oeuvre is surveyed for comparable accessory movements. In one instance, the Crucifixion scene from the *Engraved Passion* series, we find gusts of mountain air tossing Christ's hair backward while his body hangs immobile—like the wind-tossed loincloth, this was a more or less conventional way of conveying the atmospheric disturbances that accompanied the great event.[62] Dürer also knew that hair streams backward, counter to the body's facing direction, when figures lunge forward through space: a good example is the jawbone-wielding fury in his 1496 "Ercules" woodcut. (See figure E.2). Attention might be called to the natural laws of momentum and air by violating them: in Dürer's backward-riding witch of ca. 1500, for example, the hag's undulating mop is driven backward from the body by a supernatural blast in the sky, even as her mount flies her in the opposite direction.[63] In contrast to the two latter examples, the animating wind in the Bremen sheet strikes an immobile body, and unlike the crucified Christ, the force of air comes from behind. Feeling it pass over his naked shoulders, the Bremen sitter turns warily toward its source, yielding a novel form of *contrapposto* that Dürer invests with tremendous psychological power.

Quattrocento art theory had made natural wind effects and the corresponding movement of the body's accessories—principally hair and garments—important touchstones for the imitation of bodies in space. In *Della pittura* (1436), Alberti praises the variety of devices for rendering these transitory movements, explaining: "It is pleasing to see some movement in hair, locks, boughs, leafy fronds, and garments. As I said, I myself take pleasure in seeing different movements of the hair: hair should twist as if trying to break loose from its ties and rippling in the air like flames, some of it weaving in and out like vipers in a nest, some swelling here, some there."[64] Aby Warburg, though not the first to draw the connection between this passage and Sandro Botticelli's alighting wind gods in his *Birth of Venus* (ca. 1485), recognized in Alberti's advice a "compromise" characteristic of Renaissance thinking about art generally. While giving rein to his fantasies of flux and mutation, he writes, "Alberti expressly insists that in depicting such motifs the painter keep his analogical wits about him sufficiently to avoid being tempted into unnatural excess, and that he set his accessory forms in motion only where the wind really might have caused such motion."[65] To this end, Alberti recommended adding "the heads of the winds, Zephyrus or Auster, among the clouds, blowing the garments."[66]

If Dürer ever came close to following Alberti's advice to the letter, it was in the 1511 woodcut of the *Holy Trinity* (see figure 6.15), where puffing heads representing the Four Winds toss the drapery below

Chris's feet. As for the stricken draughtsman of 1522, surely he could not have forgotten the ill effects of Boreas, the north wind, after his encounter two years earlier on the North Sea, or the cosmological association with melancholia, which he allegorized in the woodcut frontispiece for Celtis's *Quatuor libri amorum*, where the deity took his place in the fourfold scheme including Zephyr (the west wind), Eurus (east), and Auster (south) that surrounds *Philosophia* (see figure 4.12).[67] The staging of the seated figure in the Bremen sheet offers little by which to infer the wind's source or cause. Nevertheless, a case can be made for the likelihood that Dürer identified this disturbance of air with another pagan deity familiar to humanists, the Roman wind goddess Fortuna, and thus with the interconnected problems of free will and fate, merit and determinism, providence and fortune current among the intellectuals of his day. Two areas of evidence, iconographic and personal, establish Dürer's close acquaintance with the goddess.

Battling Fortune

As a printmaker, Dürer's very first foray into classical subject matter was the "Little Fortune," a small engraving of circa 1496 depicting the coy goddess perched upon a globe with wind-tossed hair, holding a sprig of the aphrodisiac Eryngium and resting the same hand upon a slender staff (figure 5.12).[68] It is a work of self-conscious classical styling and—not coincidentally—considered to be the artist's first female nude in a print medium.[69] About five years later (1501–1502), Dürer depicted another goddess associated with fortune and fate, Nemesis, as a powerful winged figure floating high above a landscape. She holds out a golden chalice, symbolizing the reward she brings to some, and a bridle, referring to the punishment she prepares for others (see figure 2.8).[70] As a diarist, we will recall, Dürer had invoked Fortuna as a figure of instability, recognizing her dominion over things both great and trivial—as when his Netherlands traveling party missed the opportunity to see a giant whale because "Fortuna had carried it away again." Earlier in life, a younger, more optimistic Dürer had entrusted himself to providence, or to Fortune herself. In his first painted self-portrait, the Louvre oil-on-parchment—made when Dürer was a journeyman, probably as a token of his betrothal to Agnes Frey—he included the inscription: *My sach die gat / Als es oben schtat* (My affairs will go as ordained on high). No doubt hoping to be lucky in begetting children, the artist shows

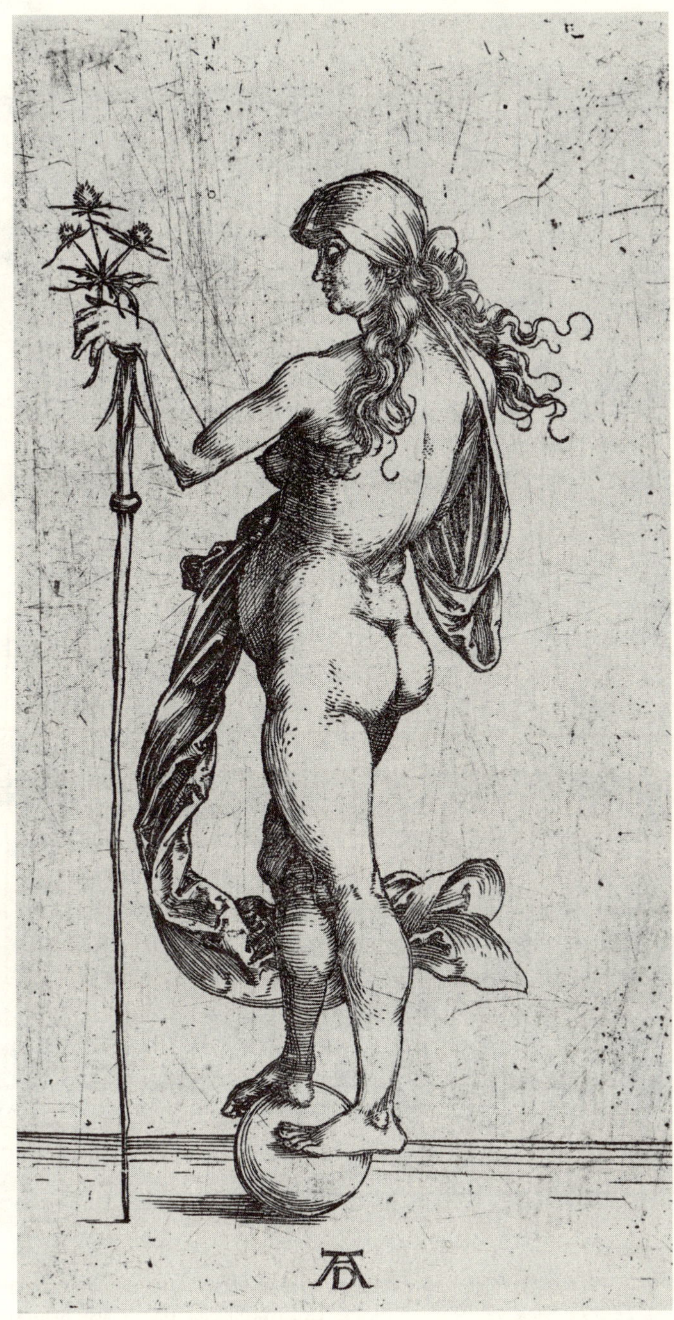

Figure 5.12. Albrecht Dürer, *Fortuna Holding Eryngium* (*"The Little Fortune"*), engraving, 12.0 x 6.7 cm (Washington, D.C., National Gallery of Art, Rosenwald Collection).

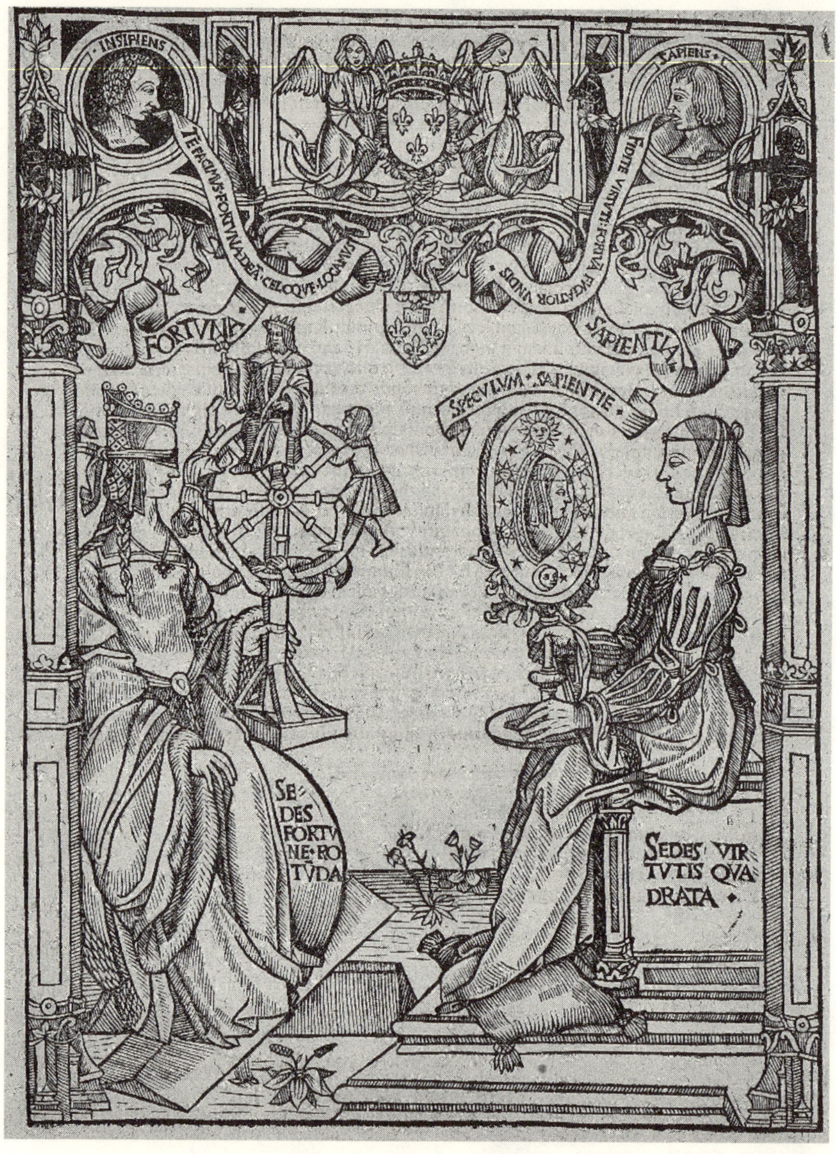

Figure 5.13. Parisian, *Fortune versus Wisdom*, woodcut from Charles de Bovelles (Carolus Bovillus), *Liber de Sapiente* (Paris, 1510), fol. 116v (Washington D.C., Folger Shakespeare Library. Used by permission of the Folger Shakespeare Library.)

himself holding the aphrodisiac Eryngium that he would later link directly to the pagan goddess.[71]

Taken together, Dürer's artistic engagements with the antique goddess and his personal experiences enduring her caprice leave little doubt that he had the resources and the motivation to associate the movements of fate with the movements of air coming from the left in the Bremen self-portrait. But wind per se was not the foremost vehicle of Fortuna's action in ancient days, nor the foremost symbol of her dominion, at least in the Middle Ages, which allegorized her mutability with the image of the wheel (figure 5.13).[72] The close association with wind was a product of the humanist renovation of the Roman Fortuna (from the Greek goddess Τύχη, whose name means "luck") as a personification of fate and man's powerlessness.

How can man get the upper hand in his dealings with fortune? Again it was Warburg who, in his 1907 study, "Francesco Sassetti's Last Injunctions to His Sons," revealed this question to be a flashpoint for diverse efforts by quattrocento literary and artistic figures to attain a "positive balance" for the individual at a time of conflicting attachments and colliding forces.[73] Warburg was captivated by the way the Florentine merchant and art patron Sassetti could express to his sons in one breath their collective subjection to Fortune's caprice—"Where Fortune intends us to make landfall, I know not, in view of the upheavals and changes amid which we now find ourselves (may God grant us safe haven)"—and in the next entreat them to engage the goddess as steadfastly as he had done: "Even if I were to leave you more debts than assets, I want you to live and die in that same state of Fortune; for this I regard as your duty."[74] The material counterpart to Sassetti's conception Warburg spotted in the *impresa* conceived for the family crest of another Florentine merchant-humanist, Giovanni Rucellai (1403–81), author of the *Zibaldone*, a collection of Greek and Roman wisdom. Placed atop his family armorial, "Fortune with the Sail" appears on the surviving relief (Florence) as a nude woman standing in a ship, holding aloft its billowing sail, similar to that found on the contemporary bronze medallion now in New York (figure 5.14).

For Rucellai, however, none of the worthies quoted in his book—Aristotle, Boethius, Seneca, Epictetus, Dante, Saint Bernard—had a satisfying answer to the question his *impresa* articulates: "Have human reason and practical intelligence any power against the

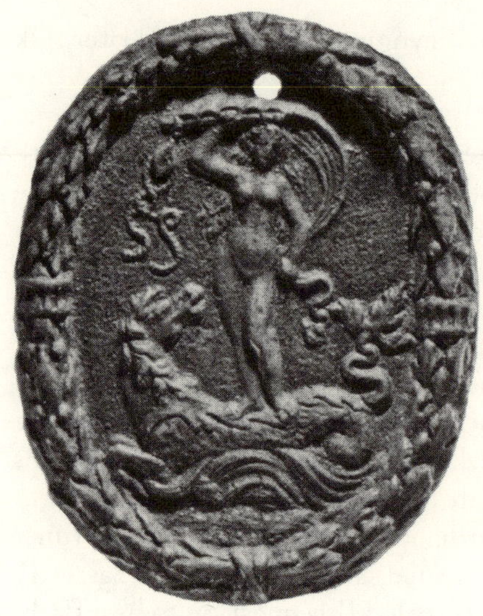

Figure 5.14. Italian (Florence?), *Fortune with Sail*, fifteenth–sixteenth century, bronze medallion, 5.2 x 4.1 cm (New York, Metropolitan Museum of Art, The Erich Lederer Collection. Gift of Mrs. Erich Lederer; photo courtesy of the Metropolitan Museum of Art, www.metmuseum.org).

accidents of fate, against Fortune"? For a better answer, he turned to Marsilio Ficino, whose long reply exemplifies the Renaissance balancing of polarities, according to Warburg. At the letter's conclusion, Ficino renders his judgment on the three options available to "the provident man" as he seeks the right remedy for misery in the face of all that can not be foreseen:

> It is good to do battle with Fortune, wielding the weapons of providence, patience, and noble ambition. It is better to withdraw, and to shun such a combat—from which so few emerge victorious, and then only after intolerable labor and effort. It is best of all to make peace or a truce with Fortune, bending our wishes to her will and willingly going the way she directs, lest she drag us by force. All this we shall do, if we can combine within ourselves the might, the wisdom, and the will.[75]

This acceptance of nature and fate in hard times, essentially Stoic in its outlook, Renaissance men such as Sassetti, Rucellai, and Ficino converted into "an emblem of energy" (*Energiesymbol*) according to Warburg, "a stimulus to bold and decisive action."[76] This balancing of antithetical impulses, this reconciliation of pagan and Christian ethics, found expression in the two mottoes Sassetti appended to his manuscripts: the aggrandizing French formula, "À mon pouvoir" (To my power), and the consolatory Latin prayer, "Mitia fata mihi" (May fate be merciful to me).[77] These same impulses, Warburg showed, carried over into the image programs Sassetti commissioned for his tomb and family chapel in Santa Trinita, each one expressive of "the organic polarity that existed within the capacious mind of one cultivated early Renaissance man."[78]

Wind metaphors inform each of these conceptualizations of fortune, reflecting their appearance in contemporary usage, where the Latin *fortuna* meant not only "chance" and "wealth" (that is, *buona fortuna*), but also "storm wind," according to Warburg. Rucellai himself used the phrase *mirabil fortuna* in describing a destructive cyclone that struck in 1456. Fifteenth-century vernaculars expressed the same equivalences: for the Italian *la fortuna*, the German term was *Ungebyter*, an older word with the same meaning as *Ungewitter*, "tempest."[79] For Italian merchant capitalists, ever-reliant on sea transport, these metaphors came together as "attributes of a single being: Storm-Fortune, whose uncanny ability to switch from daemon of destruction to bountiful goddess fostered the atavistic imagery of her single, anthropomorphic, mythical identity."[80] When Dürer, in another extraordinary exercise in self-therapy, later recorded his dream vision from the night of 7–8 June 1525 (figure 5.15), it was the image of a great tempest overpowering the earth that struck such terror in his heart, a deluge, he wrote in the sheet's lower zone, that "drowned the whole land . . . with wind and roaring, and I was sore afraid that when I awoke my whole body trembled and for a long while I could not recover myself."[81]

Storm winds were also a choice metaphor in Stoic psychology: the tempestuous "passions" of the mind were precisely what had to be calmed in order for reason to reclaim her dominion in the soul. This principle of human distress united philosophers as different in their outlooks as Petrarch and Ficino. Throughout his Latin prose works and letters, in particular, the great collection of dialogues, *De remediis utriusque fortunae*, Petrarch reminded readers that the passions include not only fear and sorrow, our natural responses to misfortune, but also hope and joy, which are equally bound to the experience of fortune. Virtue was opposed to Fortune, but also forged in confrontation with her. Only with a proper conversion to reason could the storm of the passions be calmed, and only in this way can the swings of fortune, good and ill, be withstood. Urging the magistrate and soldier Giovanni

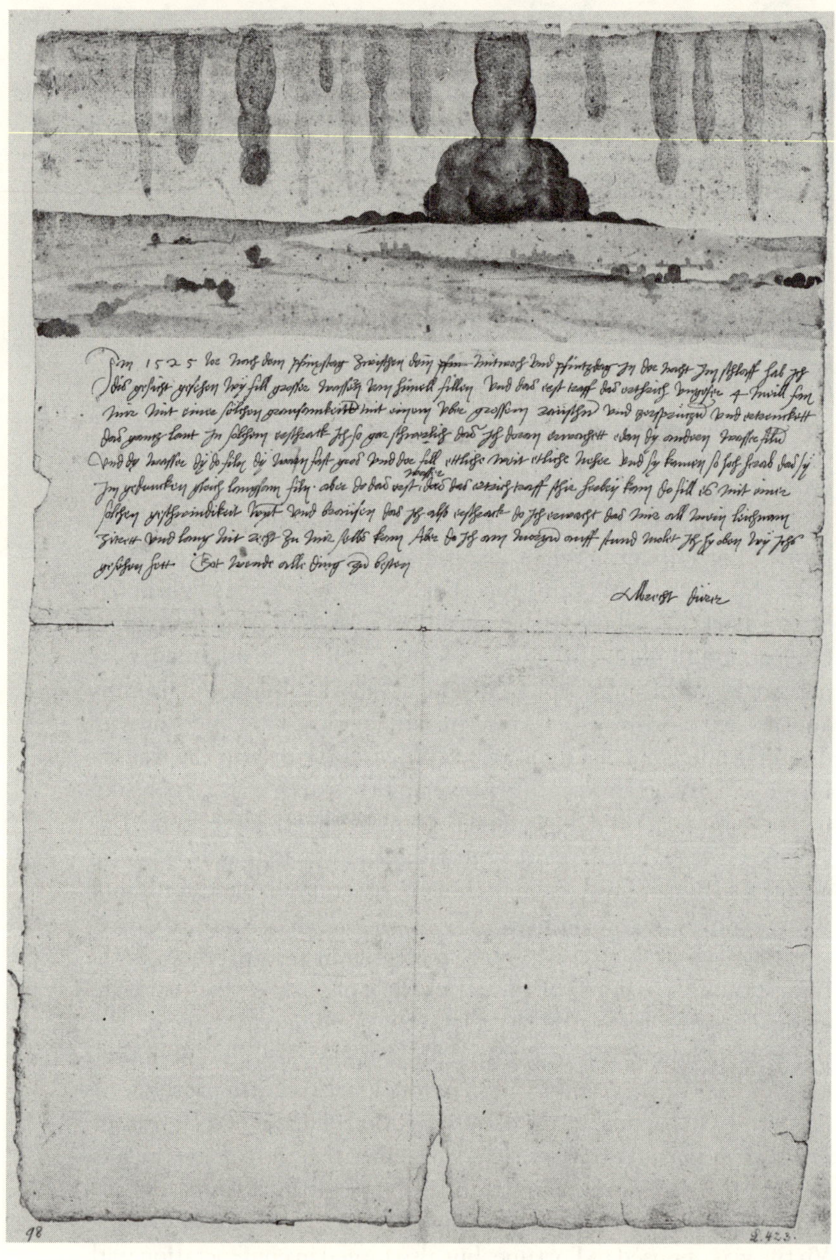

Figure 5.15. Albrecht Dürer, *Record of a Dream*, 1525, watercolor on paper, 30 x 43 cm (Vienna, Kunsthistorisches Museum).

Barrili of Capua to replace anger with peace and let reason dispel the "mists of passion" in a time of troubles, Petrarch framed the challenge in terms of a Stoic "conversion to self" (*conversio ad se*), requesting of his friend "that you subject your mind to your reason, or, to express it differently, you to yourself."[82]

In the Bremen self-portrait, Dürer appears to have struck upon an entirely novel way to visualize Fortuna's double significance for Christian ethics and for his own situation. Gathering force behind the lonely penitent tried by the world and anxious about the future, fortune comes upon the individual as a quasi-physical force, invisible and nearly demonic, putting all human endeavor in jeopardy. Yet the inward attitude of the sufferer and the weary vigilance he displays—like Christ contemplating the Passion from a place of repose outside of time—reminds us that the greater threat posed by fortune is to virtue itself. It is the project of returning to the self, of being converted to reason as a guide for the conduct of life, that the "tempest" of the passions imperils most. The picture that portrays pensiveness becomes a mirror for the beholder's own meditative stance, the state of vigilant repose he must adopt for a proper examination of self. The artist stakes out a position in a therapeutic relationship. He does so as representative man. In this role, he poses a question to the beholder-interlocutor, and to himself as well. It is the same question that Rucellai had asked his philosophical avatars in the *Zibaldone*: "Have human reason and practical intelligence any power . . . against Fortune"? The image is open enough, indeterminate enough, that we can project any one of Ficino's three options onto its protagonist: take up arms against Fortune, retreat from her, or declare a truce.

Without a straightforward answer, Dürer's picture refuses easy consolation: instead, by mobilizing reason, the mind's own healing power, the work casts Renaissance misery back upon its own inner resources. This allows it to become therapeutic in a different sense than interpretation has so far recognized. Vigilant attention to the self, the tempering of the creaturely passions by reason, the inclining of the will toward humility, the cultivation of virtue—to the Renaissance humanist, these were long-term imperatives for the conduct of life. And at the moment of reckoning, when the body's frailty and the soul's sickness reassert themselves, it is reason again that guides the embattled self in uttering its prayer: *Mitia fata mihi.*

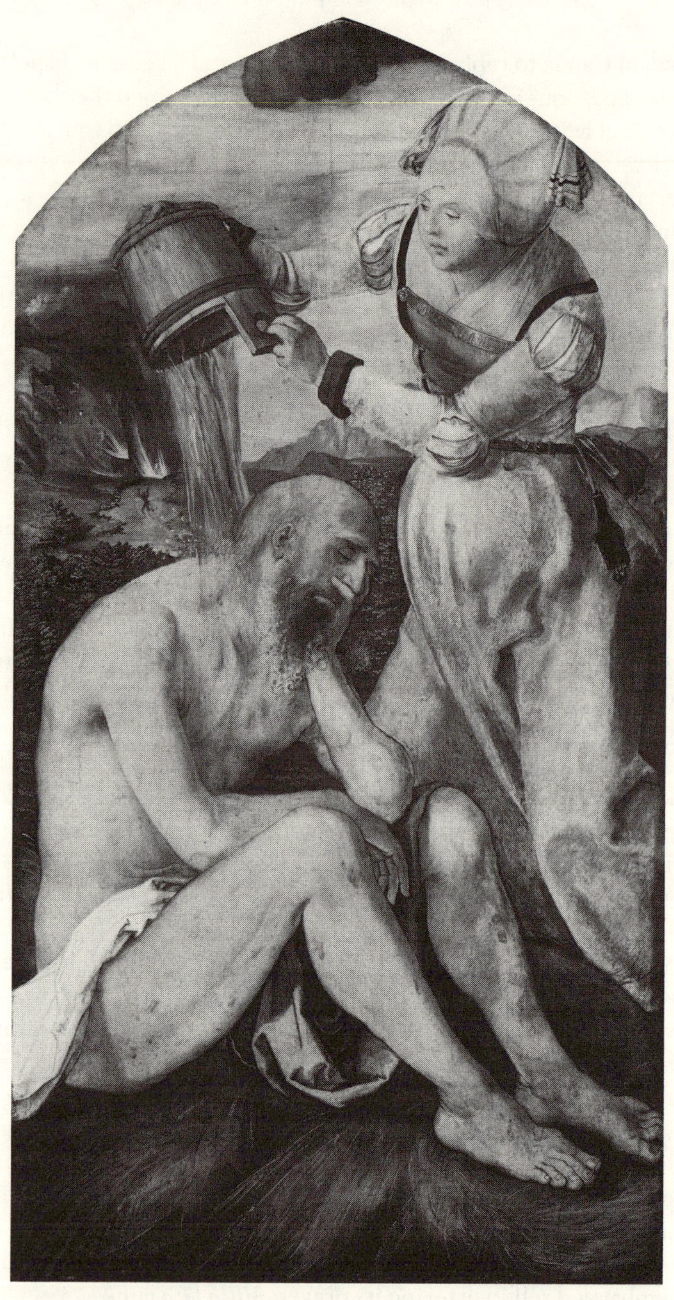

Figure 6.1. Albrecht Dürer, *Job Attended by His Wife*, left outer wing panel from the *Jabach Altarpiece*, ca. 1503-1505, mixed technique on limewood panel, 96 x 51 cm (Frankfurt am Main, Städel Museum) (photo © Städel Museum—ARTOTHEK).

CHAPTER SIX

The Artist as *Medicus*, Part Two:

Soul Service

Dürer's art is neither an art of self-expression nor an art bound to political considerations. The essence of his art is service, service not to the state but to fellow man. Dürer was his brother's keeper when he wrought his prints as much as when he wrote his treatises.
—Wolfgang Stechow

"Into The Deep Recesses of the Mind"

In the Hebrew Bible's story of Job, a simple and god-fearing man, rich in worldly blessings, is stripped of everything and, bit by bit, reduced to misery. His numerous flocks, his lands, his many sons and daughters, and finally his good health are all torn from his grasp, leaving him naked, destitute, and diseased, ulcerous "from the sole of the foot even to the top of his head" and perched on a dunghill, where he passes the time scraping the "corrupt matter" from his body (Job 2:7–8). Satan had defied God to show him a man who, once despoiled of every blessing, would persevere in his faith and reverence; in reply, God offered him his humble servant and the opportunity to put the man's faith to the test. Mocked by his wife and ridiculed by the friends—those who had first come to comfort him—Job holds fast, utters no blasphemy, and shows no pretense in questioning God's justice. Alone in his suffering and isolated in his submission to providence, he exemplifies the man who, in losing the world, gains his soul (cf. Mark 8:36). Vindicated in his perfect penance, Job is eventually redeemed, his worldly goods restored a hundredfold. As the tale ends, readers are told he "lived after these things, a hundred and forty years, and he saw his children, and his children's children, unto the fourth generation, and he died an old man, and full of days" (42:16).

In Dürer's rendition of the Job story, painted on pendant panels now divided between Frankfurt and Cologne (figures 6.1 and 6.2), Job appears as the archetypal man of sorrows, naked but for a loincloth and sitting on a pile of straw. Disconsolate and absorbed in his grief, he is attended by his wife, who douses his shoulders with water from a wooden pail, while two musicians, one of whom bears Dürer's own features (figure 6.3), pipe and drum from the opposing panel.[1] Back-story misfortunes appear in the distance: behind Job and his wife, Dürer has depicted the "fire of God from heaven" (2:16), combined with the destruction of Job's house, and in the valley behind the musicians we see the Chaldean assault on the camels and the slaying of the servants (2:17). But for these details and the instantly recogniz-able protagonist, little in Dürer's rendition derives from the bibli-cal account—not the violent gush of water, not the jaunty minstrels playing out a tune.

Dated by scholars to between 1503 to 1505, the two panels were once the folding wings of a larger ensemble still referred to as the *Jabach Altarpiece*, named for the Cologne merchant family in whose townhouse the work was displayed until around 1800. Originally, when the altarpiece was closed (*Werktagsseite*), the panels would have appeared side by side; when open, their reverse sides, which Dürer painted with two standing male saints each (Joseph and Joachim on the left, Simeon and Lazarus on the right), would have flanked the altar's central image.[2] Various proposals have been put forward for the patron's identity and the work's original location. In one recon-struction, the commission came from Dürer's patron in Wittenberg, the duke of Saxony and imperial elector Friedrich the Wise (1463–1525), who would have destined it for the high-profile castle church (*Schloßkirche*), home to family epitaphs and the duke's spectacular relic collection.[3] Alternatively, the original setting may have been Augsburg, specifically the Carmelite church where the three wealthy Fugger brothers, Georg, Ulrich, and Jacob, had laid their plans for a costly family funerary chapel, a project that brought Dürer impor-tant commissions between 1506 and 1508. This scenario would have made Georg (1453–1506), Nuremberg representative of the family firm, the altar's likely patron.[4] A third proposal places the altar in the chapel consecrated on the site of a thermal bath founded in 1505 in Annaberg (in Saxony), valued for the treatment of skin diseases and named, appropriately, "Job's Bath."

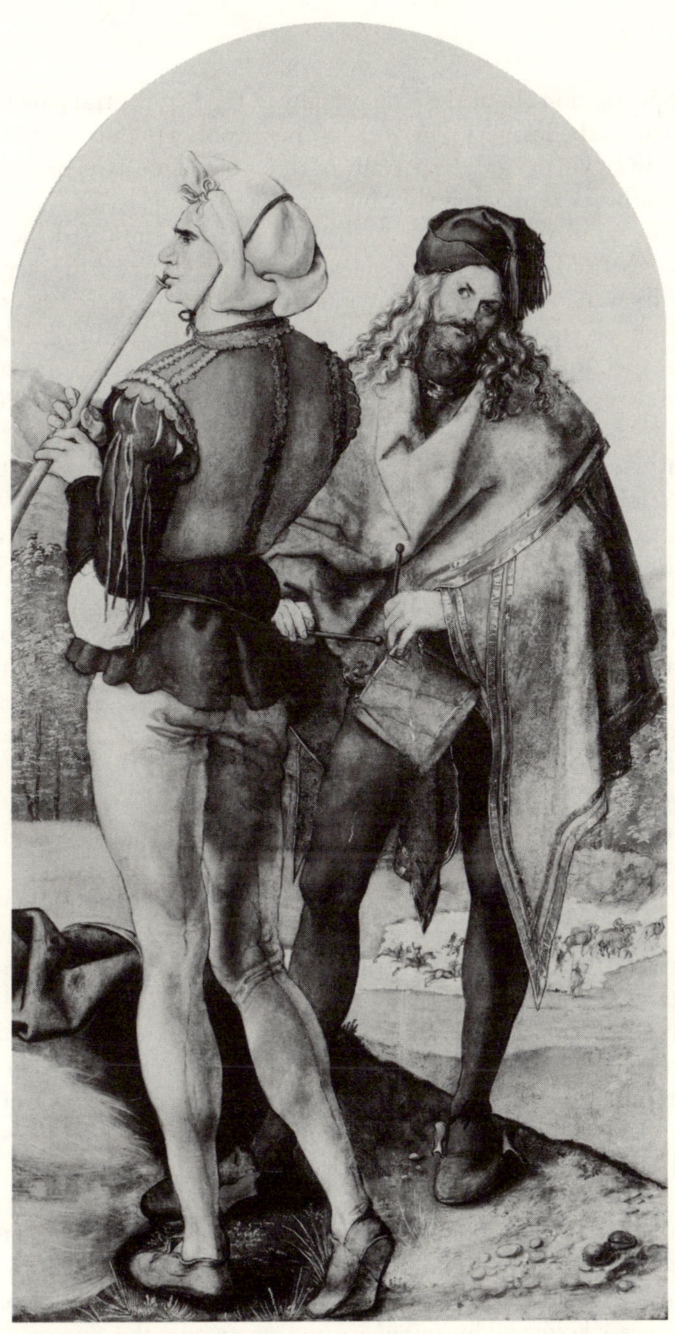

Figure 6.2. Albrecht Dürer, *Two Musicians*, right outer wing panel from the *Jabach Altarpiece*, ca. 1503–1505, mixed technique on limewood panel, 94 x 51.2 cm (Cologne, Wallraf-Richartz Museum) (photo: © Rheinisches Bildarchiv Köln).

Speculation about the iconography of the lost central panel has settled on the imagery of Mary's mother, Anne, a popular protector saint in German lands, especially in times of plague. (Germany saw one outbreak at precisely this time, between 1503 and 1506.)[5] A dedication to Saint Anne—that is, to the popular "Trinitarian" depiction of her with Mary and the baby Jesus, called *Anna Selbdritt*—argues equally well for an original location in Wittenberg, where Friedrich actively promoted Anne's cult, Augsburg, where the Fugger family chapel, formally begun in 1509, found its home in the Carmelite Church of St. Anne, and the thermal bath at Annaberg.[6] The stronger proposals—the first two—assume a mortuary context for the altar. Centuries of tradition had recast the Jewish Job into the Christian Saint Job, a type for Christ and a prophet of the Resurrection. His image decorated sarcophagi and catacomb walls in late antiquity and routinely appeared in association with the Office of the Dead in late medieval books of hours.[7] Here his image becomes the focal point for a well-heeled penitent's prayers for a future Resurrection. Both our prime candidates, Duke Friedrich in one scenario and Georg Fugger in the other, struggled with illness around this time, and Georg had even withdrawn from all business affairs in the six years before his death in 1506, probably for health reasons. In short, the *Jabach Altar* seems to be a votive altar in which both Anne and Job assume the role of protector saints, thus a work symbolically and ritually tailored for "a patron foreseeing his own death."[8]

Dürer's distinctive take on the legendary and visual traditions of the Job story—the gush-of-water motif, the presence of the musicians, and the artist's self-identification with one of these—has proved tantalizing for scholars. One guiding question has been this: Have Dürer's supporting characters come to heap further abuse on the tormented Job, or do their actions convey comfort? Hewing closely to the biblical text, Panofsky read into the picture a sharp opposition between the "friendly spirit of the strangers" and the "spitefulness of his [Job's] wife"—none of it of much consequence, however, since the grieving Job, in Panofsky's view, seems not even to notice the "well-meant efforts" of the former or the "cruel action" of the latter.[9] Fedja Anzelewsky, in a different kind of Panofskyian moment, claimed the tableau to be an allegory of the four temperaments. In this, Job plays the melancholic and his impulsive and angry wife the choleric[10]—a willful conclusion, given that Dürer endows the woman's expression

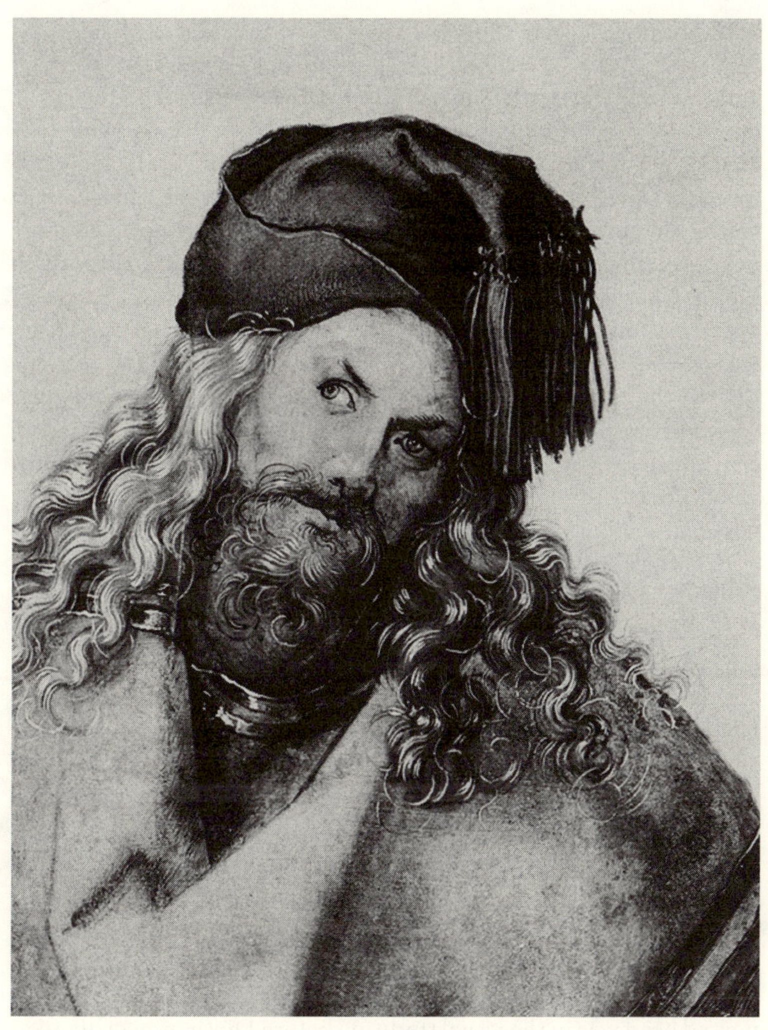

Figure 6.3. Detail from the *Jabach Altarpiece* (Cologne): Dürer as drummer. (See figure 6.2.)

with nothing more passionate than a determined focus on her task. And what of the water? Does the gush inflict greater agony on Job, scalding or infecting the sores spread over every inch of his body,[11] or does it cool and cleanse, bringing relief and healing? Observing that "a gush of water meant to bring relief to the sick has . . . all the signs of folk medicine," Joachim Jacoby has traced the positive endorsement of this, the simplest form of hydrotherapy, from the Hippocratic corpus through prescriptions found in the Arabic medical authorities such as Rhazes (Abū Bakr Muhammad ibn Zakariyyā al-Rāzī, 854–925) down to Dürer's own time and place. In the view of Dirk van Ulsen (ca. 1460–1508), the Dutch humanist physician brought to Nuremberg by the city council in 1495 to help manage the syphilis epidemic, whose poem-pamphlet on the disease was illustrated by Dürer in 1496 (see figure I.2), feverish patients should be treated with baths or with water poured over their heads—a technique especially effective, he notes, in dealing with headaches.[12]

Centuries earlier, another leading medical writer, Avicenna, prescribed a similar form of hydrotherapy specifically for the treatment of melancholia. From the point of view of humoral medicine, the dryness and danger of overheating associated with the preponderance of black bile in the gut—capable of producing a dangerous combustion, as we've seen (Chapter 4)—could be mitigated with bathing. The patient should bathe before eating or have slightly warm water poured over his head, while music or some other cheerful entertainment works to lighten the spirits.[13] Whether or not Ulsen, Dürer, or whoever might have advised the artist during the creation of the *Jabach Altar* had this or similar advice in mind, the reference to melancholia's wearied state is clear in the figure of Job, who catches his sunken head with an open hand and splayed fingers. Readers of this book will already know how pervasive the gesture of the supported head was in the visual tradition before Dürer, especially as an attribute of the seated Christ (*sessio Christi*), who patiently endures humanity's ingratitude from a thought-space abstracted from the Passion's violence.[14] Dürer's "melancholic" Man of Sorrows in Karlsruhe (see figure 4.3) and the title page of the *Small Passion* (1511) are the prime examples.[15] And that same gesture, we know, would be immortalized in the *Melencolia*.

That Job's state of dejection and sorrow approached the conditions of melancholia in its worst clinical manifestation, making him a victim of *melancholia adusta*, is one of the themes Thomas Aquinas developed in his influential commentary *Expositio super Iob ad litteram* (The literal exposition of Job), written around 1260.[16] In a particularly powerful passage resonant with the desolate imagery of Psalms, the sufferer who sought the "light" of consolation only to find the "darkness" of misery laments his wretchedness with somatic metaphors of blackened skin, burned and parched bones:

> I expected good things and evil things came to me. I waited for the light and darkness rushed in. My bones are inflamed without any rest, and days of affliction came upon me. I walked along grieving; rising up without fury. I cried out in the crowd. I was the brother to snakes and the companion of ostriches. My skin turned black on me and my bones dried out from the heat. My lyre was turned to mourning and my tongue to the voice of those who weep. (Job 30:26–31)

With the humoral pathophysiology of melancholia clearly in mind, Aquinas explains that Job

> begins [this part of his lament] with interior evils when he says, "My bones are inflamed without rest." This can refer to the weakness of the interior powers coming from too much heat, and also to the affliction of the heart proceeding from the intensity of the heat of pain. To show this kind of turmoil is too early, he says, "Days of affliction have anticipated me." For all men suffer in their old age from ill health, but he has been anticipated with afflictions in his youth. Then . . . he continues, "I was the brother of snakes," because those who should have loved me as a brother, bit me like snakes, "and the companion of ostriches," who usually forget even their own offspring (39:15). So they were so forgetful of me that they did not help me. His adversity was also partly the result of weakness of the body, and so first as to exterior infirmity he says, "My skin turned black on me," from the interior corruption of the humors. Then, as to the interior infirmities he continues, "and my bones dried out from the heat," so great an amount of inordinate heat rested on [him] that it dried up the marrow of bones.[17]

Judging from this, from the visual evidence (ambiguous as it is), and from Dürer's clear association of Job's distress with melancholy, it seems reasonable to see the gush of water as a medical treatment, alleviative, refreshing, and appropriate to the organic corruption brought on by atrabilious imbalance.[18] Yet the combined visual, textual, and dramatic tradition of depicting Job's wife as his tormentor is too expansive to ignore. Scolding her husband, shaking keys in his face, beating him with a spoon, and throwing water at him—the angry wife appears as a stock motif in woodcuts, altar predellas, miniatures, and genrelike panels from the Bosch circle and by the Master of the Legend of Saint Barbara (ca. 1485). The latter work draws narrative connections between the minstrels' concert and the wife's anger.[19] Behind all of these interpretations is the notion that Job's Christlike patience is tested by his wife, whose effort to seduce him away from wisdom allies her with Satan.

Do the same ambivalences apply to the playing of the minstrels? Despite Hans Kauffmann's judgment more than a century ago that, in Dürer's panels, "water and music alleviate physical and spiritual pain,"[20] and Panofsky's sympathetic view of the strangers, scholars have continued to attribute malice to their music. Rudolf Preimesberger, for example, presents the negative conception of drumming and piping as "delights of the godless" and Luther's exegesis of Job as twin keys to understanding the mocking intent.[21] Yet already in 1954, Kathi Meyer's research revealed a consistently benevolent role for these characters in the visual tradition from the fourteenth century onward. Job's minstrels are often shown as a professional ensemble brought expressly to cheer the suffering man; often replacing the "three friends" of the biblical story, they are frequently shown being rewarded by their patron with pieces of skin that, once plucked from his body, turn miraculously to gold. Each of these "unofficial" motifs, Meyer showed, can be traced to the apocryphal *Testamentum in Job*.[22]

The healing power of music and its unique enlivening or purgative effect on the soul are long-lived topoi in the Western philosophical and medical traditions—from Plato's *Timaeus* and Aristotle's *Politics* onward to Ficino's *De triplici vita* and many other texts—as well as in the Hebrew Bible's story of David and Saul (1 Samuel 16:23) and the imagery of Psalm 42.[23] Let us listen to Ficino's analysis of how music reacts upon the faculties. Replying to his Florentine colleague Antonio Canisiano on the question of why one should study medicine and music together, the philosopher first recalls the biblical example of David and Saul, then continues:

> Nor is this surprising; for, since song and sound arise from the cogitation of the mind, the impetus of the phantasy, and the feeling of the heart, and, together with the air they have broken up and tempered, strike the aerial spirit

of the hearer, which is the junction of the soul and body, they easily move the phantasy, affect the heart and penetrate into the deep recesses of the mind.[24]

Needless to say, the jaunty minstrels of the *Jabach Altar* are not agents of Ficino's divine "astrological music," striving for harmonic consonance with the heavenly spheres and mobilizing planetary spirits through imitative vibrations. For Ficino, the special power of music to move the soul arose both from this inherent, imitative movement and from a kind of consubstantiality between music's natural medium, air, and the *spiritus* of listeners.[25] This made it especially effective in easing distresses of the mind and soul. The melancholic Ficino looked specifically to stringed instruments and voice to achieve this vibratory consonance with *spiritus*, and evidently accompanied his own therapeutic singing with a so-called *lyra orphica*, a recreation of sorts of Orpheus's lyre.[26] Dürer's gay entertainers, by contrast, arrive at the dung heap with something cheerfully profane, uplifting, and amusing—just right for banishing melancholy's gloom.

Something like this mixture of sacred and profane music is exactly what Dürer himself prescribed for the relief of work-related depression—the one and only time, as we remarked in the Introduction, that he invoked the term "melancholy" (*Melecoley*) in his writings. It was in his manual for the education of young artists, *Ein Speis der Malerknaben*, begun around 1512–13, that the master noted the remedy for those occasions when the apprentice "exerted himself too much" and risked falling "under the hand of melancholy." Learning to play stringed instruments not only provided a practical diversion, but fostered a therapeutic rebalancing of the humors, which Dürer terms a "pleasuring of his blood" (*ergetzlikeit seins geplütz*).[27] A similar approach to banishing gloom was prescribed for Dürer's famed Netherlandish predecessor, Hugo van der Goes (c. 1430/40–1482), when the monks of the Rood Klooster, the monastery outside Brussels where he resided as a lay brother, were convened to play music to soothe his mania.[28]

I have opened with the *Jabach Altarpiece* for what it reveals about Dürer's agency in a different kind of therapeutic situation than the one we examined in the previous chapter—not the healing and consolation of the self, but a consoling address to fellow Christians. This mode allowed the artist to take up the "Petrarchan" office of the *medicus animorum*, the healer of souls, with the techniques specific to his discipline, making his painting practice a form of soul service. To see this dynamic at work in the altarpiece itself, contrast it with the conventional way Job's saintly suffering would function for the beholder of a conventional votive altar. As a protector saint (*Schutzpatron*), Job's sacrificial merit would have guaranteed that any devotion directed toward him be repaid in the form of security and refuge—refuge from plague, from syphilis, from the fear of sudden death, and so on.[29] Visible in the central shrine with the altar open, the altar's patron saint would typically have fulfilled this role. Dürer's frozen mystery play on the altar's *exterior*, however, demands and offers something more. From the tableau's brittle emotional center, the suffering servant appears to the beholder as an object of pity, a Christlike tragic hero enduring an undeserved fate with equal measures of stoic reserve and disbelieving sorrow. Already this psychological complexity tells us that Dürer's interpretation is no traditional episode from a saint's *vita*. Contriving to make Job the model for a novel form of identification, Dürer anticipates the magnetic intensity of Dame Melancholy's meditation in the great engraving of 1514 (see Chapter 4).

Contrasting forms of therapeutic attention and the tension their opposition imposes on the beholder become the real drivers of identification in the *Jabach Altar*. Centering our attention, Job appears in the crossfire of two distinct and possibly opposed efforts to "effect" or "persuade" or "move" him from one state of being to another—the player's efforts to soothe him, to move him from distress to relief, and his wife's taunting efforts to get him to renounce God, "to curse God and die" (2:9), a different kind of release from suffering. In showing Job's subjection to these countervailing forces, Dürer is able to thematize all the more intensively the seated thinker's silent, meditative stance. Marguerite Brown was quite correct in 1941 when she wrote that the three figures around him "express the conflict in Job's mind,"[30] but this is too spare a conclusion. To "attend" sympathetically to Job's torment, to enter the inner struggle of the hero poised on the razor's edge of a dangerous imbalance—psychological, spiritual, and physical—means, in this context, allowing the suffering man's silent cognition to mirror our own, and vice versa. Taking up a position in the therapeutic encounter, face to face, as it were, with the suffering Job, the beholder, like the physician or the philosopher, gauges the patient's pain and judges his disposition toward health. Dürer's tableau compels the beholder toward a reflexive compassion that is at once spiritual, ethical, and medicinal. Finally, by depicting himself in the role of the "Trommler," Dürer offers himself as a special kind of delegate figure within the composition: calling the beholder's attention back to itself, prompting us toward self-examination as we reflect on what we see.[31]

With this conceit, the painter stakes out a privileged position within a network of attention and care—a position, I wish to emphasize again, that is uniquely empowered by his representational craft. Self-positioned in the scene, Dürer stands "behind" the work professionally and artistically: he is the guarantor of its daring conception and persuasive power. He also stands "within" the work ethically, posing the challenge of Job's situation as a philosophical question to viewers. Painter, musician, physician, philosopher—by fusing these roles, notional and real, Dürer clears an extraordinary new space within the religious image for a nascent claim, namely, that the pious Christian artist might assume the office of the rhetorical healer.

Before proceeding, we need to develop both parts of this claim: first, that the artist can thematize and realize a form of soul service akin to rhetorical healing, and second, that he can do so specifically as a Christian painter. (Later Catholic writers, asserting a necessary link between the painter's piety and his capacity for depicting divinity, extolled the character of the *pictor christianus*.)[32] This, in turn, demands that we revisit the connections between the ethical, sacramental, and spiritual care for others that Christian theology long identified with the virtue of *caritas*, charity.

The historical sweep of Christian *caritas*, its theory and its practice, can, for obvious reasons, only be touched upon here.[33] Envisioned as an imperfect, earthly reflection of God's perfect, infinite love, *caritas* unfolded across an ever-expanding network of reciprocal support, mutual assistance, and care that made all believers part of an expanded human family. Paul's first letter to the Corinthians, which established the "theological virtues" (faith, hope, and charity) for the church, declares charity to be the greatest (13:13) of the three. Augustine of Hippo, whose thought stamped all subsequent discussions of Christian love down to Dürer's time, described the dynamic intersection of a "vertical" love between God and people and a "horizontal" love connecting neighbors, family members, and friends.[34] That Augustine developed these ideas in the context of his great treatise on the Trinity should not escape our attention. Dürer's own treatment of the theme, which we will pick up later in this chapter, is deeply informed by it. When we get there, we will catch another glimpse of the Nuremberg master in his role as a healer, in this case, a universal healer, placing the medicine of his art at the disposal of the whole "community of love" (*consortium amoris*), as the Benedictine Richard of St. Victor called the Trinity and its earthly counterparts.[35]

Between these two poles, between the soul service Dürer offered the patron of the *Jabach Altar* and the universal medicine he distributed farther afield—and, through his prints, farther still—Dürer's practice as a Christian painter-physician found fertile soil in the context of another key horizontal relationship, a relationship that, in the age of humanism, Renaissance, and Reformation, was undergoing rapid reformulation: the love between friends.

"Not Only Writing Will I Do!"

Dürer's male friendships brimmed with jocular humor, insults, and witty displays of one-upsmanship. And yet the surviving correspondences with Willibald Pirckheimer, like his relationships with other leading figures on the Nuremberg scene, men such as Lazarus Spengler, also betray a touching desire on Dürer's part to be taken seriously as an intellectual fellow traveler in addition to the famous artist they acknowledged him to be. It was in the context of these relationships that Dürer tried his hand at poetry and, half-ironically, advanced the case for his right to do so. The contest for proper recognition began, according to Dürer's own account, when Pirckheimer rebuked him on technical grounds for the pious ode to divine wisdom he penned in 1509 ("he laughed at me and said that no rhyme ought to have more than eight syllables").[36] Following this, Dürer, evidently with complete seriousness, appealed to Spengler for mentoring—but the jest, it seems, was already in full swing. Pirckheimer's poem satirizing Dürer's pretensions as a poet made its way back to him via Spengler, who had in the meantime composed his own *Spottgedicht*, a satirical poem lampooning the painter's hubris.[37] This prompted the following riposte from "the hairy, bearded painter" (Dürer's beard had already become the butt of wisecracks among Germany's humanist elite). Addressing Spengler, the poet grouses:

> But as he likes my verses not,
> He makes a laughing stock of me,
> And says I'm like the Cobbler, he
> Who criticized Apelles' art.
> With this he tries to make me smart,
> Because he thinks it is for me
> To paint, and not write poetry.
> But I have undertaken this
> (And will not stop for him or his),
> To learn whatever thing I can,
> For which will blame me no wise man.

To devote the mind to only a single art, the poem goes on to declare, needlessly constrains the creative individual, rendering him no better than a notary who knows only "to write one form and one alone" (a thinly veiled jab at Spengler's bureaucratic "art"). Vowing never to let the same fate befall him, Dürer embraces the vision of the *uomo universale*—likely gleaned from his readings of Vitruvius—when he writes, "Something of all things I will know."[38]

It is at this point in the same poem that the painter, flaunting the prerogative gained from the equality of painting and poetry (see the Prologue to Chapters 5 and 6), enlarges his vocation still further. Binding his office and art to that of the physician, Dürer now boasts of real-world therapeutic know-how:

> Not only writing will I do,
> But learn to practice physic too;
> Till men surprised will say, 'Beshrew me,
> What good this painter's medicines do me!'
> Therefore hear and I will tell
> Some wise receipts to keep you well.
> A little drop of Alkali,
> Is good to put into the eye;
> He who finds it hard to hear,
> Should mandel-oil put in his ear;
> And he who would from gout be free,
> Not wine but water drink should he;
> He who would live to be a hundred,
> Will see my counsel has not blundered.[39]

It is significant that, within the context of the poem, though it may be "mocked and jeered" by real men of letters, the painter-poet's self-declared right to rhyme is vindicated by the efficacy of his specialized "medicines," which, Dürer surely knew, were more powerful than anything his amateurish verses could accomplish. An elision of healing figures and substances occurs in that transitional image, "this painter's medicines" (*die Arznei'n des Malers*), and this elision effects a shift, however clumsy, in the poem's imagery. Each item in the little catalogue of remedies is now cast as metaphor: the alkali that keeps the eyes healthy are the painter's means for stimulating vision and "clarifying" sight. The mandel oil for improved hearing is suggestive of an higher predisposition toward wisdom, an opening to the Word that is ethical philosophy's proper task. Even the prescription to avoid wine in favor of water sounds like an art-theoretical trope: wine, the ancient symbol of licentiousness, gateway to unbridled passions, was long associated with the wrong kinds of inducements made by mimetic art's mainstay, illusion. (The recommended austerity is also a personal jab at the self-indulgent Pirckheimer, who suffered from gout.)

Claims about painting's persuasive powers have, in other words, suddenly jumped discursive tracks: rather than being conveyed exclusively by the *paragone* with poetry, it is now the medical analogy—more specifically, the Ciceronian and Petrarchan view of rhetorical healing as medicine for the soul—that drives the poem's language. A serious claim bubbles up through the posturing and jest. Shut out from the innermost circle of "divine" poetry by his best friends, Dürer stakes his own, distinctive claim to be a kind of amateur *medicus*, a physician of the soul, with his own tried-and-true remedies: nonverbal potions and plasters for clearing the channels of perception, stimulating health, affecting the mind, and moving souls where they need to go.

Revealingly, Dürer's self-assertion in this private context would not be the last time his name was invoked to strengthen the parallel of painting and medicine. To convey the exceptional rank achieved by the radical physician-philosopher-astrologer-alchemist Theophrastus Paracelsus (1493–1541), commemorative engravings dedicated to him drew the comparison to Dürer with verses such these:

> As is Dürer in painting
> So too is this one [Paracelsus] in the healing arts,

> No one before or since has come close to matching his powers.
> Must he have gotten them from the devil?
> Certainly not. Heavens no, heavens, no![40]

Of course, neither Dürer's playful poetry nor the broadsheets for Paracelsus offer more than a limited kind of evidence for the equality of visual and healing arts. Set within the larger constellation of therapeutic concerns surveyed in this and the previous chapter, however, they shine bright as reference points for understanding Dürer's self-conception as an artist with the power to heal.

Renaissance Friends

What did the men who assembled on the Winklerstrasse for conversation and collaboration mean to one another? What benefits flowed from those relationships into Dürer's art, and what did Dürer's art offer in turn to sustain them? With little hope of reconstructing the actual discussions that took place among the humanist vanguard of the *Poetenschule*, we have the choice of taking the narrow, instrumental view of the benefits it brought Dürer or a broader one. The immediate benefits have been in plain view for a long time. Scholars often remark that Dürer's engagements with mythological themes and classical allegories are neatly concentrated in the years between 1494 and 1505, that is, between the time of his first pen-and-ink tracings of Andrea Mantegna's engravings, the *Battle of the Sea Gods* and the *Bacchanle with Silenus* (an encounter that coincided closely with the opening of his Nuremberg workshop in the spring or summer 1495) and his departure for Venice in late summer 1505. Surely Celtis and Pirckheimer were never short on suggestions for antique myths and medieval legends that would be amenable to reinterpretation by the "German Apelles," and so would have provided their admired friend mentoring as well as the translation help that Dürer, who lacked Latin, needed.

Typical of the erudite, allusive, and eclectic mode of treating classical myths in these years is the *Death of Orpheus* (figure 6.4).[41] Its theme was almost certainly chosen by Pirckheimer, perhaps also the picture's ironic reference to the martyred hero's defiant turn to same-sex desire. A banderole winding through the tree tufts above the violence reads: *Orfeus der erst puseran* (Orpheus, the first lover of boys). Also from this period is the so-called *Sea Monster* of ca. 1497–98,

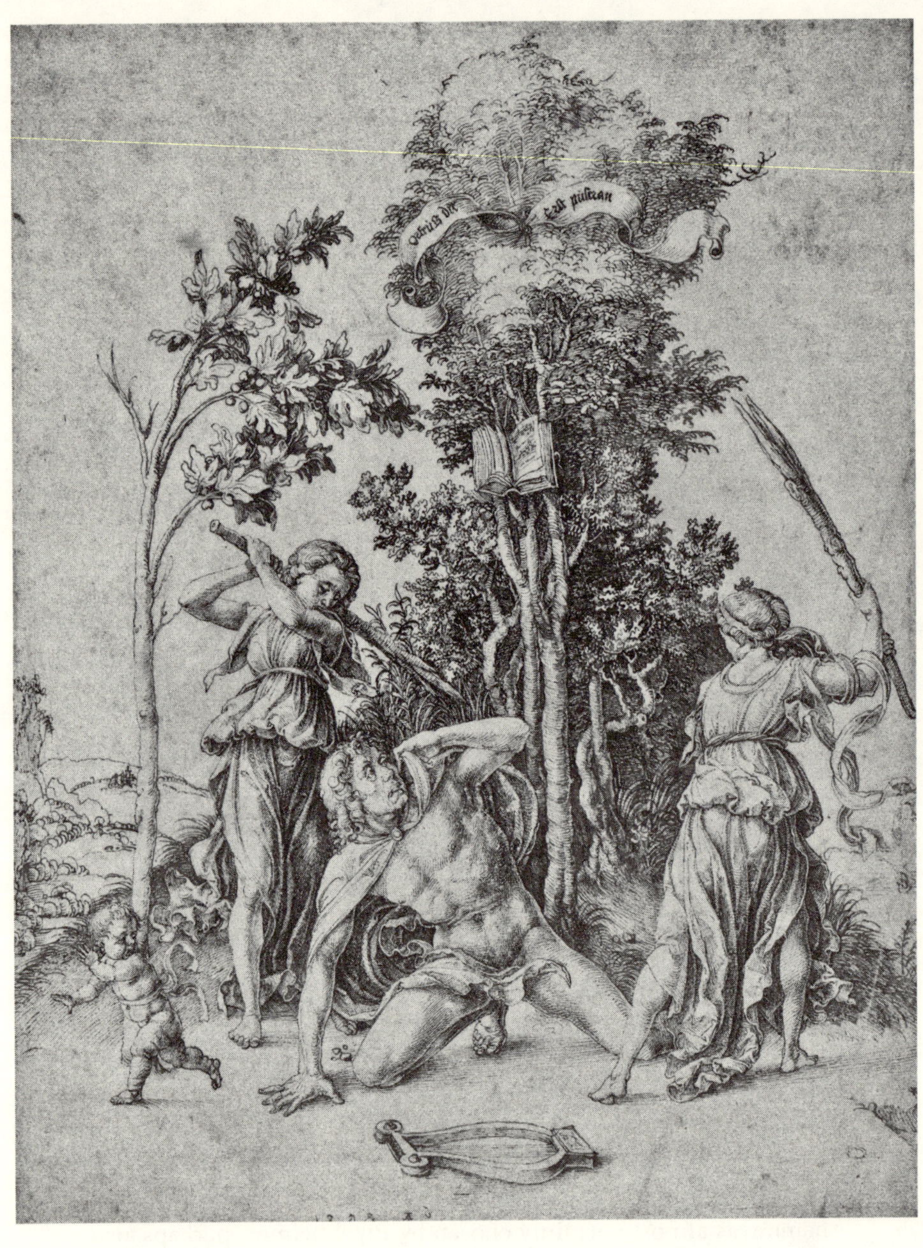

Figure 6.4. Albrecht Dürer, *Death of Orpheus*, 1494, pen-and-ink drawing, 28.9 x 22.5 cm (Hamburg, Kunsthalle) (photo: bpk Bildagentur / Christoph Irrgang / Art Resource, NY).

whose source lies either in Athenaeus's tale of Syme's abduction by the sea god Glaucus, as recounted in the *Deipnosophistae* (Banquet of the learned), or, as more recently suggested, in Kaspar von der Rhön's fifteenth-century telling of the Langobard Queen Theudelinde's rape by a sea monster in the *Dresdner Heldenbuch*.[42] That nearly all of the printed works arising from Dürer's collaborations during these years are engravings—the exception here is the woodcut "Ercules" (see figure E.2)—suggests a concerted effort to cultivate a dedicated audience of scholars, adepts, and collectors within Nuremberg and beyond.

For all we might say about the sources and research behind them, each of these projects share a programmatic link with the humanists' research agenda and its implicit patriotic mission: to redeem German culture from its negative associations with barbarism—a trope of Italian cultural chauvinism since Petrarch and a sore spot for German intellectuals. This makes the works we have cited compelling documents of an intellectual partnership within a specific context. By 1509, however, that context would already be unraveling. There would be no more occasional visits to Nuremberg from Konrad Celtis, who died in February 1508, apparently of syphilis, one of several factors that doomed the *Poetenschule*. Whatever intellectual associations the school fostered would henceforth be carried on in other settings, for example, the evenings Pirckheimer sponsored at his large house on the Herrenmarkt (now the Hauptmarkt), praised by Celtis in his *Norimberga* as a choice gathering place for scholars and artists.[43] That Dürer's forays into poetry took place while the Nuremberg *Poetenschule* was in decline is in one sense not surprising. One detects behind those efforts a desire to maintain the bonds this experimental academy had forged, and once sustained, for the ambitious artist. At any rate, Dürer had already begun refocusing his print production to concentrate almost exclusively on religious themes—at least since early 1507, following his return from Italy.[44] This makes his deep commitment to the *Meisterstiche* in 1513 and 1514, and to the *Melencolia* in particular, with its dense layering of scientific, humanist, and literary motifs, all the more remarkable.

Understanding the complex relationships fostered within these humanist sodalities means more, of course, than simply taking stock of the texts the men read together, the models of poetic composition they examined, or the myths and legends they discussed. It also means accounting for the social and spiritual bonds these activities engendered. Along with classical thought itself, Renaissance men of letters actively revived the ancient cult of *friendship*. They did so within the framework of an eudaimonistic ethics that insisted on the irreducible goodness of friendship, its status as a natural activity of social and political man, its value within a life ordered by reason, and its necessity for human health and flourishing. These principles were rooted in Aristotle's close examination of friendship in the *Nicomachean Ethics*, a theory that overturned Plato's insistence (articulated mainly in the *Lysis*, but also in the *Symposium*) that even when friendship appears most reciprocal, it remains rooted in human neediness and is ultimately directed toward our own good, not the good of the other. For Aristotle, by contrast, the inherent selfishness found in friendship does not determine the relationship's whole complex nature. In fact, a paradox attends the experience of true friendship. Lorraine Pangle summarizes this view: "In seeking and choosing friends, we seek the good for ourselves, and apparently only love another if and so long as he seems good for us; yet we are persuaded that we are not real friends unless we wish one another good apart from what is good for ourselves."[45]

This mutual recognition of goodness in the other, coupled with a mutual wish for the good of the other, sets the stage—emotionally, aesthetically, spiritually—for the experiences peculiar to friendship. Shared activities become steeped in a particular kind of shared awareness. Amidst their common pursuit, we might say, friends conjoin their powers of attention in a way that sharpens perception and deepens the love of things both sensible and intelligible. "Friendship is important for Aristotle for much the same reason that virtue and philosophy are," Pangle writes. "Each in a different way is a perfection of man's potential as a rational being."[46]

Above all it was Cicero—both his Stoic arguments for the value of friendship as a good chosen for its own sake, prominent in the dialogue *Laelius de amicitia* (Laelius on Friendship), and the example of his letters—that Northern humanists looked to when cultivating their own friendships. Erasmus and Thomas More, for example, carried on an epistolary friendship that was self-consciously Ciceronian in spirit, and it was the Prince of Humanists who, in a note placed inside his own edition of the *Laelius*, exclaimed, "How much holier this man is, than certain theologians who teach the rule of charity!"[47] Ancient

Stoicism had developed a theory that resolved the apparent contradiction between the image of the passionless sage who has, in Seneca's words, "retired into himself, and is with himself" (*Epistles* 9.16) and the reciprocal sympathy demanded by genuine friendship. Paradoxical as it may sound, only the sage who, in the spirit of austerity, has removed himself from emotional attachments can be a true friend. For only a fully realized moral agent—one who "grasps the intrinsic value of what is fully in accordance with nature, namely, the moral virtues"—can recognize the virtue of friendship for its own sake and cultivate it on that basis alone.[48] Stoics make the best friends, the reasoning goes, because they are susceptible neither to flattery nor to the disruptive passions that can make friends unreliable. Nor is Stoic self-sufficiency endangered by the mutual reliance that conventional forms of friendship assume. Drawing upon Aristotle's description of the friend as an other self, Cicero claimed to hold the friend's moral virtue and reason as dearly as his own.[49] Genuine friendship for Cicero, then, would always be fully grounded in philosophy and be carried on as a practical, therapeutic art—an "art of healing for the soul."[50]

Christianized over the course of centuries by avid readers of Cicero such as Jerome, Augustine, and Isidore of Seville, this stoical form of soul service survived by coexisting with the clerical *cura animarum* and the sacramental therapies offered by the church. Imbued with the theological virtue of *caritas*, this ethic of mutual assistance evolved into a kind of "verbal and rhetorical ministry of consolation" undertaken between equals.[51] Pirckheimer, whose voluminous letters include correspondence with Erasmus and More, expressed the ideal in its modern Christian form in the dedication of his first published translation of Plutarch, which itself took the form of a long letter to his learned sister Caritas (1467–1532), then abbess of the Convent of St. Klara in Nuremberg:

> Therefore the Stoics assert that it is a gift of God that we live, but of philosophy that we live well. Nor is it astonishing since nothing greater or more excellent has been given by God to men.... [I speak] of that philosophy which (as Cicero says) heals the mind, removes useless cares, frees from desires, drives out all fears. Instructed and armed with this philosophy, most worthy sister, we bravely bear all misfortunes, sorrows, calamities and labors.[52]

Pirckheimer's was a religious philosophy, grounded in philological scholarship, indebted to the church fathers, and concerned primarily with the conduct of life; as a collaborative and accumulative endeavor, it demanded of the individual a labor of self-reform, but one that was always situated within a network of mutual aid and care.

Dürer and Pirckheimer

At first glance, Dürer's friendship with Pirckheimer, as reflected in what survives of their correspondence, looks less like a treasury of moral virtue than a race to the bottom of locker-room vulgarity. "You stink so much of whores that it seems to me I can smell it from here!" Dürer wrote to his friend from Venice, on 8 September 1506, recalling Pirckheimer's student days. "When you go courting, they tell me here, you pretend to be no more than 25 years old. Ocha! Double that and I'll believe it. God's body! there are so many Italians here who look exactly like you; I don't know how that happens!"[53] Smutty insults such as these are interspersed throughout the ten letters Dürer sent to Pirckheimer from Italy, otherwise invaluable documents that rank as "the first truly personal letters written by an artist to a friend."[54] Other topics naturally took priority over such banter while Dürer was in Venice: the commission to paint an altarpiece for the Fondaco dei Tedeschi, for instance; Dürer's observations about the city; his complaints about Italian artists and their treatment of him; and so on. And since the trip had been made possible by a loan from Pirckheimer, there was more than usual pressure on Dürer to gratify his friend's collecting mania. Updates on the purchase of jewels on Pirckheimer's behalf, for example, were expected aspects of these communiqués. (Also on the shopping list were books and paper, two large carpets, crane feathers for Pirckheimer's hat, and Venetian glass.)[55] But the verbal pranks, boasting, and crass adolescent humor in the correspondence—especially on the topic of one another's wives—is striking. Another letter from Venice, this one from mid-October 1506 and notorious among Dürer biographers, offered the following riposte to Pirckheimer's apparent promise to "clyster" (that is, sodomize) Dürer's wife, Agnes, if he didn't return home to Nuremberg soon: "It's off limits to you," Dürer warns his heavy-set friend, "you would screw her to death."[56]

No doubt the thought had crossed the self-indulgent patrician-scholar's mind. Few of Dürer's biographers have entertained doubts that Agnes Dürer loathed Pirckheimer deeply or that the humanist playboy, a widower since 1504, "cordially reciprocated,"[57] although the constructed contrast between Agnes as the shrewish, mean-spirited wife who dragged Albrecht down at every turn and Willibald as the visionary who single-handedly "elevated Dürer out of his Gothic captivity and made him into a modern Renaissance artist" has been crudely overdrawn in the literature.[58] It is true, as Colin Eisler has stated, that "Dürer's precocious role as the most conspicuously 'Renaissance' of Germany's artists would be unthinkable without a relationship of extraordinary intimacy with that country's leading humanist."[59] But it's also true that this elevated stature, as well as the friendship that fostered it, put the artist at odds with more traditional duties and roles. Futile as it may be to try to disentangle Pirckheimer's genuine love and sympathy for his friend from his misogynist judgment of Agnes, or the bitter feelings engendered by his gout, it is safe to say that an abiding wish for the good of the other was a constant feature of this Renaissance friendship. "With Dürer I have truly lost the best friend I had on earth," Pirckheimer confesses in a letter written two years after the painter's death and sent to the imperial architect, Johann Tschcrttc, who had known Dürer personally and professionally, "and I regret nothing more than that he died such a hard death. For God's sake, I can blame no one other than his wife, who made his heart heavy and tormented him, to the extent that he took leave of this life all the more quickly. He was dried up like a bundle of straw."[60]

Pirckheimer's conflicted state after his friend's death, as much as the banter found in the letters from Venice while Dürer was still vital and strong, betray glimmers of a homoerotic as well as a homosocial bond. Although no piece of Pirckheimer's side of the correspondence has survived, and we have to imagine the tenor of his letters and reconstruct what we can of their content from Dürer's references, there is plenty else in Pirckheimer's portfolio as "the lustiest of bisexuals" to suggest it.[61] We have already mentioned the inscription that Dürer, no doubt acting under his mentor's advice, added to the *Death of Orpheus* drawing, referring to the tragic hero's love of boys. Equally recondite, but cruder in its humor—and certainly more personal—is the Greek inscription Pirckheimer himself added to the silverpoint portrait Dürer made of him in 1503: *Arsenous te psole es ton prokton*, roughly meaning "with the erect penis in the anus of the man" (figure 6.5).[62] Earlier scholars struggled to find a classical citation to help them better stomach the prank, or at least to

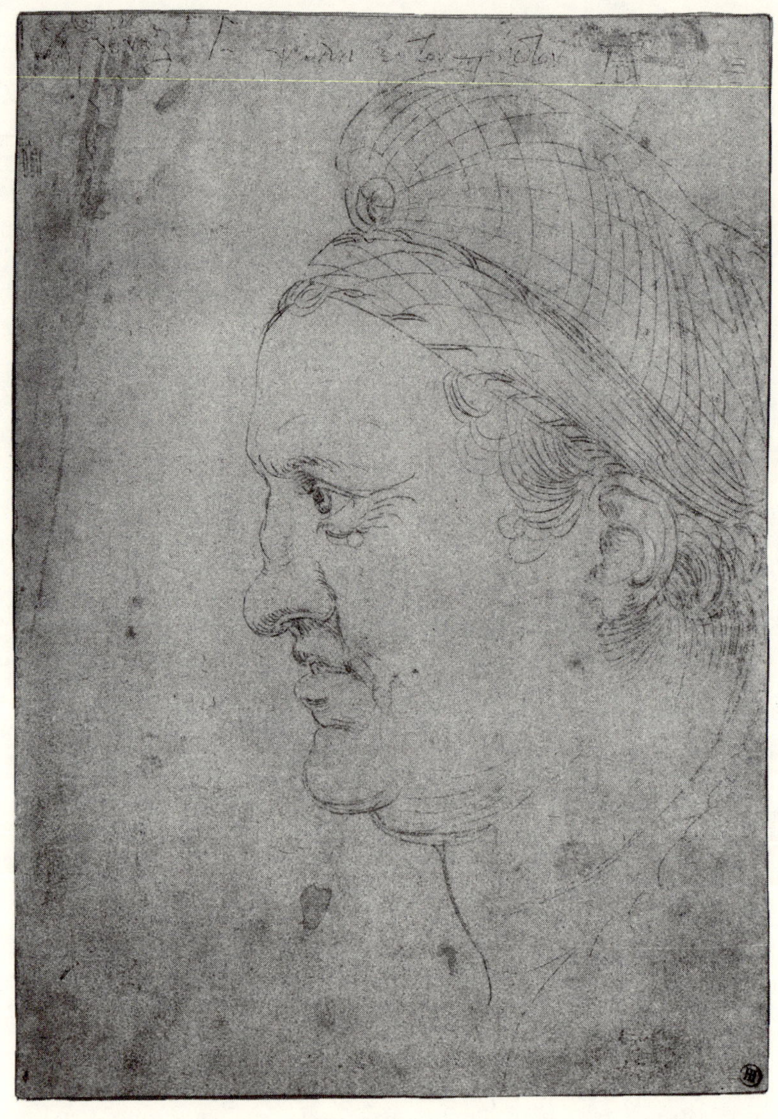

Figure 6.5. Albrecht Dürer, *Portrait of Willibald Pirckheimer*, ca. 1503, silverpoint drawing, 21.5 x 15 cm (Berlin, Staatliche Museen, Kupferstichkabinett) (photo: bpk Bildagentur / Jörg P. Anders / Art Resource, NY).

clear Dürer from any suspicion of being, one way or another, on its receiving end. Dürer may well have been bisexual, as Eisler believes and as others have confessed in more hushed tones,[63] but most indications are that the "intimate space of friendship that Dürer and Pirckheimer had created for themselves" was platonic.[64] For most commentators, the impulse to satisfy one another's egos was more important to the men than anything their bodies could offer. "Pirckheimer believed in the existence of genius," Jane Hutchison observes, "and had recognized it in Dürer early on, and more importantly, had enabled Dürer to recognize it in himself. The two friends, therefore, were mutually delighted in one another's steadily increasing fame, viewing it as the just reward for extraordinary achievement."[65] That sense of mutual support in intellectual achievement and personal mythmaking comes across in the larger, and more dignified, portrait likeness Dürer produced in charcoal in 1503 (figure 6.6), possibly as a design for a commemorative medal.[66] Culminating Dürer's project of portraying his friend and contemplating the qualities of his mind is an engraving dated 1524 and inscribed "We live by the spirit, the rest belongs to death."[67] Brilliantly enlivened by crisp light reflections on the eyes, the commemorative likeness conveys a spiritual pathos that breaks through the outer trappings of a self-satisfied, fifty-three-year-old patrician scholar. Curiously, we have no evidence that Dürer ever *painted* Pirckheimer's portrait.[68]

Witty displays of erudition were never incompatible with emotionally genuine expressions of care in Renaissance friendships, even in mournful times. The beautiful and tender portrayal of Crescentia Pirckheimer's death-bed scene, which Dürer made in watercolor on parchment for his widowed friend, shows how these impulses mingled. Lost in its original form after being sold by Pirckheimer's heirs in the seventeenth century, the composition survives in four fairly exact copies (figure 6.7).[69] Crescentia had died on 17 May 1504, immediately after giving birth to the couple's sixteenth child, and Dürer portrays her recumbent in bed, holding a death candle and a crucifix, surrounded by a circle of mourners kneeling in prayer. Befitting the sorrow of a humanist and proving Pirckheimer's involvement in the design, the picture features an epitaphlike inscription that extols the incomparability of the deceased wife and the boundless affliction of her husband.[70] Together, text and image draw inspiration from Pliny the Elder's description of a famous painting by Timanthes of Cythnus

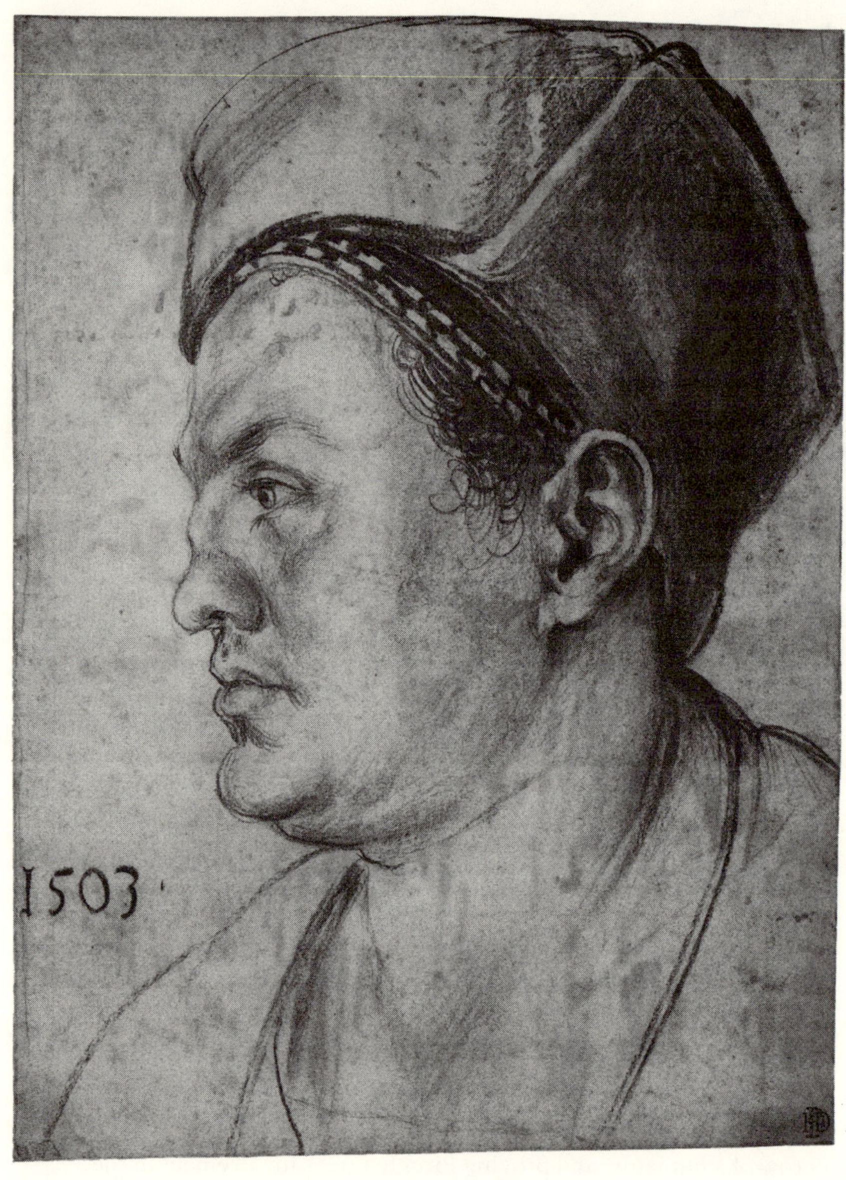

Figure 6.6. Albrecht Dürer, *Portrait of Willibald Pirckheimer*, dated 1503, charcoal, 28.1 x 20.8 cm (Berlin, Staatliche Museen, Kupferstichkabinett) (photo: bpk Bildagentur / Jörg P. Anders / Art Resource, NY).

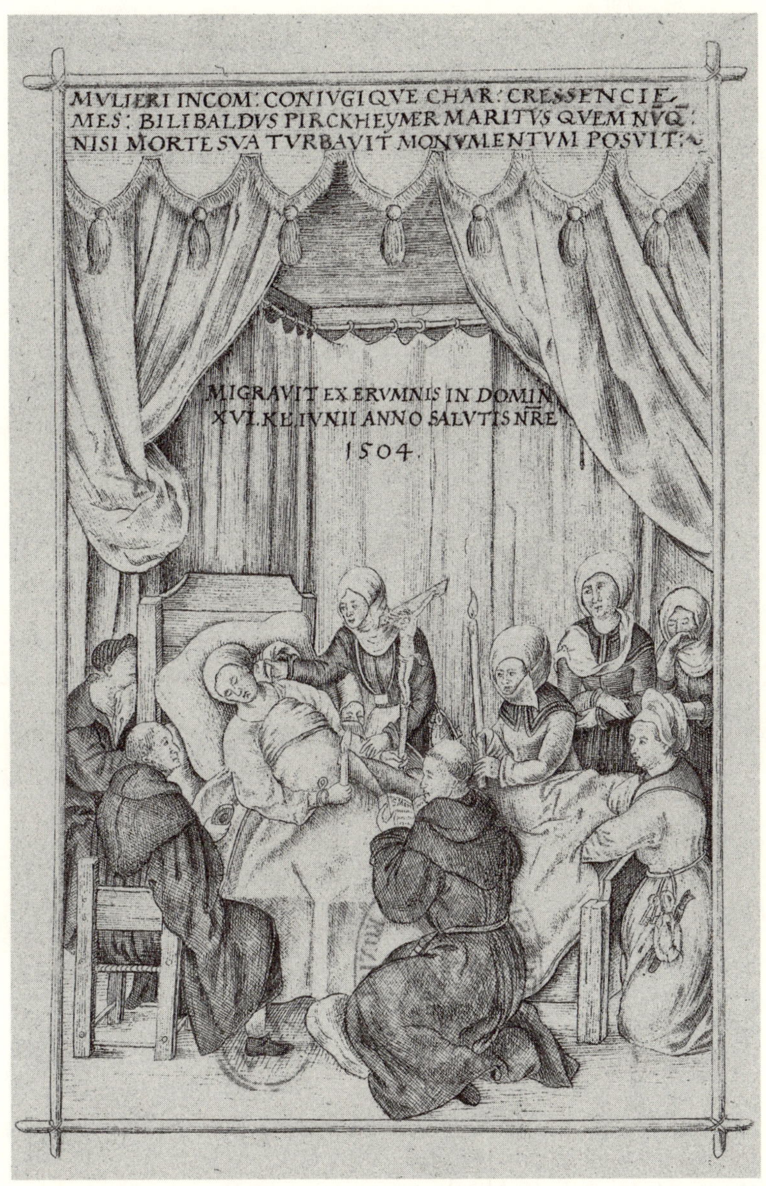

Figure 6.7. Albrecht Dürer (after), *Deathbed Scene of Crescentia Pirckheimer*, original date 1504, pen and brown ink on parchment, 20.3 x 13.9 cm (Berlin, Staatliche Museen, Kupferstichkabinett) (photo: bpk Bildagentur/Jörg P. Anders/Art Resource, NY).

that depicted the sacrifice of Iphigenia: Timanthes "depicts Iphigenia standing by the altar ready for death. Having presented all the
onlookers—especially her father's brother—as plunged in sorrow,
and having thus exhausted every presentment of grief, he has veiled
the face of her father, for whom he had reserved no adequate expression."[71] Consoled in his sorrow, flattered in his piety, and implicitly
praised in his erudition by Dürer's art, Pirckheimer appears in the
picture standing behind his wife's headboard, isolated in grief, a cloth
pressed up against his face. The classical allusion redounds to the
virtue of both men, each on one side of the therapeutic encounter.
As if to further sanctify the death of the long-suffering Crescentia,
Dürer models the scene upon a chestnut of Christian iconography:
the Dormition of the Virgin, the traditional death-bed scene depicting the ascent of Mary's soul to heaven. Drawn-aside curtains further
establish the setting as a morally edifying spectacle for the beholder.
Crescentia's death-vigil is the closest thing in Dürer's oeuvre to a
consolatory address to his friend Pirckheimer, who never had occasion, it seems, to commission a painting from Dürer (though Dürer
did illustrate several books in Pirckheimer's library).

"By Charity of the Spirit Serve One Another"

Dürer's friendship with Lazarus Spengler (1497–1534), first city council secretary in Nuremberg, precipitated a very different kind of personalized *Trostbild*. I am referring to the pendant sheets preserved
today in the British Museum (figures 6.8 and 6.9).[72] Both are done in
black ink on parchment with red lettering in decorative cartouches
at the bottom, with touches of gilding around the framed inscriptions at the top. One sheet depicts the solitary Christ carrying his
Cross and looking over his shoulder; he is crowned with thorns and
surrounded by an aureole of clouds, the lines of which spiral upward
into the kind of calligraphic fantasy Dürer enjoyed adding to his
drawings. The second sheet portrays a solitary Christian in patrician
garb; surrounded by an arched vine stock heavy with grapes where it
springs from the ground, the man bears his own cross in imitation,
following along with hands clasped in prayer. As Jesus turns to look,
the words taken from Matthew 10:38 proclaim the truest test of discipleship: "And he that taketh not up his cross, and followeth me, is
not worthy of me." From the corresponding cartouche on the second
sheet comes the disciple's faithful vow: "For though I should walk in

the midst of the shadow of death, I will fear no evils, for thou art with me" (Psalms 22:4). Although the identification of the good disciple with Spengler can not be proven absolutely, the coat of arms added (by someone other than Dürer) to the second sheet, in the upper left, are indeed those of the Spengler family (albeit with the tinctures reversed). Friedrich Winkler proposed early on that the London sheets form a coherent group with a *Stifterbild* (now in Weimar) depicting a man kneeling in prayer before a prie-dieu and displaying the same coat of arms; two mythological drawings Dürer completed for Spengler in pen and ink around 1515; and the miniatures formerly in the Spengler family chronicle (*Geschlechtbuch*).[73]

Spengler was sworn in alongside Kaspar Schmutterherr to the prestigious post of city council secretary (*Ratsschreiber*) on Easter Day 1507. The timing of this appointment and the scope of his responsibilities ensured that he would be involved with every aspect of the council's business during the critical early years of the Reformation. Together with his personal commitment to Luther's teachings, his advantageous legal and administrative position truly made him "the man who was destined to implement the Reformation in Nuremberg."[74] Like Pirckheimer, Spengler hailed from a wealthy patrician family and took a deep interest in the progress of humanism; he got to know Konrad Celtis and participated in the post-*Poetenschule* dining club that met at Pirckheimer's house. In the winter of 1516, this same group, which included Dürer, formed the target audience at a momentous event: a series of Advent sermons on the theme of "true repentance," delivered by the Augustinian vicar-general for Germany, Johann von Staupitz (ca. 1460–1524), Luther's mentor and confessor. Galvanized by Staupitz's teachings, which fused mysticism and practical piety, the group began calling themselves the "Sodalitas Staupitziana." Later, through the efforts of another Augustinian prior, Wenzeslaus Linck (1483–1547), the group deepened its familiarity with Luther's own teachings and began calling itself the "Sodalitas Martiniana."[75] Spengler also participated as a layman in the pamphlet wars of the early Reformation, albeit reluctantly at first. In 1519 his little treatise championing Luther, *Defense and Christian Reply of an Honorable Lover of the Divine Truth of Holy Scripture against Several Opponents with Reasons Why Doctor Martin Luther's Teaching Should Not Be Rejected But on the Contrary Be Considered Christian*, was published anonymously in Augsburg, apparently against its author's will;

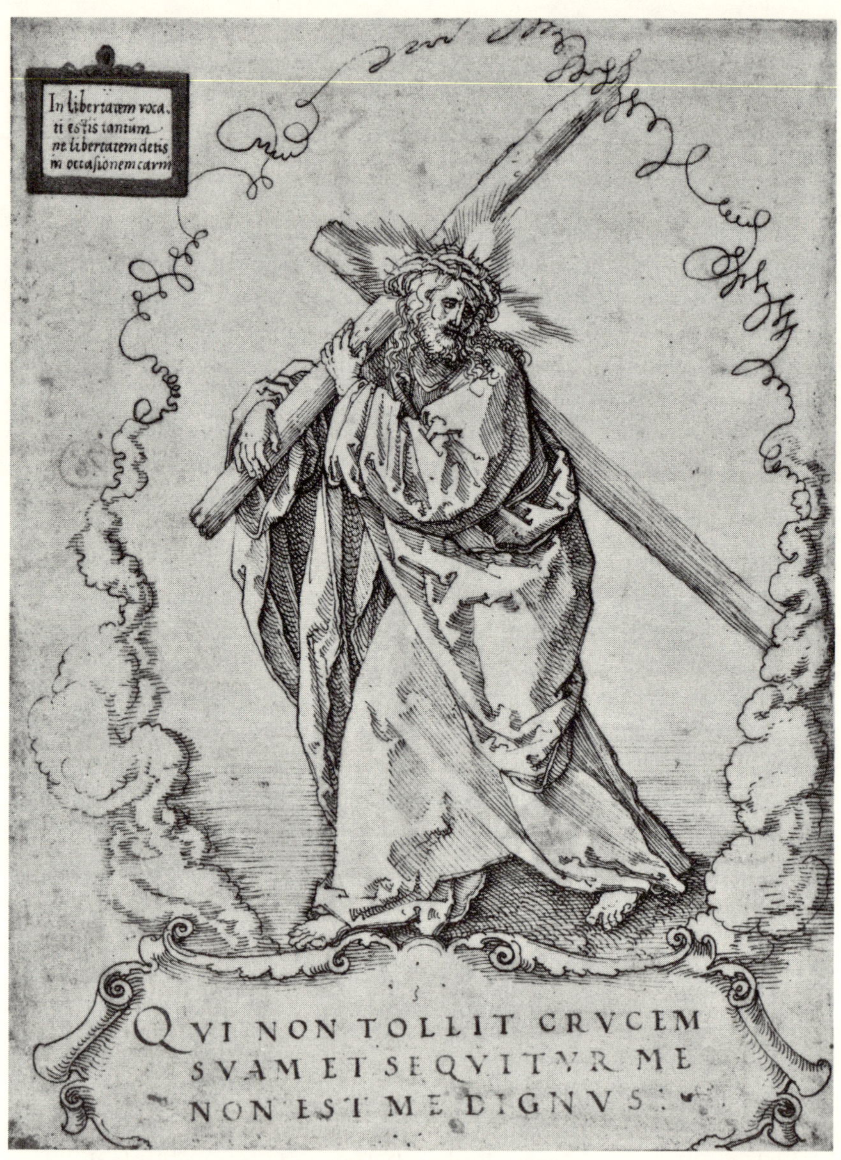

Figure 6.8. Albrecht Dürer, *Christ Carrying the Cross*, ca. 1520–25, pen, black and red ink, and gilding on parchment, 13.8 x 10.4 cm (London, British Museum) (photo: © The Trustees of the British Museum London).

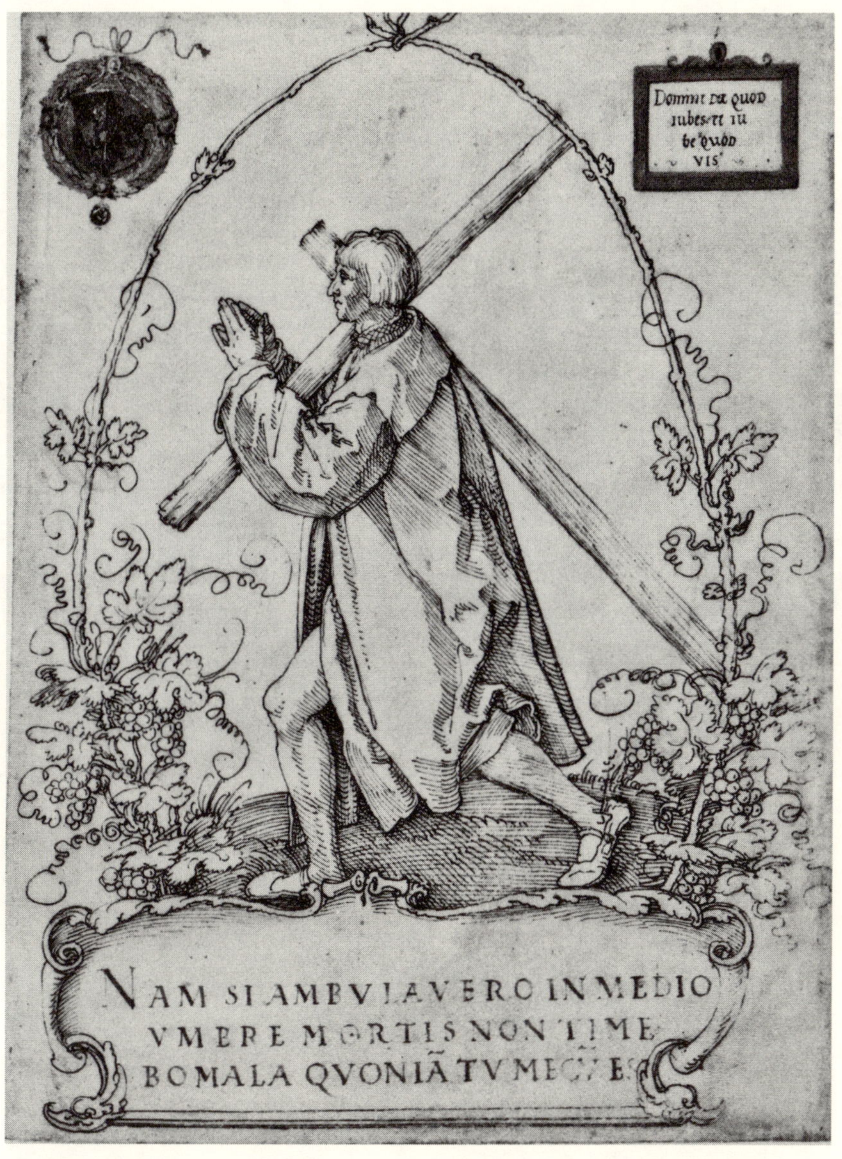

Figure 6.9. Albrecht Dürer, *Lazarus Spengler Carrying the Cross*, ca. 1520–25, pen, black and red ink, and gilding on parchment, 13.7 x 10.4 cm (London, British Museum) (photo: © The Trustees of the British Museum London).

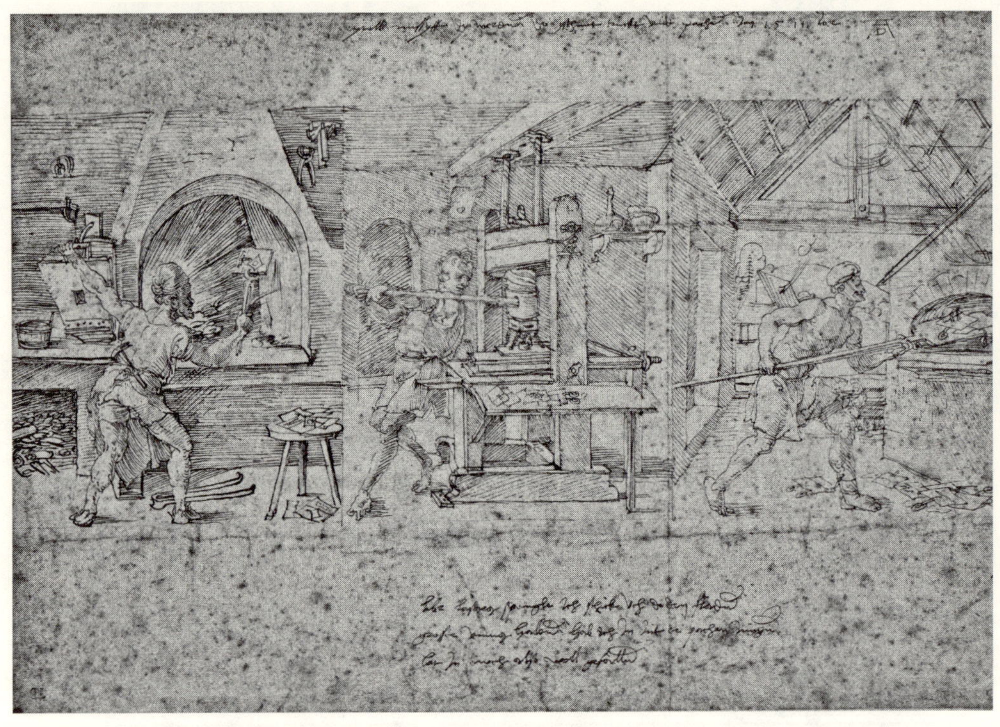

Figure 6.10. Albrecht Dürer, *New Year's Sheet for Lazarus Spengler*, 1511, pen and ink, 20.4 x 29.8 cm (Bayonne, Musée Bonnat) (photo: © RMN-Grand Palais/Rene-Gabriel Ojeda/Art Resource, NY).

several editions followed in 1520.[76] The work earned him the wrath of Luther's archenemy, the Dominican controversialist Johann Eck, who personally anathematized Spengler (along with Pirckheimer) in the list of heretics mentioned in the papal bull *Exsurge domini* (15 June 1520), which famously called for Luther's excommunication should he refuse to recant.[77]

Though their acquaintance surely began earlier, Spengler and Dürer's friendship took on more definite contours after 1509, when Dürer was made a *Gennanter*, or member of the Great Council (a second governing body composed of representatives from *ehrbar*, "honorable," families).[78] Public duty and private fun seem to have mixed well in their friendship. "Many a merry day" did the friends enjoy together when, for instance, Dürer accompanied Spengler and the councilman Kaspar Nützel (ca. 1471–1529) on official business to the imperial diet in Augsburg in 1518. The expense sheet submitted to the council for their twenty-one-day stay, which amounted to 300 gulden—the equivalent of a high city official's annual salary—certainly confirms it.[79] We have already observed some of the waggish hilarity of the poems that the men exchanged, and to this comic corpus Dürer would soon add a visual mockery of the bureaucrat's profession. A drawing sent as a New Year's greeting in 1511 parodies the work of Spengler, along with his colleagues Nützel and Hieronymus Holzschuher (ca. 1469–1529), both of whom evidently piled on Spengler's head all of their report-writing duties when away on diplomatic missions (figure 6.10). A smith, a printer, and a baker (or possibly a glassmaker) are shown hammering and forging, pressing and printing, and then baking (or annealing) their mind-numbing reports. "Superb missives are here cast," Dürer jests in the inscription, "printed and baked in the year 1511—Dear Lazarus Spengler, I am sending you herewith the cake that for lack of leisure I could not bake before. Enjoy it!"[80]

But it was the friends' common interest in religious matters, their mutual cultivation of Christian virtue, and their spiritual kinship that made the intimate conception of the London pendant sheets possible. Religious identities are notoriously hard to pin down for the period before 1530—confessional divides were still porous—but Spengler's partisan commitment to Luther's cause and the new evangelical doctrines is impossible to question. Far less agreement surrounds the question of "Dürer's Protestantism" among biographers;

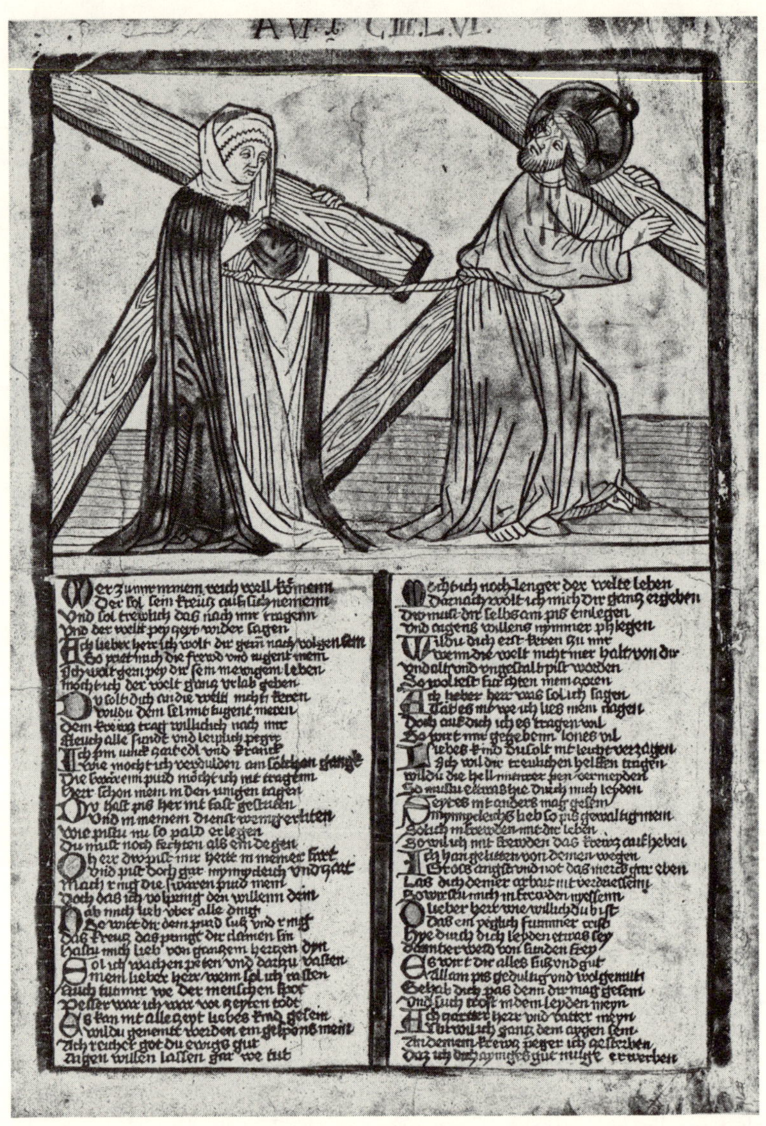

Figure 6.11. South German, *Love Bearing the Cross*, second half of fifteenth century, hand-colored woodcut broadsheet, 37.9 x 25.5 cm (image) (Nuremberg, Germanisches National-museum).

we'll steer around this overgrown thicket of opinion. What can be affirmed is the very real concern the men shared for searching out an ethical-spiritual orientation compatible with civic identity. Both seem to have understood that improvement in their city's moral life would come from the top down and find equal nourishment in a classical (that is, Stoic) pursuit of virtue and a traditional Christian idealization of neighborly love. In 1520, amidst heightening tensions between Wittenberg and Rome and surely inspired by his contacts with Erasmus, Spengler published his own little guide to Christian living, the *Admonition and Instruction for a Virtuous Life*. The book, a collection of biblical passages, folklore, and classical quotations, the author dedicated to Dürer, his "special, intimate, and brotherly friend."[81]

Are the London drawings a reciprocal gift? Despite the difficulty of dating them precisely, the ballpark guess of "circa 1525" often seen in the Dürer literature is probably a few years too late.[82] If we are justified in putting the drawings in closer proximity to Spengler's *Admonition*, and interpret them as a return expression of ethical-spiritual care from one Christian to another, their personalized character comes through more clearly. Late medieval devotional culture furnished the basic formula for an image in which personifications of love or humility take up the labor of the Cross in imitation of Christ, enacting a symbolic pilgrimage of the soul and becoming a focal point for penitential identification. A hand-colored broadsheet from Bavaria, for example, presents a female figure of *Minne* (spiritual love), hefting her cross along a virtual *via crucis* and tethered by a rope to Christ, who turns to address her (figure 6.11). Rhymed couplets, beginning with a variation on Mark 8:34, form the two columns of text below, a dialogue between Christ and the soul known as "Love Bearing the Cross."[83] On behalf of his friend, Dürer updates this allegory of the soul's vocation and, speaking to the new evangelical conviction, "horizontalizes" the ethical chain of love connecting the Christian to Christ. In the gilded frame of the first London drawing are set the words from Galatians 5:13, which resonate with Luther's call for a new form of Christian liberty: "For you, brethren, have been called unto liberty: only make not liberty an occasion to the flesh, but by charity of the spirit serve one another" (*Vos enim in libertatem vocati estis, fratres: tantum ne libertatem in occasionem detis carnis, sed per caritatem Spiritus servite invicem*). And in the corresponding frame above the penitent's head: "Lord, grant what you command and command what thou wilt" (*Domine da quod / iubes at iu / be quod / vis*). This famous prayer, repeated three times in Augustine's *Confessions* (10.29.31, and 10.29.37) is often referred to as the spark that lit the debate over predestination and free will in Augustine's day, the so-called Pelagian Controversy. In dialogue with the rubricated words of Psalm 22, inscribed by Dürer beneath the disciple's feet, their expression of a radical submission to providence again proclaims the emergence of a new, specifically Lutheran model for the care of souls.[84] Superimposed on the mutual consolation of the suffering Christ and the penitent soul, updated within a humanistic ethics, and transformed by the new evangelism, Dürer's agency as a rhetorical healer is here set in dialogue with that of his spiritual brother, the author of a consolatory address to all Christians. Both inside and outside the space of the picture, therapeutic agency is defined by a special form of *attending*, a soul service at once philosophical, medical, and spiritual.

Universal Medicine

Less than a decade after casting himself as the agent of a merry musical therapy in the *Jabach Altarpiece*, Dürer pictured himself as the purveyor of a universal heavenly medicine in the *Landauer Altarpiece*, a work dubbed by Moritz Thausing "a perfect jewel of art" and now in the Kunsthistorisches Museum in Vienna (figure 6.12).[85] Standing on the crest of a hill overlooking a glistening landscape and seascape that arcs toward the horizon, a diminutive Dürer appears *in assistenza* in the lower right corner. Dressed in patrician finery, he is recognizable by the shoulder-length blonde hair that cascades over his fur collar (figure 6.13). An oversized placard declaring his authorship is propped up by his side: *ALBERTUS DVRER NORICVS FACIEBAT ANNO A VIRGINIS PARTV 1511* (Albrecht Dürer of Nuremberg was making this in the year of the Virgin's offspring, 1511).[86] High above him, and yet right before our eyes, an otherworldly vision explodes into an exhilarating spectacle of color and form. A rotating retinue of female saints and martyrs behind the Virgin Mary on the left, Old Testament prophets and worthies behind John the Baptist on the right, genuflect, gesture, and gaze toward the Trinity, which gleams out from the composition's center, a perfect epiphany suspended before parting clouds. God the Father, crowned, implacable, and

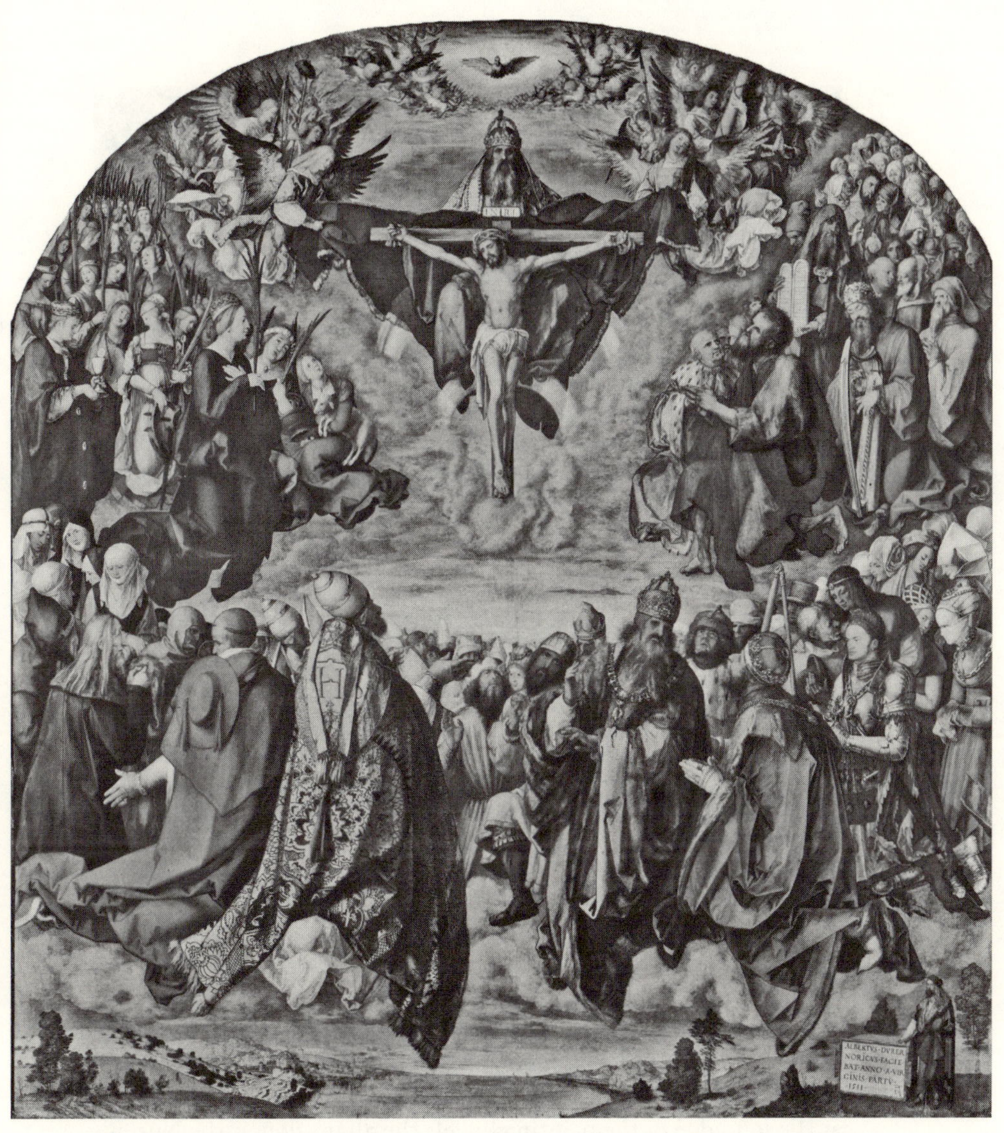

Figure 6.12. Albrecht Dürer, *Adoration of the Holy Trinity*, panel for the *Landauer Altarpiece*, 1511, oil on poplar, 135 x 123 cm (Vienna, Kunsthistoriches Museum) (photo: HIP/ Art Resource, NY).

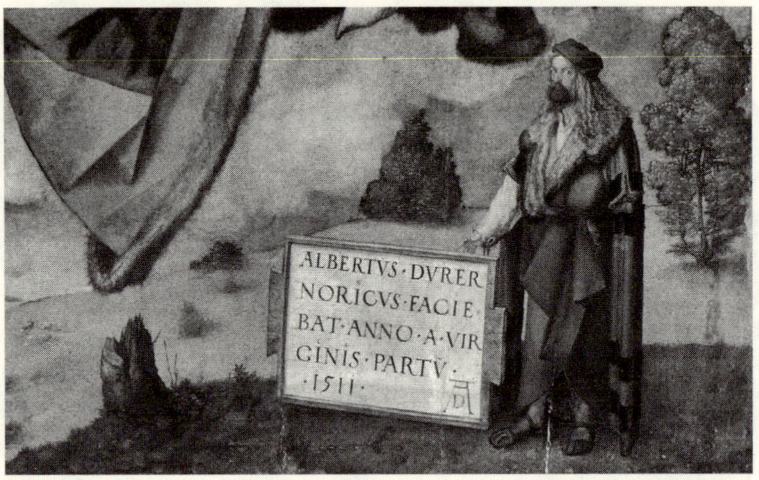

Figure 6.13. Detail from Dürer, *Adoration of the Holy Trinity*: self-portrait *in assistenza*. (See figure 6.12.)

enthroned on a double rainbow, holds his crucified Son before his lap, while the edges of his great mantle are parted by angels to reveal the Cross. More angels converge upon this heavenly "Throne of Grace" and display the *arma Christi*, while the dove of the Holy Spirit hovers motionless before a tunnel of light. Below them, and likewise borne aloft, is an even greater multitude—saints and emperors, kings and queens, male and female religious, laymen of all ranks, and several of Dürer's contemporaries—all captured in states of dawning awareness: a visionary communion of saints in a heavenly theater beyond space and time. Only the author of this great *chori beatorum*, only Dürer, remains with his feet planted in the terrestrial world.

Nestled among the popes, cardinals, bishops, abbots, and abbesses at the left edge of the painting kneels the altar's donor, the Nuremberg ore magnate, Matthäus Landauer (1451–1515). Shown in profile, he is recognizable from the study drawing Dürer made of him, which is today in Frankfurt.[87] It was in 1501, the year of his wife's death, that Landauer, together with Erasmus Schiltkrot, founded the charitable institution called the House of the Twelve Brethren (*Zwölfbrüderhaus*), a hospice designed for the care of twelve aging artisans, impoverished and needy through no fault of their own. Several years later, between 1506 and 1508, the donors saw to the furnishing of the hospice's chapel, dedicated to All Saints (*Allerheiligenkapelle*). Their architect, the Nuremberg master Hans Behaim the Elder (1455/60–1538), framed the view of the altar with elegant grooved columns that spiral upward to join the decorative rib vaulting enclosing the space.

Dürer's altar for the late Gothic chapel displays a similar boldness of design: in an unprecedented move for a German sanctuary, Dürer conceived a wingless, single-panel altarpiece of the Italian type, its painted spectacle visible through an elaborate architectural frame carved by the Nuremberg sculptor Ludwig Krug. Long ago separated from its painted panel, the original frame survives today (in Nuremberg), as does the *modello* of the integrated altarpiece that Dürer prepared for Herr Landauer's approval (in Chantilly) (figure 6.14).[88] Crowned by a Last Judgment distributed across the lintel frieze (with processions of the Blessed and the Damned) and the tympanum (showing the Dëesis), the frame bears a dedicatory inscription on the lower bar, flanked by the Landauer family coats of arms: "Matthäus Landauer has finally completed the house of worship of the Twelve Brethren together with the charitable foundation and this panel. After Christ's birth, the year 1511."[89] To complete the sanctuary's design, three stained-glass windows were set into the eastern wall, while the north and south walls received one window each. In the central window, the Holy Trinity is presented using the then-controversial motif of an enthroned God with three faces. Thus did the windows complement the themes of the altarpiece. Adjacent to a scene of God greeting the Wise and Foolish Virgins (left east window), Landauer appears again in devotion, this time with his family; while the Fall of the Rebel Angels is paired with the Sacrifice of Isaac on the right.[90] Executed in the workshop of Veit Hirschvogel the Younger (1485–1553) on the basis of Dürer's designs, the windows have been considered the premier works of Nuremberg glass art for this period.[91]

Eschatological themes of resurrection and judgment appear frequently in the visual programs designed for hospices such as Nuremberg's *Zwölfbrüderhaus*, many of which had large, open wards with adjoining chapels to allow patients to attend Mass from their beds. Well-known examples include Rogier van der Weyden's *Last Judgment Altarpiece*, commissioned in 1443 for the hospice in Beaune (Hôtel-Dieu) by the Burgundian chancellor Nicholas Rolin and his

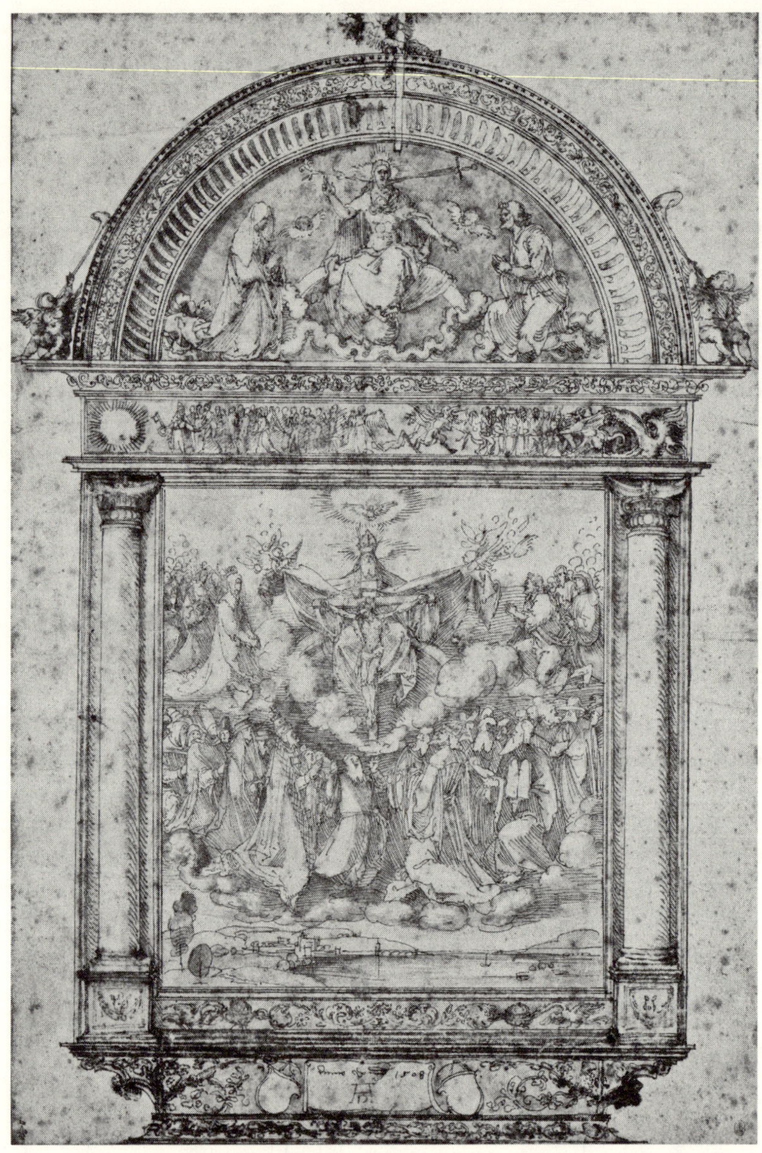

Figure 6.14. Albrecht Dürer, *Modello for the Landauer Altar with Frame*, dated 1508, pen with blue, green, and red washes, 39.1 x 26.8 cm (Chantilly, Musée Condé) (photo: © RMN-Grand Palais/Gérard Blot/Art Resource, NY).

wife Guigone de Salins; Matthias Grünewald and Nicholas Hagenauer's *Isenheim Altarpiece* of ca. 1512–16, made for the monastery of St. Anthony near Colmar, where monks specialized in the treatment of plague and ergotism; and the high altarpiece of ca. 1517–20 placed in the hospital church of the Holy Spirit (Spitalkirche Heilig Geist) in Laatsch, South Tirol, the combined work of sculptor Jörg Lederer and painter Jörg Mack.[92] Their purpose of consoling sufferers, inspiring penance in preparation for a good death, and placing the delights of the next life squarely before the eyes is easy enough to comprehend. Dürer naturally found room for innovation within this functional genre, though the iconographic solution he arrived at remains the subject of some debate. Panofsky pointed to Augustine's *De civitate dei* (specifically the last chapter of book 22) to account for Dürer's thematic integration of picture and frame. According to his account, the novelty lay in the effort to imagine the heavenly city "as it will exist after time has come to an end." No longer half-beholden to the terrestrial world—as all Christians, in Augustine's scheme, must be before final judgment—the faithful are portrayed proleptically, "accepted among the beatified."[93] This comingling in heaven of the already perfected with the boundless "surging sea of humanity," in Panofsky's view, makes the picture a very special sort of *Allerheiligenbild*—an eternal and blissful vision of God after the Last Judgment, historical time's final act. Thus the frame's aesthetic function as a "gateway" to this vision, he could conclude, works in "perfect harmony with its doctrinal content."[94]

Yet Panofsky did not take seriously enough the symbolic implications of Dürer's recourse to the "Throne of Mercy" (*Gnadenstuhl*), one of several distinct ways the Trinity had been visualized since the twelfth century. Its distinctiveness lay in the emphasis given to the Father's eternal offering of the Son as an expiatory sacrifice to rescue humanity from sin. Consequently, as a sign of redemption—the redemption that will be perfectly realized only on the Day of Judgment—the image would have held strong Eucharistic associations for its viewers. In recovering these associations, Carolyn Carty has argued that what the multitude depicted in Dürer's painting has come to adore is "the analogue of Christ on the altar"; the picture, in other words, stages the Father's invitation "to pass through the portal of the frame and to approach the Eucharistic sacrificial table."[95]

By declaring himself the impressario of this universalizing welcome, Dürer steps into a privileged role in relation to the altar sacrament, the greatest heavenly medicine. Inviting humanity to the eschatological meal, the painter's perfect vision participates in God's perfect offering. A surrogate Eucharist for the inmates of the *Zwölfbrüderhaus*, the altarpiece proffers a "foretaste" (as theologians described the altar sacrament)[96] of the manna served at the heavenly banquet. Like all other ordinary Christians on the eve of the Reformation, Dürer knew that, as a variation on sacramental eating (*manducatio per gustum*), Eucharistic wholeness could be accessed through vision alone (*manducatio per visem*);[97] to extend the artist's presence *in assistanza* from the scene of visual adoration into the territory of sacramental communion, then, is not an unorthodox gesture. With the earthbound Eucharist as one's touchstone, it is but a small step to orient the office of the *medicus animorum*, the healer of souls, toward the indivisible, the infinite, the metaphysically perfect.

When it came to distributing the therapeutic agency claimed in the *Landauer Altar* beyond the frame of the picture, beyond the space of the chapel, even beyond the city walls of his native Nuremberg, Dürer knew he could rely on the medium of print. In 1511, the very year the altar was completed and set in place in the *Allerheiligenkapelle*, he published his large woodcut version of the *Gnadenstuhl* as a single devotional sheet (figure 6.15).[98] Now, in the hands of the beholder, the vision has been brought closer: the Throne of Mercy hovers in the chilly ether above the swirling atmosphere created by the Four Winds, which toss the drapery around Christ's feet. The hieratic presentation of the Crucified *before* the Father is now replaced with the dead Christ's intimate embrace *by* his Father, whose look betrays a familial tenderness, whose mercy consoles and heals the world.

It is fitting, I think, to end this trio of case studies with an image of universal healing and heavenly perfection. When the problem of human flourishing is catapulted into the next world, the fundamental oppositions that define all therapeutic projects—sickness and health, suffering and happiness, distress and peace, misery and relief—are abolished and overcome. Likewise transcended are all the anxieties that attend the human quest for perfection. Over the

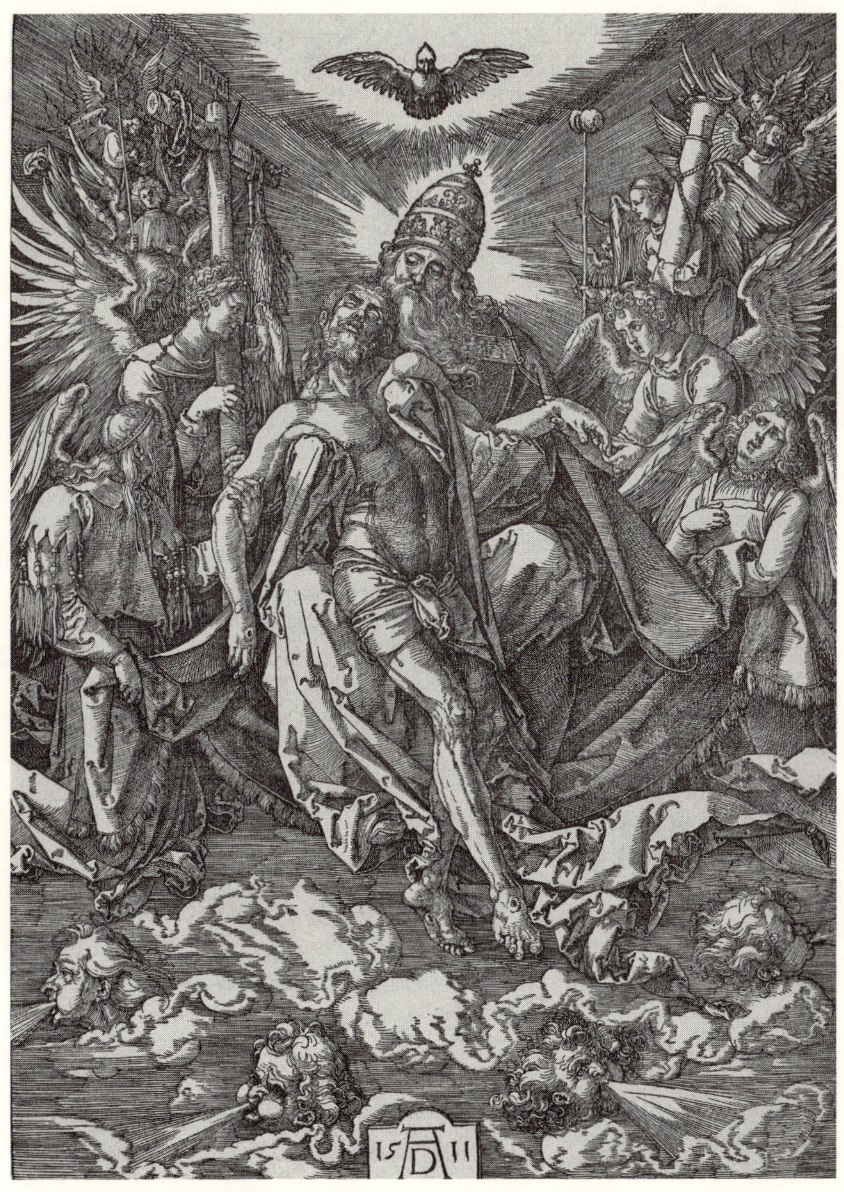

Figure 6.15. Albrecht Dürer, *Holy Trinity*, 1511, woodcut, 39.7 x 28.6 cm (Washington, D.C., National Gallery of Art, Rosenwald Collection).

course of his career as a Christian image maker, Dürer, we have seen, cultivated a unique sensibility for discerning and "attending to" the particular needs of the audiences he addressed. This chapter and the one preceding it revealed the fundamental ways the artist used the means afforded by his art—his imitative, inventive, and imaginative *pictorial* art—to offer care and consolation to himself, to his patrons and friends, and then to the extended human family united under Christ. A century and a half before him, Petrarch had innovated a humanist model for such a threefold therapeutic project, and had developed the poetic and philosophical language appropriate to each context in which he encountered souls in distress. For a poet to assume the office of the *medicus animorum* was new. In antiquity, that role had been the exclusive preserve of the philosopher; in the long Christian era following, soul service was a shared obligation, undertaken reciprocally within the context of the cloistered life or as a function of the clergy's pastoral mission to the laity. In his vernacular poetry and Latin prose works, Petrarch modeled the possibility of a "modern" therapy of the passions. It has been the work of these two chapters to reveal a parallel ambition in Dürer's work across media, across genres, and across the functional contexts his art served.

My purpose in writing this book has been to reveal how that ambition informed Dürer's art generally and how it found singular realization in the *Melencolia*, a perfect work of art singularly geared to remedy Renaissance misery, a therapy for the world-weariness and spiritual sorrow attending the mind and the soul's quest for perfection. With all that said, one fundamental question remains unanswered: For whom were the therapeutic resources of the engraving intended?

Epilogue

In the final line of his learned commentary appended to the monumental woodcut project known as the "Arch of Honor" (*Ehrenpforte*), made for Emperor Maximilian I by a team of designers, artisans, and advisors that included Dürer, Jörg Kolderer, Hans Springklee, Wolf Traut, and Albrecht Altdorfer, the court historian, cartographer, and royal astronomer Johannes Stabius (1468–1522) invited the beholder to collaborate in prizing loose meaning from the gargantuan pile of symbols, signs, figures, and forms before him: "And there are still many other ornaments in this Arch of Honor, about which so much more could be said, [and] which the observer may explain and interpret [better] for himself, [but] which I omit for the sake of brevity."[1] Stabius's stance on the beholder's interpretative freedom may sound like a postmodern primer in decentered meaning, but it is better understood as the distillation of German humanist convictions about the nature of the curious picture signs spread across the architectural zones of the *Ehrenpforte*—picture signs rooted in the humanist study of hieroglyphs.

Profound reverence for the esoteric character of "the old Egyptian letters originating with the god-king Osiris" (*alten Egiptischen Buchstaben, herkumend von dem künig Osyris*) united Stabius with other leading humanists such as Pirckheimer, the intelligence behind the *Ehrenpforte*'s conception. To these men, the symbolic language of hieroglyphs transported thought to something like the primordial ground of all philosophical and theological wisdom—a coded container for the *prisca theologia*, waiting to be unlocked by those in possession of its key. A step toward the discovery of that key was taken with Pirckheimer's Latin translation of the Greek treatise known as the *Hieroglyphica*, written by the "Egyptian" adept Horus Apollon (possibly a

Roman author of the second or fourth century; possibly a medieval forger), a project the Nuremberg humanist undertook around 1512 or 1513. Though never published, the work in manuscript, featuring illustrations by Dürer—figural interpretations of "hieroglyphic picture signs" meant to engage the reader's speculative thought through paradoxes and *impossibilia*—was presented to the emperor in April 1514 by its translator and illustrator. This was precisely the time work on the *Ehrenpforte* was nearing its conclusion. During this same period of intense work, Dürer brought out his *Melencolia I.*

"Astro-medical-philosophical esoterica" may be an appropriately ponderous term for the overlapping works produced during this heady moment in Dürer's career. More important than any organizing label, of course, is what the convergence of these projects tells us about the imperatives of German humanism in the service of Maximilian in the decade before his death in January 1519. Backed by scholarly pretensions of his own, the emperor's reliance on genealogy, mythology, and astrology for articulating his grandest political ambitions, as well as the sophisticated use of printed propaganda to project them, are striking. Divine providence and political fortune were intimately bound up with personal virtue in Maximilian's self-conception. As a Christian philosopher-king and chivalric warrior in the Burgundian mold, his noble dream was that of a perfect Christian world empire based on the union of mitre and sword. (He planned someday to rule as emperor and pope.) It was the combined task of the Nuremberg, Augsburg, and Vienna humanist elite, along with their eager counterparts in the visual arts, to give persuasive political shape to the intersections of knowledge underlying these claims.

Maximilian's destiny as a world-emperor is summed up in the overlapping cosmological, mythological, genealogical, and biographical imagery of the *Ehrenpforte*, a totalizing program that culminates at the base of the central tower's cupola. There, in the "mystical tabernacle" above a monumental inscription, Dürer's hieroglyphic portrait of Maximilian holds pride of place (figure E.1). According to Stabius's commentary, this emblematic royal image is a "misterium," a rebus to be unpuzzled "word by word" according to the logic of Egypt's venerable picture-sign language. The ruler's divinity, his virtues of power, strength, and magnanimity, the praise and glory that are his eternal due, his noble ancient lineage and natural gifts in art and learning, his dominion over great expanses of the globe and his

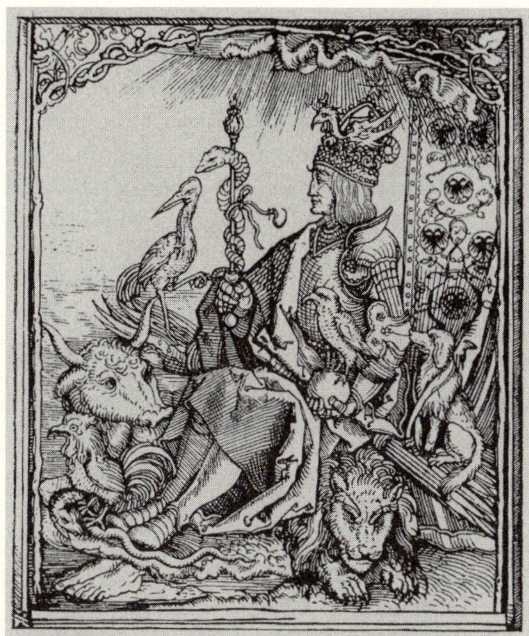

Figure E.1. Albrecht Dürer, *Hieroglyphic Portrait of Maximilian as Hercules*, detail from the *Triumphal Arch of Maximilian*, 1515 (photo: Karl Möseneder, *Paracelsus und die Bilder: Über Glauben, Magie und Astrologie im Reformationszeitalter* [Tübingen: Max Niemeyer, 2009], fig. 56).

awesome potential to realize the impossible—all of this is symbolized in the menagerie with which Maximilian is posed.[2] A summa of virtue, the image expresses an ideal balance of earthly achievement and spiritual wisdom, physical valor and intellectual insight. In his person, Maximilian embodied a perfect equilibration of the passions (his motto, *Halt Maß*, short for "Halt Maß in allen Dingen" and borrowed from the ancient precept "moderation in all things," is emblazoned on a banderole held by a griffin atop the right tower of the arch). To capture this balance of qualities in a single image, he wished to be represented as a "new Hercules."[3] Specifically, because Dürer's hieroglyphic image combines Hercules's attributes (such as the lion) with the serpent-coiled scepter and winged helmet of Mercury, it has been proposed that Maximilian is represented here as a "mercurial Hercules," an image of grand spirit and physical strength in perfect proportion.[4]

A constant fixture of imperial propaganda during his reign, Maximilian's identification with the hero Hercules was not confined to humanist fiction or political mythmaking. Court genealogies encouraged him to trace his family origins back to the son of Osiris, Hercules Aegypticus. (The papyrus bundle on which he sits in Dürer's woodcut may refer to this.) With this identification we arrive at one imperative behind the *Hieroglyphica-Ehrenpforte-Melencolia* convergence that scholars have so far not recognized—an imperative, this study has argued, that Dürer built into the very fabric of his great image of images: the therapeutic. Recall the Pseudo-Aristotelian *Problemata physica* (no. 30, section 1) and the impetus it gave to Renaissance equations of black bile with extraordinary achievement. Its famous opening passage, which we may now quote in full, meshed perfectly with what humanists already knew from Senecan tragedy about "Hercules furens" (figure E.2),[5] the heroic prototype of the gifted melancholic:

> Why is it that all those who have become eminent in philosophy or politics or poetry or the arts are clearly of an atrabilious temperament, and some of them to such an extent as to be affected by diseases caused by black bile, as is said to have happened to Heracles among the heroes ? For he appears to have been of this nature, wherefore epileptic afflictions were called by the ancients the sacred disease after him. That his temperament was atrabilious is shown by the fury which he displayed towards his children and the eruption of sores which took place before his disappearance on Mount Oeta; for this often occurs as the result of black bile.[6]

The powers and dangers associated with the "atrabilious temperament" that Maximilian shared with his divine ancestor were also the subject of a memorandum sent to the emperor in March 1514 by Dürer's friend in Augsburg, the humanist diplomat Konrad Peutinger (1465-1547). In reply to Maximilian's queries about a silver coin bearing the image of Hercules, supposedly unearthed on the Greek island of Thasos, Peutinger, at precisely the same time Dürer was portraying Maximilian as a "hieroglyphic Hercules," appealed to the authority of the *Problemata* in discussing the emperor's descent from the mythological hero, the special health challenges associated with the melancholic humor, and also its privileges.[7] Maximilian's condition was a matter of serious concern to his court astrologers, his doctors, and no doubt to the emperor himself. From 1497 he suffered from gallbladder attacks, and the imperial horoscope showed the malignant influence of Saturn in 1518, when Maximilian fell seriously ill. Georg Tannstetter (1482-1535), who attended Maximilian on his death bed in

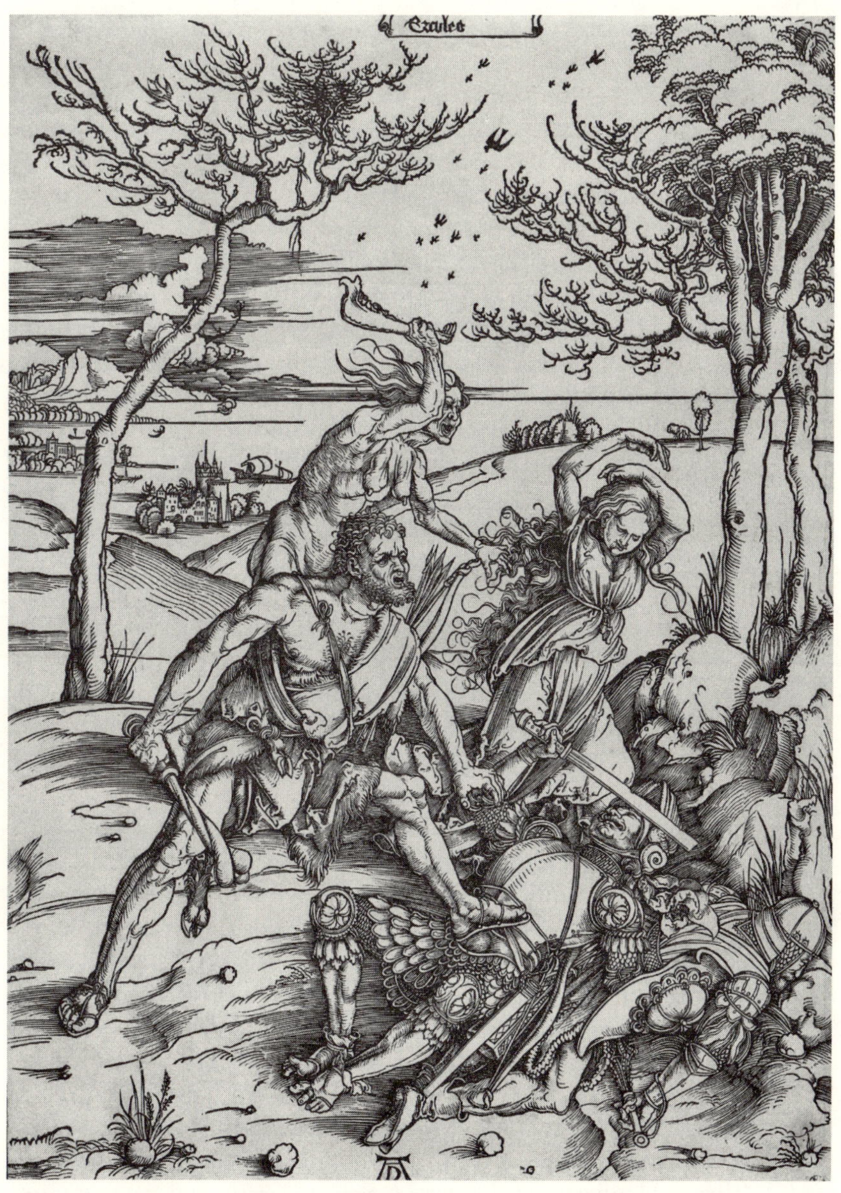

Figure E.2. Albrecht Dürer, *Hercules Punishing Cacus* (*"Hercules furens"*), ca. 1496, wood-cut, 38.8 x 28.2 cm (Washington, D.C., National Gallery of Art, Rosenwald Collection).

Wels, would later conjecture that an escalation in bile, wrought by a solar eclipse in that year, contributed to his patron's fate.[8] Already in 1514, the year Dürer completed *Melencolia I*, Maximilian was greatly preoccupied with his demise and his resting place; everywhere he traveled, reports tell us, he brought his coffin, prepacked, as it were, with documents and his personal treasury.[9]

It would be no overstatement to say that modern scholarship's recognition of these convergences—the Peutinger memo, the *Ehrenpforte*, Pirckheimer and Dürer's work on the *Hieroglyphica*, the realization of the *Meisterstiche*—constitutes something like the primordial dawn of *Melencolia* research itself, beginning with Karl Giehlow's emphatic situation of that work in the "maximilianische Humanistenkreis," the humanist circles of Maximilian's Vienna.[10] Placing the Peutinger memo at the forefront of his analysis, Giehlow drew together all the right threads, but stopped short of grasping the true purpose of Dürer's engraving. To make good on this promise, Peter-Klaus Schuster, ever the encyclopedist, detailed the correspondences between Dürer's allegory of humanist virtue and the "Geheimbild" of Maximilian, his mystery image, and, following Warburg, suggested that *Melencolia* might be taken as a consoling image for a royal melancholic, a *Trostblatt* to aid a humanist emperor in counteracting the baleful effects of dark Saturn with the "jovial" light of Jupiter. Was *Melencolia* conceived as a special dedication to Maximilian?[11] Was Dürer chasing royal patronage with an image expressly designed for his appreciation? Attractive as this thesis may be, the ambivalence and "contradictoriness" of its signs, so essential to the character of *Melencolia*, won't allow us to pin such a narrow rap on the engraving—nor will the essentially public nature of the printed image.

Why the qualifying "I" in *Melencolia*'s title? Perhaps Dürer had planned, but never realized a second image, a *Melencolia II*, to diagnose and remedy that form of melancholia peculiar to great rulers and statesmen, as the doctrine of the *Problemata* had defined it?[12] Conjectures that the most famous allegory of frustrated achievement in European art was conceived as but one image in a series will never lose their allure. With Agrippa's hierarchical scheme of the "threefold capacity of the soul" (*imaginatio*, *ratio*, and *mens*) in mind, Frances Yates, for example, saw in *Melencolia I* the lowest of three different "stages of inspired vision" and even proposed that Dürer's *St. Jerome* may be the missing *Melencolia III*.[13] The interpretation put forward here suggests there's no real need to conjure up missing pieces; *Melencolia* is complete in its incompleteness, perfect in its studied aesthetic imperfections. Perplexity is the picture's therapeutic gift, its diagnosis and its cure; the speculative labor it sets in motion is, after all, exactly what the soul's physician has prescribed in order to alleviate the "cold" torpor and weariness of melancholia, but also to moderate the potential for "hot" frenzy and madness. With the engraving in hand, the subject's own natural activity yields, of its own accord, a "pleasuring" of the blood and a return to flourishing.

Why did posterity never receive a *Melencolia II* or a *Melencolia III* from the master's hand? Had Dürer come to the realization that the species of picture Thomas Schauerte has called the "thought-and-puzzle image" (*Denk- und Rätselbild*) could admit of no further development?[14] Perhaps. Or perhaps it was instead the species we have been calling the allegorical-speculative therapeutic image that had reached its furthest extension in the engraving. Only one thing will ever be certain when these questions are raised, as they surely will be, again and again. If a *Melencolia II* and a *Melencolia III* were never completed, it can't be because Dürer didn't think it worth the effort.

Enigmatic things abound in *Melencolia I*, and prominent among them is the object directly concerned with mitigating the debilitating power of the illness: the Jupiter square (*mensula Iovis*) set into the wall above Melancholy's head (see figure 4.13). Amidst all the fanfare the magic square has garnered, one thing has tended to escape notice: its implied materiality. In antiquity, the Middle Ages, and even as late as the eighteenth century, astrological amulets—whether bearing the effigy of the personified planet or inscribed names and characters or a magic square—were struck from the planetary metals appropriate to them,[15] and according to Panofsky, the astrological talisman inspired by Dürer's contact with Ficinan and Agrippan white magic is portrayed here as if engraved upon a slab of tin.[16] Though Panofsky overestimated the correspondence between Agrippa's writings on melancholy and the picture's overall conception,[17] *De occulta philosophia* is not improbable as the source for the requirement that talismans be made of the right metal in order to attract the right planetary radiance and thus realize their therapeutic potential.[18] Occultists such as Ficino, Johannes Trithemius, and Leonard

Thurneisser likewise reported such correspondences in the making of astral talismans: silver with the moon, lead with Saturn, tin with Jupiter, iron with Mars, and copper with Venus.[19] This reflected an age-old faith in the material and spiritual connections between the seven "intelligent bodies" dwelling in the heavens (the planets) and their seven "embodied intelligences" (the metals) here on earth.[20]

To attract and intensify the healing influence of Jupiter, the *temperator Saturni* that drives away the dark planet's gloom, Melancholy could have been shown *wearing* a talisman, but instead the slab is fixed in the wall, where it confronts the beholder directly, like a picture. Did Dürer grasp, did he intend to convey, something of the analogy between the healing power of metal talismans and the therapeutic value of his own art, in particular the specialty of making pictures with engraved copper and iron plates? When we attune ourselves to the humanist aspirant's need for a special kind of relief from the burdens of achievement, when we remember that it was only the "well-balanced" melancholic who could return to creativity and persist in the Sisyphean striving toward perfection in the face of ever-renewing frustrations—only then does the possibility to which Dürer is alerting us become clear. The talisman *in* the picture figures the talismanic function *of* the picture. Melancholics could dream of a relief that descends from planetary forces. Yet Dürer's perfectly imperfect image has already proffered something down-to-earth and closer at hand, an alternative therapy for the afflictions of genius and fate. Thrown back upon its own resources, Renaissance misery could discover in *Melencolia I* its most efficacious remedy.

Acknowledgments

Freud and Marx should have sat for a double portrait by Dürer, a famous German writer once quipped, thinking of the dialectic of melancholy and utopia, thinking that modernity's Janus face is already perfectly captured in the form of our meditating goddess. In turn, we who spend time meditating on that form risk stumbling into the same affliction, or curing ourselves of it—nobody's quite sure which. Faced with the choice of spending either four years or forty years down the rabbit hole of *Melencolia* studies and choosing the former, I seem to have steered clear of melancholy and her sister syndromes, if only because the anxieties of modern academic life can stand in so well for existential boredom. Given this confession and this psychological profile, I doubt Dürer will ever seat me for a double portrait with Panofsky or with Saxl. And yet, I still like to think he would appreciate the efforts of a fellow self-therapist both to understand him and to do his part in preventing his masterpiece from being, once again, "cast in lead as a cute souvenir," as Günter Grass wrote, this time thinking of the work's historic overproduction—a phenomenon as continually fascinating as it is embarrassing to those of us guilty of perpetuating it.

In addition to the formidable *Dürerforschern* whose thoughts and labors fill these pages, a number of people close to me deserve credit for helping make this essay possible. For her unfailing support, I want to thank, first and foremost, Jacqueline Jung. Our cocktail-hour conversations brought clarity where there had been confusion, reassurance where there had been doubt. Jackie consulted with me on translations, lent me her books, and grudgingly made room on her shelves for mine. Above all, she strengthened my sense of purpose by believing in the project from start to finish. Equally therapeutic were my adventures inside the speculative microverse of the video game *Botanicula*, where there is no better guide than Klaus Jung. Sincere, or sincerely puzzled, expressions of interest from August Merback, Felix Merback, Theo Merback, and Alice Merback provided timely reminders that readers beyond the hermetic enclosures of Dürer studies were expecting me to write for them, too.

Despite too short a gestation for a book on so canonical a subject, I have incurred my share of debts, and I relish the chance to acknowledge them. Various forms of advice and assistance, input and insight, were graciously given by Joaquin Dominguez Arduengo, Michele Asuni, Shane Butler, Stephen Campbell, Christopher Celenza, Colin Eisler, Marian Feldman, Hal Foster, Yu Na Han, Marius Hauknes, Christopher Lakey, Leonardo Lisi, James Magruder, Jürgen Müller, Keith Moxey, John Ricco, Ronald Rittgers, Larry Silver, Jeffrey Chipps Smith, Peter Starenko, and Nino Zchomelidse. As a critical reader of an earlier draft, Shira Brisman could not have been more openhanded or more intuitively right about what the argument needed to make it better. Peter Parshall offered characteristically sage counsel, keen provocations, friendly consolation, and a willingness to share his work in progress on Dürer's inexhaustible "image of images." All readers, but especially those inclined to check my footnotes, will recognize an immeasurable debt to his learning and example. Outstanding research assistance was provided at various stages by Elizabeth Bernick, James Pilgrim, Rachel Danford, and especially Orsolya Mednyánzsky. Amidst a chronic need for books, articles, photographs, and tips on where to get them, I benefited from the generosity of Tim Barringer, Nina Gockerell, Tim Healing, Don Juedes, Gerhard Lutz, Miriam Said, Freyda Spira, and the wonderful staff of Yale's Divinity School library.

Surely it was Fortuna herself who guided me to Zone Books and my collaboration with Jonathan Crary, who has shown unfading enthusiasm for the project and has offered nothing but good counsel. I am also grateful to Meighan Gale for keeping things so neatly on track to our finished product, Julie Fry for the dazzling cover design, and Bud Bynack for his humane, hilarious, and skillful copyediting.

Nearly all the material between these covers is being presented in print for the first time. Opportunities to test drive the therapy thesis before an audience came, first, at a symposium held by the Metropolitan Museum of Art on the occasion of *Melencolia*'s quincentennial in 2014, and second, at the Renaissance Society's Annual Meeting in Berlin in 2015. For kind invitations to participate in these respective events, I am grateful to Nadine Orenstein and Lorenzo Pericolo. A small section of Chapter 3 will appear in longer form in *The Primacy of the Image in Northern European Art, 1400-1700: Essays in Honor of Larry Silver*, edited by Debra Cashion, Ashley West, and Henry Luttikhuizen (Leiden: Brill, 2017). For supporting a sabbatical leave in 2016–17, a grace that permitted me to complete the writing, I thank my department colleagues at Johns Hopkins, the dean's office of the Krieger School of Arts and Sciences, and the John Simon Guggenheim Memorial Foundation. Additional support came from the National Endowment for the Humanities.

New Haven, April 2017

Notes

INTRODUCTION

The epigraph is from Sigmund Freud, *Beyond the Pleasure Principle* (1920), in *The Standard Edition of the Complete Psychological Works of Sigmund Freud*, trans. James Strachey et al., vol. 18 (London: The Hogarth Press and the Institute of Psycho-Analysis, 1953–74), p. 42.

1. My literary recreation, based on a story I misremembered from Chungliang Al Huang, *Quantum Soup*, 2nd ed. (London: Jessica Kingsley Publishers, 2011); it bears some affinity with a Buddhist parable John Cage liked to quote, saying he got it from Shunryu Suzuki (whose *Zen Mind, Beginner's Mind* was beloved in the 1960s counterculture). A discussion on Ask Meta-Filter.com on May 12, 2012, http://ask.metafilter.com/215112/Now-that-Im-enlightened-Im-just-as-miserable-as-ever, suggests that Cage, too, misremembered it, since the passage can't be found in any of Suzuki's works. One discussant believes it to be a narrative variation of a well-known Zen proverb: "Before enlightenment: chop wood, carry water. After enlightenment: chop wood, carry water." Another claims the kōan Cage misattributed goes as follows: "One day the Master [Joshu] announced that a young monk had reached an advanced state of enlightenment. The news caused some stir. Some of the monks went to see the young monk [Kyogen]. 'We heard you are enlightened. Is that true?' they asked. 'It is,' he replied. 'And how do you feel?' 'As miserable as ever,' said the monk."

2. Though he singles out *Melencolia*, Vasari's judgment evidently applies to all three *Meisterstiche*: Dürer "executed some copper plates that put the world in awe" (*fece in rame alcune carte che feciono stupire il mondo*), adding that "it would not be possible to do more delicate engraving with the burin" (*che non è possibile col bulino intagliere più sotilmente*); see Rainer Schoch, Matthias Mende, and Anna Scherbaum, *Albrecht Dürer: Das druckgraphische Werk*, 3 vols. (Munich: Prestel, 2001–2004), vol. 1, no. 71; also Norbert Wolf, *Albrecht Dürer, 1471–1528: The Genius of the German Renaissance* (Cologne: Taschen, 2010), p. 48; Andrew Robison et al., *Albrecht Dürer: Master Drawings, Watercolors, and Prints from the Albertina*, exhibition catalogue (Washington, D.C.: National Gallery of Art / Munich: Delmonico Books, Prestel, 2013), no. 80, p. 210. Vasari's conception of *perfezione* is among the topics

treated in Lorenzo Pericolo and Elisabeth Oy-Marra (eds.), *Perfection: The Essence of Art and Architecture in Early Modern Europe*, forthcoming (Turnhout: Brepols, 2018). I thank my colleague Nino Zchomelidse for discussing the Vasari translation with me.

3. The acknowledgement that life as well as culture in Renaissance Europe had its "dark side" was fairly novel before the 1970s; a programmatic awakening is announced in Robert S. Kinsman (ed.), *The Darker Vision of the Renaissance: Beyond the Fields of Reason* (Berkeley: University of California Press, 1974).

4. Schoch, Mende, and Scherbaum, *Albrecht Dürer*, vol. 2 (2002), no. 103; see esp. Colin Eisler, "Who Is Dürer's 'Syphliitic Man'?," *Perspectives in Biology and Medicine* 52.1 (Winter 2009), pp. 48–60.

5. Schoch, Mende, and Scherbaum, *Albrecht Dürer*, vol. 2, no. 115.

6. Elliott M. Simon, *The Myth of Sisyphus: Renaissance Theories of Human Perfectibility* (Madison: Fairleigh Dickinson University Press, 2007), p. 136.

7. See Alina N. Feld, *Melancholy and the Otherness of God: A Study in the Hermeneutics of Depression* (Lanham: Lexington, 2011), whose critical genealogy gives depression, taken as "a privileged locus of significant metaphysical, existential, and anthropological unveilings" (p. xvii), a central role in the development of Western consciousness; also see Jeremy Schmidt, *Melancholy and the Care of the Soul: Religion, Moral Philosophy and Madness in Early Modern England* (Aldershot: Ashgate, 2007).

8. Distinctions between these, as well as other models of "perfectibilism," are laid out by John Passmore, *The Perfectibility of Man* (New York: Charles Scribner's Sons, 1970), pp. 11–27.

9. Blaise Pascal, *Pensées*, quoted in translation in Ioan P. Couliano, *Eros and Magic in the Renaissance*, trans. Margaret Cook (Chicago: University of Chicago Press, 1987), p. 52.

10. Because Dürer gave up the original project of which this was a part (a treatise covering all aspects of the aspiring painter's training), what survives is a draft outline; this passage comes from the sixth article. See Chapter 6 for the full passage and references.

11. "So wir nun zu dem aller besten nit kumen mögen, sol wir nun gar von vnser lernung lassen? Den fihischen gedancken nem wir nit an"; quoted in Jaya Remond, "Perfection," in Daniel Hess and Thomas Eser (eds.), *The Early Dürer*, exhibition catalogue (Nuremberg: Germanisches National Museum; New York: Thames and Hudson, 2012), p. 521; translation from Albrecht Dürer, *The Writings of Albrecht Dürer*, ed. and trans. William Martin Conway (New York: Philosophical Library, 1958), p. 245.

12. From the biographical preface to Camerarius's Latin translation of Dürer's *Four Books on Human Proportions*, published posthumously, in *The Writings of Albrecht Dürer*, p. 139. Cf. Panofsky's more ornate translation and his suggestion that Erasmus, when composing his eulogy of Dürer, drew from Camerarius's idea that the painter's sole shortcoming was "exaggerated diligence" (the two humanists exchanged letters between 1524 and 1528). See Erwin Panofsky, "Erasmus and the Visual Arts," *Journal of the Warburg and Courtauld*

Institutes 32 (1969), p. 227. On the biography and its criteria for artistic achievement, see Peter Parshall, "Camerarius on Dürer—Humanist Biography as Art Criticism," in Frank Baron (ed.), *Joachim Camerarius (1500–1574): Beiträge zur Geschichte des Humanismus im Zeitalter der Reformation / Essays On the History of Humanism during the Reformation* (Munich: Wilhelm Fink, 1978), pp. 11–29.

13. Petrarch, *Secretum*, quoted in Siegfried Wenzel, *The Sin of Sloth: Acedia in Medieval Thought and Literature* (Chapel Hill: University of North Carolina Press, 1967), p. 156.

14. Passmore, *The Perfectibility of Man*, p. 13.

15. Simon, *The Myth of Sisyphus*, p. 137; Petrarch quoting Augustine, p. 140.

16. The classic statement of this thesis is Theodor E. Mommsen, "Petrarch's Conception of the 'Dark Ages,'" *Speculum* 17.2 (April 1942), pp. 226–42: "With this change of emphasis from things religious to things secular, the significance of the old metaphor became reversed: Antiquity, so long considered as the 'Dark Age,' now became the time of 'light' which had to be 'restored'; the era following Antiquity, on the other hand, was submerged in obscurity" (p. 228). Although Petrarch may be credited with the founding conception, the term *medium aevum* was not coined until later.

17. Giuseppe Mazzotta, *The Worlds of Petrarch* (Durham: Duke University Press, 1993), p. 4; discussed in Gur Zak, *Petrarch's Humanism and the Care of the Self* (New York: Cambridge University Press, 2010), p. 9.

18. Zak, *Petrarch's Humanism*, p. 10.

19. Mommsen, "Petrarch's Conception of the 'Dark Ages,'" p. 228.

20. Frank Ankersmit, *Sublime Historical Experience* (Stanford: Stanford University Press, 2005), p. 177.

21. Petrarch, *Africa*, bk. 9; quoted in Mommsen, "Petrarch's Conception of the 'Dark Ages,'" p. 240.

22. A modern translation is Francesco Petrarca, *Petrarch's Remedies for Fortune Fair and Foul: A Modern English Translation of De Remediis Utriusque Fortune, with a Commentary*, trans. Conrad H. Rawski, 5 vols. (Bloomington: Indiana University Press, 1991). Petrarch's place in the *consolatio* tradition is fully laid out in George W. McClure, *Sorrow and Consolation in Italian Humanism* (Princeton: Princeton University Press, 1991), pp. 46–72. On the Christianization of consolation and its renewal in the age of Reformation, see Ronald K. Rittgers, *The Reformation of Suffering: Pastoral Theology and Lay Piety in Late Medieval and Early Modern Germany* (Oxford: Oxford University Press, 2012).

23. Zak, *Petrarch's Humanism*, pp. 79–80.

24. *Ibid.*, p. 81, citing Seneca's *Moral Letters to Lucilius*. On Petrarch's efforts to demonstrate the "interrelationship between his style and inner life," see Ronald G. Witt, *In the Footsteps of the Ancients: The Origins of Humanism from Lovato to Bruni* (Leiden: Brill, 2000), p. 240.

25. See the Prologue to Chapters 5 and 6.

26. Pierre Hadot, *Philosophy as a Way of Life: Spiritual Exercises from Socrates to Foucault,* ed. Arnold I. Davidson, trans. Michael Chase (Oxford: Blackwell, 1995), p. 82.

27. Letter to Giovanni Barrili, in Francesco Petrarch, *Letters on Familiar Matters,* trans. Aldo S. Bernardo, 3 vols. (Albany: State University of New York Press, 1975–85), vol. 2, pp. 162–63; discussed in Zak, *Petrarch's Humanism,* p. 37 n.27, who argues for an indissoluble link between Petrarch's humanism and his ethical-spiritual therapeutic project.

28. William J. Bouwsma, "The Two Faces of Humanism: Stoicism and Augustinianism in Renaissance Thought," in *A Usable Past: Essays in European Cultural History* (Berkeley: University of California Press, 1990), pp. 19–64.

29. Schoch, Mende, and Scherbaum, *Albrecht Dürer,* vol. 1, no. 102.

30. Desiderius Erasmus, *Manual of a Christian Knight (Enchiridion milites Christiani),* ch. 38 ("Against Wrath and Desire of Vengeance"), online translation (with my stylistic modifications), available at http://oll.libertyfund.org/index.php?option=com_staticxt&staticfile=show.php%3Ftitle=191&layout=html - toc_list.

31. Erwin Panofsky, *Albrecht Dürer,* 2 vols. (Princeton: Princeton University Press, 1943), vol. 1, pp. 151–52, though preceded by Paul Weber, *Beiträge zur Dürers Weltanschauung: Eine Studie über die drei Stiche Ritter Tod und Teufel, Melancholie und Hieronymus im Gehäus* (Strassburg: Heitz & Mündel, 1900), pp. 13–18. For basics on the print, see Walter Strauss, *The Complete Engravings, Etchings and Drypoints of Albrecht Dürer* (New York: Dover, 1973), no. 71; and Schoch, Mende, and Scherbaum, *Albrecht Dürer,* vol. 1, no. 69.

32. Heinrich Wölfflin argued that the *Melencolia* and *St. Jerome* engravings may be seen as "conscious opposites" but warned that "they are not meant to be studied simultaneously, for they are not formal counterparts. Both are pictures of certain moods." Wölfflin, *The Art of Albrecht Dürer,* trans. Alastair Grieve and Heide Grieve (London: Phaidon, 1971), p. 196; cf. Martin Büchsel, "Die gescheiterte 'Melancholia generosa': *Melencolia I,*" *Städel-Jahrbuch,* new series 9 (1983), p. 110. Most authorities follow Wölfflin in regarding the *Knight, Death, and Devil* as occupying a distinctive place in Dürer's oeuvre, unconnected to the two other *Meisterstiche,* despite the relatively close similarity of sizes. For a useful overview of the issue, see Robert Grigg, "Studies on Dürer's Diary of His Journey to the Netherlands: The Distribution of the 'Melencolia I,'" *Zeitschrift für Kunstgeschichte* 49.3 (1986), pp. 398–409, esp. pp. 398–400.

33. Peter Parshall, "Graphic Knowledge: Albrecht Dürer and the Imagination," *Art Bulletin* 95.3 (September 2013), p. 404.

34. *Ibid.*

35. From 1504 onward, Dürer demonstrated a strong preference for left lighting; the most significant exception among the early works, as Parshall has pointed out, is the *Nude Self-Portrait* of ca. 1502, pen and ink and brush on green paper, 29.1 x 15.3 cm (Weimar, Staatliche Kunstsammlung, inv. KK 106), whose right-handed lighting "carries a distinctly ominous and unsettling tone," possibly related to the illness Dürer was battling at the time

(see Chapter 5); Peter Parshall, "Albrecht Dürer and the Axis of Meaning," *Bulletin of the Allen Memorial Art Museum* 50.2 (1997), p. 19, and Parshall's useful remarks on *Melencolia*'s lighting on pp. 21–22.

36. See Chapter 4 for discussion of this criss-crossing of natural medicine, demonology, and theology in early modern theories of melancholia.

37. For that history, see Peter-Klaus Schuster, "Das Bild der Bilder: Zur Wirkungsgeschichte von Dürers Melancholiekupferstich," *Idea: Jahrbuch der Hamburger Kunsthalle* 1 (1982), pp. 72–134, and my more delimited account in Chapter 1.

38. Passmore, *The Perfectibility of Man*, p. 26.

39. This in the judgment of his preeminent Nuremberg colleague, Dirk van Ulsen (1460–1508; who published under his latinized name Theodoricus Ulsenius), in his 1496 edition of the Hippocratic *Aphorisms*; see Ewald Lassnig, "Dürers 'Melencolia-I' und die Erkenntnistheorie bei Ulrich Pinder: Versuch einer Interpretation aus einer Naheliegenden Quelle," *Wiener Jahrbuch für Kunstgeschichte* 57 (2008), pp. 56–57.

40. *Ibid.*, p. 64, where the author (Ewald Lassnig) reads Dürer's *Melencolia* as a figural-diagrammatic interpretation of the four "beams" of Pinder's allegorical crucifix, each of which stands for one kind of Christian discipleship, one kind of striving for virtue, and one kind of potential for knowing God—a fascinating hermeneutic confection that the engraving can hardly sustain.

41. Here and throughout, my use of the rhetorical concept of *ductus* (something that leads, guides, or conveys) is adapted from Mary J. Carruthers, *The Experience of Beauty In the Middle Ages* (Oxford: Oxford University Press, 2013), esp. pp. 53–54: "*Ductus* models an artefact as *iter*, journey, with an overall intention or *tenor* towards its end."

42. Parshall, "Camerarius on Dürer," p. 18. For Petrarch's use of medical terminology in delineating the craft of the moral philosopher, see the Prologue to Chapters 5 and 6.

43. Francesco Petrarch, *Letters of Old Age—Rerum senilium libri I–XVIII*, trans. Aldo S. Bernardo, Saul Levin, and Reta S. Bernardo, 2 vols. (Baltimore: Johns Hopkins University Press, 1992), vol. 2, p. 381; also quoted and discussed in Zak, *Petrarch's Humanism*, p. 99.

44. Ernst Cassirer, *The Individual and the Cosmos in Renaissance Philosophy*, trans. Mario Domandi (Oxford: Basil Blackwell, 1963), pp. 37–38, a reflection on Petrarch as a transitional subject that deserves to be quoted in full. That subject, for Cassirer, is found "struggling to achieve a balance between the requirements of ancient humanism and of medieval religiosity. But he never reaches a resolution, an inner balance between the conflicting forces. Petrarch's dialogues place us in the midst of the battle itself. They show the Ego, harassed and unsteady, at the mercy of opposed intellectual forces.... Petrarch's inner world is divided between Cicero and Augustine. He must reject on the one hand what he seeks on the other.... This duality applies to all the worldly human ideals—fame, beauty, love—to which he was attached with every fibre of his Ego. From this is born that schism within his mind, that sickness of the soul which Petrarch depicted in his most personal

and most profound work, the dialogue *De secreto conflictu curarum suarum*. The only result of this conflict is resignation, surfeit with the world, *acedia*. In Petrarch's own depiction of his mood, life becomes a dream, a phantasm; it sees its own nullity without being able to escape it."

45. Here and in what follows, readers will recognize the debt to Foucault's fourth type of "technology," understood as a "matrix of practical reason": the "technologies of the self, which permit individuals to effect by their own means, or with the help of others, a certain number of operations on their own bodies and souls, thoughts, conduct, and way of being, so as to transform themselves in order to attain a certain state of happiness, purity, wisdom, perfection, or immortality"; Michel Foucault, "Technologies of the Self," in *Ethics: Subjectivity and Truth*, ed. Paul Rabinow, trans. Robert Hurley et al. (New York: New Press, 1997), p. 225.

CHAPTER ONE: AN "ALLEGORY OF DEEP, SPECULATIVE THOUGHT"

The epigraph is from Dan Brown, *The Lost Symbol* (New York: Doubleday, 2009), p. 68.

1. In Rainer Schoch, Matthias Mende, and Anna Scherbaum, *Albrecht Dürer: Das druck-graphische Werk*, 3 vols. (Munich: Prestel, 2001–2004), vol. 1, no. 71, p. 179, Matthias Mende expresses the dominant view in calling it "ein fallender Komet"; the case for Saturn is made by David Pingree, "A New Look at *Melencolia I*," *Journal of the Warburg and Courtauld Institutes* 43 (1980), pp. 257–58, who also points out that the planet does not cast light rays, but "rays of divine energy." Cf. Martin Büchsel, *Albrecht Dürers Stich* Melencolia I: *Zeichen und Emotion—Logik einer Kunsthistorischen Debatte* (Munich: Wilhelm Fink, 2010), pp. 53–60.

2. Heinrich Wölfflin, *The Art of Albrecht Dürer*, trans. Alastair Grieve and Heide Grieve (London: Phaidon, 1971), p. 200.

3. British Library, London, Sloane 5229, fol. 60r; Peter-Klaus Schuster, *Melencolia I: Dürers Denkbild*, 2 vols. (Berlin: Gebr. Mann, 1991), fig. 8. Discussed in Giulia Bartrum et al., *Albrecht Dürer and His Legacy: The Graphic Work of a Renaissance Artist*, exhibition catalogue, British Museum (Princeton: Princeton University Press, 2002), cat. 129. See also Patrick Doorly, "Dürer's *Melencolia I*: Plato's Abandoned Search for the Beautiful," *Art Bulletin* 86.2 (June 2004), pp. 255–76, fig. 7.

4. Kupferstichkabinett, Berlin, KdZ 3876; Friedrich Winkler, *Die Zeichnungen Albrecht Dürers*, 4 vols. (Berlin: Deutscher Verein für Kunstwissenschaft, 1936–39), vol. 3, no. 621; Schoch, Mende, and Scherbaum, *Albrecht Dürer*, vol. 1, no. 71, pp. 179–80.

5. The phrase is from Michael Camille's incisive essay, "Walter Benjamin and Dürer's *Melencolia I*: The Dialectics of Allegory and the Limits of Iconology," *Ideas and Production: A Journal in the History of Ideas* 5 (1986), p. 59.

6. The term is from Schuster, *Melencolia I*, vol. 1, p. 84, with further discussion below.

7. Translation from William S. Heckscher, "*Melancholia* (1541): An Essay in the Rhetoric of Description by Joachim Camerarius," in Frank Baron (ed.), *Joachim Camerarius*

(1500–1574): Beiträge zur Geschichte des Humanismus im Zeitalter der Reformation / Essays On the History of Humanism during the Reformation (Munich: Wilhelm Fink, 1978), p. 33; cf. Philip L. Sohm, "Dürer's *Melencolia I:* The Limits of Knowledge," *Studies in the History of Art* 9 (1980), p. 31.

8. See esp. Doorly, "Dürer's *Melencolia I*."

9. The vocabulary of esoteric concealment and protected meaning—symbol, enigma, riddle, hieroglyph, lock and key, knowledge and ignorance—is prevalent in the literature; for a recent example, see the otherwise brilliant interpretation by Doorly in "Dürer's *Melencolia I*."

10. Walter Benjamin, *Ursprung des deutschen Trauerspiels* (1925 *Habilitation*, first published in 1928), translated as *The Origin of German Tragic Drama*, trans. John Osbourne (London: Verso, 1977), p. 184; cited in Camille, "Walter Benjamin and Dürer's *Melencolia I*," p. 60 and discussed below.

11. See my discussion in the Epilogue of Pirckheimer and Dürer's collaboration on an illustrated manuscript of the *Hieroglyphica* by Horapollo (1514), presented to Maximilian I.

12. Schoch, Mende, and Scherbaum, *Albrecht Dürer*, vol. 1, no. 71, p. 179, where Mende calls it "a batlike fantasy-creature" (*ein fledermausähnliches Fantasiewesen*).

13. In his description of *Melencolia I*, which Klibansky, Panofsky, and Saxl called a "mixture of minute observation and subtle psychological interpretation, and of pure fantasy," Melanchthon writes of "Dürer's most noble melancholy" (*melancholia generosissima Dureri*); see Raymond Klibansky, Erwin Panofsky, and Fritz Saxl, *Saturn and Melancholy: Studies in the History of Natural Philosophy, Religion, and Art* ([London]: Nelson, 1964), p. 319 n.117. Cf. Hans Rupprich (ed.), *Dürer: Schriftlicher Nachlass*, 3 vols. (Berlin: Deutscher Verein für Kunstwissenschaft, 1956–69), vol. 1, p. 319 (no. 27), Melanchthon's remarks in the *Commentaria de anima* (Wittenberg 1548); also Erwin Panofsky, *Albrecht Dürer*, 2 vols. (Princeton: Princeton University Press, 1943), vol. 1, p. 171; and Joseph Leo Koerner, *The Moment of Self-Portraiture in German Renaissance Art* (Chicago: University of Chicago Press, 1993), p. 27.

14. Klibansky, Panofsky, and Saxl, *Saturn and Melancholy*, p. 304, quoted and discussed in Wojciech Bałus, "Dürer's *Melencolia I:* Melancholy and the Undecidable," *Artibus et historiae* 15.30 (1994), p. 9.

15. Karl Giehlow, "Dürers Stich Melencolia I und der maximilianische Humanistenkreis," *Mitteilungen der Gesellschaft für vervielfältigende Künste* 26.2 (1903), pp. 29–41; 27.3 (1904), pp. 6–18; and 27.4 (1904), pp. 57–78; a useful overview is Schuster, *Melencolia I*, vol. 1, pp. 29–32.

16. Erwin Panofsky and Fritz Saxl, *Dürers 'Melencolia I': Eine quellen- und typengeschichtliche Untersuchung* (Leipzig and Berlin: B. G. Teubner, 1923); overview in Schuster, *Melencolia I*, vol. 1, pp. 34–36. After Giehlow's untimely death (at age forty-nine) in March 1913, Saxl and Panofsky were recruited by Arpad Weixlgärtner to bring his unfinished book, then in manuscript, to publication, using their latest research on astrological sources as

an appendix; they instead synthesized Giehlow's research with their own and published it under their own names. For an account of the book's genesis, see *ibid.*, pp. ix–xv ("Zum Geleite" by Weixlgärtner). Giehlow's study of hieroglyphics in the Renaissance is now republished as *The Humanist Interpretation of Hieroglyphs in the Allegorical Studies of the Renaissance*, trans. Robin Raybould (Leiden: Brill, 2015). Before Panofsky and Saxl completed their work, the conversation was joined by Aby Warburg, who originally was to receive the Giehlow commission but could not, due to "manifold circumstances," take it on—a veiled reference, it seems, to Warburg's mental health problems. His 1919 publication is discussed below.

17. Panofsky was not the first to recognize a self-reflexive element in Melancholy's "faustian" striving for impossible knowledge; it was anticipated by the physician and painter Carl Gustav Carus (1789–1869) in his 1835 essay, "Briefen über Goethe's *Faust*"; see Schuster, *Melencolia I*, vol. 1, pp. 22–23, with references. Panofsky, however, irrevocably stamped the idea with both the appearance of empirical certainty and unequaled sympathetic conviction.

18. See my discussion in Chapter 4.

19. In his text Isidore expressly calls for seven *figurae*, all but one of them *rotae*, setting the stage for the widespread use of wheel diagrams in scientific manuscripts; see John E. Murdoch, *Album of Science: Antiquity and the Middle Ages* (New York: Charles Scribner's Sons, 1984), pp. 52–61; also Robert Herrlinger, *History of Medical Illustration: From Antiquity to 1600*, trans. Graham Fulton-Smith (New York: Editions Medicina Rara, 1970), p. 31 (fig. 30) and p. 53 (figs. 74–75); and Simona Cohen, *Transformations of Time and Temporality in Medieval and Renaissance Art* (Leiden: Brill, 2014), pp. 66–71.

20. Klibansky, Panofsky, and Saxl, *Saturn and Melancholy*, pp. 15–41. For recent studies of the *Problemata*, see Eckart Schrütrumpf, "Black Bile as the Cause of Human Accomplishments and Behaviors in *Pr.* 30.1: Is the Concept Aristotelian?"; and Jason G. Rheins, "Homo numerans, venerans, or imitans? Human and Animal Cognition in Problemata 30.6," both in Robert Mayhew (ed.), *The Aristotelian Problemata Physica: Philosophical and Scientific Investigations* (Leiden: Brill, 2015), pp. 357–80 and 381–412, respectively.

21. Marsilio Ficino, *Three Books On Life*, ed. and trans. Carol V. Kaske and John R. Clark (Binghamton, NY: Medieval and Renaissance Texts and Studies, in conjunction with the Renaissance Society of America, 1989). Strictly speaking, book 1 is dedicated to health, book 2 to the prolongation of life, and book 3 to the effect of astral influences. Klibansky, Panofsky, and Saxl, in *Saturn and Melancholy*, overestimated the extent to which Renaissance medical thinking accepted Ficino's occultist extrapolation of the *Problemata*; for a corrective view, see Winfried Schleiner, *Melancholy, Genius and Utopia in the Renaissance* (Wiesbaden: Otto Harrassowitz, 1991), esp. pp. 31–56.

22. Panofsky and Saxl, *Dürers 'Melencolia I,'* p. 19; translation adapted from Benjamin, *The Origin of German Tragic Drama*, p. 149.

23. Panofsky's emphasis on the "struggle between the rational and irrational tendencies of the German national temperament" and its operative role in his Dürer monograph of 1943 is the focus of Keith Moxey, "Panofsky's Melancholia," in Moxey, *The Practice of Theory: Poststructuralism, Cultural Politics, and Art History* (Ithaca: Cornell University Press, 1994), pp. 65-78, esp. p. 74.

24. Konrad Hoffmann, "Dürers 'Melencolia,'" in Werner Busch, Reiner Haussherr, and Eduard Trier (eds.), *Kunst als Bedeutungsträger: Gedenkschrift für Günter Bandmann* (Berlin: Gebr. Mann, 1978), pp. 251-77, abridged and translated as "Dürer's 'Melencolia,'" *Print Collector's Newsletter* 9.2 (May-June 1978), pp. 33-35. For its propagandistic reach, Hoffman singles out the *Almanach* of the Swabian astronomer and mathematician Johannes Stöffler, published in Ulm in 1499. Hoffman's arguments actually reprise those of Warburg's famous essay of 1919, "Pagan-Antique Prophecy . . ." (see below, n.27).

25. Frances Yates, "Chapman and Dürer on Inspired Melancholy," *University of Rochester Library Bulletin* 34 (1981), pp. 25-44, concluding that Reuchlin's reworking of the Agrippan system in *De verbo mirifico*, a synthesis of white magic and kabbalah that Dürer could have easily accessed before 1514, "was probably the main inspiration of his engraving" (p. 32).

26. *Ibid.*, p. 32.

27. Originally published as "Heidnisch-antike Weissagung in Wort und Bild zu Luthers Zeiten," in *Sitzungsberichte der Heidelberger Akademie der Wissenschaften, Philosophisch-Historische Klasse*, 26 (1919) (Heidelberg, 1920); translated as "Pagan-Antique Prophecy in Words and Images in the Age of Luther," in Aby Warburg, *The Renewal of Pagan Antiquity: Contributions to the Cultural History of the European Renaissance*, trans. David Britt (Los Angeles: Getty Research Institute for the History of Art and the Humanities, 1999), pp. 597-697.

28. This emphasis exemplifies Warburg's deep agenda, which in Peter Gay's words was "not merely an art historian's prescription for the understanding of the Renaissance . . . but an *Aufklärer*'s prescription for life in a world threatened by unreason." Peter Gay, "Weimar Culture: The Outsider as Insider," in Donald Fleming and Bernard Bailyn (eds.), *The Intellectual Migration: Europe and America, 1930-1960* (Cambridge, MA: Belknap Press of Harvard University Press, 1969), p. 39. See also Schuster, *Melencolia I*, vol. 1, pp. 32-34; and Moxey, "Panofsky's Melancholia," p. 71. For Warburg's self-understanding as a "Bildhistoriker, kein Kunsthistoriker," see Horst Bredekamp, "A Neglected Tradition? Art History as *Bildwissenschaft*," *Critical Inquiry* 29 (Spring 2003), p. 423.

29. On this aspect of Warburg's thought, see Gay, "Weimar Culture," p. 39; and Moxey, "Panofsky's Melancholia," p. 71.

30. Panofsky and Saxl, *Dürers 'Melencolia I,'* p. 54 n.1.

31. Thomas DaCosta Kaufmann, "Hermeneutics in the History of Art: Remarks on the Reception of Dürer in the Sixteenth and Early Seventeenth Centuries," in Jeffrey Chipps Smith (ed.), *New Perspectives on the Art of Renaissance Nuremberg: Five Essays* (Austin: University of Texas Press, 1985), p. 35.

32. Benjamin, *The Origin of German Tragic Drama*, pp. 148–58, with quoted material at p. 140 and p. 158, respectively. After receiving the book, Panofsky sent back a "cold, resentment-laden letter"; see Wolfgang Bock, *Walter Benjamin—Die Rettung der Nacht: Sterne, Melancholie und Messianismus* (Bielefeld: Aisthesis, 2000), p. 69 n.29, with references. Referring to the same episode, George Steiner (introduction to Benjamin, *The Origin of German Tragic Drama*) expresses the belief that the Warburg Institute would have made a fitting intellectual home for Benjamin and accords Panofsky's rejection life-or-death implications for the struggling critic: "Panoskfy could have rescued Benjamin from isolation; an invitation to London might have averted an early death" (p. 19). See also Wolfgang Kemp, "Walter Benjamin und die Kunstwissenschaft, Teil 2: Walter Benjamin und Aby Warburg," *Kritische Berichte* 3.1 (1975), pp. 5–25; and Camille, "Walter Benjamin and Dürer's *Melencolia I*," pp. 59–60.

33. Ernst Cassirer, quoted in Michael Podro, *The Critical Historians of Art* (New Haven: Yale University Press, 1982), p. 182; discussed in Camille, "Walter Benjamin and Dürer's *Melencolia I*," p. 63. Also see Michael Ann Holly, *Panofsky and the Foundations of Art History* (Ithaca: Cornell University Press, 1984), pp. 114–57.

34. *Melencolia*'s ravishment in this regard can largely be blamed on the "magic square," which for decades has mesmerized hunters of secrets and code breakers both fictional (such as Harvard "symbology" professor Robert Langdon in Dan Brown's *The Lost Symbol*) and real (such as Würzburg philosophy professor Leonhard G. Richter, recent author of *Dürer-Code: Albrecht Dürers entschlüsselte Meisterstiche*). I discuss the magic square in Chapter 4.

35. See the conclusions of Doorly, "Dürer's *Melencolia I*," p. 272. Arguing that *Melencolia I* is based on Plato's *Greater Hippias* and that the major symbols illustrate the "value of mathematics" according to Fra Luca Pacioli's treatise *De divina proportione* (1509), the author claims that Dürer turned to the imagery of melancholy as a convenient metaphor for the abandoned search for Platonic beauty.

36. See Chapter 4.

37. For example, Thomas Schauerte, "Von der 'Philosophia' zur 'Melencolia I': Anmerkungen zu Dürers Philosophie-Holzschnitt für Konrad Celtis," in Franz Fuchs (ed.), *Konrad Celtis und Nürnberg: Akten des interdisziplinären Symposions vom 8. und 9. November 2002 im Caritas-Pirckheimer-Haus in Nürnberg* (Wiesbaden: Harrassowitz, 2004), pp. 117–39, who, drawing from Schuster's designation *Denkbild* (see below), usefully places *Melencolia* in a group of Dürerian "thought and puzzle images" (*Denk- und Rätselbilder*), a species that includes the *Philosophia* woodcut of 1502 (see figure 4.12), the *Nemesis* (see figure 2.8), the so-called *Hercules at the Crossroads*, and several others (pp. 132–33); Schauerte nevertheless assumes a more or less intelligible "symbolic picture-language" (*symbolischen Bildersprache*) requiring an act of "decryption" (*Entschlüsselung*) by the beholder.

38. Peter-Klaus Schuster, "Das Bild der Bilder: Zur Wirkungsgeschichte von Dürers Melancholiekupferstich," *Idea: Jahrbuch der Hamburger Kunsthalle* 1 (1982), pp. 72–134.

39. See Matthias Mende, *Dürer-Bibliographie* (Wiesbaden: Harrassowitz, 1971), pp. 246–51; Jane Campbell Hutchison, *Albrecht Dürer: A Guide to Research* (New York: Garland, 2000); also Kaufmann, "Hermeneutics in the History of Art"; and Schuster, "Das Bild der Bilder."

40. See esp. Michael Ann Holly, "Interventions: The Melancholy Art," *Art Bulletin* 89.1 (March 2007), pp. 7–17.

41. Schuster's *Melencolia I* is an expansion of his Göttingen dissertation of 1975; preceded by Schuster, "Bild der Bilder." Ultimately, Schuster does not escape Panofsky's shadow, in the final analysis embracing the idea of a "spiritual self-portrait" (vol. 1, pp. 402–404), understood as a function of the picture's true identity as an "kunsttheoretisches Thesenblatt." For the opposition of virtue and fortune, which led Schuster to propose a structural divide between the engraving's left and right zones, see vol. 1, pp. 163–76. A helpful critique of this proposal is offered by Rainer Hoffmann, *Im Zwielicht: Zu Albrecht Dürers Meisterstich* Melencolia I (Cologne: Böhlau, 2014), pp. 39–46. Despite all this, Schuster's study remains indispensible for Dürer research.

42. In this scheme, the 1504 *Adam and Eve* engraving supposedly represents the "sanguine" type, but this proposal introduces more problems than it solves; see the critique by Matthias Mende in Schoch, Mende, and Scherbaum, *Albrecht Dürer*, vol. 1, no. 71, pp. 166–68.

43. On the modern genealogy of the term, see Gerhard Richter, *Thought-Images: Frankfurt School Writers' Reflections from Damaged Life* (Stanford: Stanford University Press, 2007).

44. Camille, "Walter Benjamin and Dürer's *Melencolia I*," p. 68. See also in this connection Günter Grass's "modern variations" on Dame Melancholy, a lecture delivered on the occasion of the Dürer quincentennial of 1971, translated as "On Stasis in Progress: Variations of Albrecht Dürer's Engraving *Melencolia I*," in Bartrum et al., *Albrecht Dürer and His Legacy*, pp. 61–76.

45. Schuster's remarks on Benjamin in *Melencolia I* are largely confined to questions of the reception history of Dürer's print: Benjamin's projection of melancholic attributes onto Paul Klee's *Angelus Novus* watercolor (which he owned) in the "Theses on the Philosophy of History" of 1940 (vol. 1, p. 396) and the thematization of unrealizable hope in the *Einbahnstraße* of 1928 (vol. 1, p. 412).

46. Hartmut Böhme, *Albrecht Dürer, Melencolia I: Im Labyrinth der Deutung* (Frankfurt am Main: Fischer Tachenbuch, 1987). Similar questions would soon be raised with regard to that other great "enigma" of art history, Bosch's *Garden of Earthly Delights* triptych in Madrid; see Keith Moxey, "Hieronymus Bosch and the 'World Upside Down': The Case of *The Garden of Earthly Delights*," in Norman Bryson, Michael Ann Holly, and Keith Moxey (eds.), *Visual Culture: Images and Interpretations* (Middletown, CT: Wesleyan University Press, 1994), pp. 104–40.

47. Koerner, *The Moment of Self-Portraiture in German Renaissance Art*, p. 23. This "abstract" melancholic inwardness of the Renaissance Koerner contrasts with the "substantialized" inwardness of medieval thought, exemplified in the attribution of melancholy to humoral excess and its moral interpretation as an offshoot of *acedia* (p. 26).

48. Martin Büchsel, "Die gescheiterte 'Melancholia generosa': *Melencolia I*," *Städel-Jahrbuch*, new series 9 (1983), p. 110. Much commentary from 1980 onward has learned to see this symbolic *Widersprüchlichkeit*, if not its very construction, as a byproduct of the historical accumulation of interpretative receptions, scholarly and artistic, of Dürer's engraving; there is, in a sense, no other objectively valid starting point. See Schuster, *Melencolia I*, vol. 1, p. 84; also Sohm, "Dürer's *Melencolia I*": "Dürer planned disparate ideas to coincide with a single object" (p. 24); and Bałus, "Dürer's *Melencolia I*": "Melancholy is thus a state of undecidability" (p. 18).

49. Hoffman claims for *Melencolia I*, among other things, a critique of Scholasticism's overvaluation of human reason in apprehending God; see Hoffman, "Dürers 'Melencolia,'" p. 255.

50. It is easy enough to mistake the dead ends of iconographical method for the limitedness of knowledge in general, but this does not disprove the point; epistemic irresolution, after all, comes in many intellectual flavors. For a discussion of *Melencolia* as an exposure of the limits of knowing, see esp. Sohm, "Dürer's *Melencolia I*."

51. William J. Bouwsma, "The Renaissance Discovery of Human Creativity," in John W. O'Malley, Thomas M. Izbicki, and Gerald Christianson (eds.), *Humanity and Divinity in Renaissance and Reformation: Essays in Honor of Charles Trinkhaus* (Leiden: Brill, 1993), p. 24.

52. Benjamin, *The Origin of German Tragic Drama*, p. 140. It was on this basis that Benjamin could assert that *Melencolia* anticipates the Baroque.

53. See *ibid.*, pp. 180–82, and Camille's trenchant commentary ("Walter Benjamin and Dürer's *Melencolia I*," p. 67). For a recent application of Benjamin's dialectical concept of "dead" works of art, see Amy Knight Powell, *Depositions: Scenes from the Late Medieval Church and Modern Museum* (New York: Zone Books, 2012), pp. 258–60.

54. Although I share Koerner's view of the work as undecipherable and therefore as an "occasion" for a certain kind of thought, I would question the more radical insistence that *Melencolia* "seems to articulate a pivotal moment in the history of subjectivity"; see Koerner, *The Moment of Self-Portraiture in German Renaissance Art*, p. 26.

55. Bałus, "Dürer's *Melencolia I*," p. 17.

CHAPTER TWO: RESTLESS EYE, ACTIVE MIND

The epigraph is from Michel Jeanneret, *Perpetual Motion: Transforming Shapes in the Renaissance from Da Vinci to Montaigne*, trans. Nidra Poller (Baltimore: Johns Hopkins University Press, 2001), p. 82.

1. Walter Strauss, *The Complete Engravings, Etchings and Drypoints of Albrecht Dürer* (New

York: Dover, 1973), no. 77; Rainer Schoch, Matthias Mende, and Anna Scherbaum, *Albrecht Dürer: Das druckgraphische Werk*, 3 vols. (Munich: Prestel, 2001–2004), vol. 1, no. 70.

2. Erwin Panofsky, *Albrecht Dürer*, 2 vols. (Princeton: Princeton University Press, 1943), vol. 1, p. 156; Philip L. Sohm, "Dürer's *Melencolia I:* The Limits of Knowledge," *Studies in the History of Art* 9 (1980), p. 13; Wojciech Bałus, "Dürer's *Melencolia I:* Melancholy and the Undecidable," *Artibus et historiae* 15.30 (1994), pp. 12–14. On the patterns of *Melencolia*'s distribution during the Netherlands journey, with a critique of past arguments favoring a thematic association of the two engravings, see Robert Grigg, "Studies on Dürer's Diary of His Journey to the Netherlands: The Distribution of the 'Melancolia I,'" *Zeitschrift für Kunstgeschichte* 49.3 (1986), pp. 398–409.

3. Albrecht Dürer, *Underweysung der messung mit dem zirkel und richtscheyt in Linien ebnen unnd gantzen corporen* (Nuremberg, 1525), and Dürer, *Hierin sind begriffen vier Bücher von menschlicher Proportion* (Nuremberg, 1528). For the evolution of Dürer's work as an art theorist, see esp. Panofsky, *Albrecht Dürer*, vol. 1, pp. 242–84; also Patrick Doorly, "Dürer's *Melencolia I:* Plato's Abandoned Search for the Beautiful," *Art Bulletin* 86.2 (June 2004), pp. 258–59, with additional bibliography on this expansive topic.

4. Bałus, "Dürer's *Melencolia I,*" p. 12. See also William S. Heckscher, "*Melancholia* (1541): An Essay in the Rhetoric of Description by Joachim Camerarius," in Frank Baron (ed.), *Joachim Camerarius (1500–1574): Beiträge zur Geschichte des Humanismus im Zeitalter der Reformation / Essays On the History of Humanism during the Reformation* (Munich: Wilhelm Fink, 1978), pp. 54–56, who describes the visual strategy as a turning "away from the principles of artistic 'ordinatio' (the art of arranging objects as if on a depth-oriented stage)" (p. 54), with the help of "the untranslatable German word Ineinanderschachtelung" (p. 55).

5. Bałus, "Dürer's *Melencolia I,*" p. 12. On lighting effects in *Melencolia I,* also see Peter Parshall, "Albrecht Dürer and the Axis of Meaning," *Bulletin of the Allen Memorial Art Museum* 50.2 (1997), pp. 21–22.

6. David Pingree, "A New Look at *Melencolia I,*" *Journal of the Warburg and Courtauld Institutes* 43 (1980), pp. 257–58.

7. Bałus, "Dürer's *Melencolia I,*" p. 14.

8. Peter Parshall, "Graphic Knowledge: Albrecht Dürer and the Imagination," *Art Bulletin* 95.3 (September 2013), p. 404.

9. Luigi Toccacieli, *Melencolia I di Albrecht Dürer: Un modo di leggere un'opera d'arte incisoria* (Milan: Silvana Editoriale, 2008), p. 28 (pl. 9). For an earlier and more cautious "reconstructive analysis" of *Melencolia,* see Eberhard Schröder, *Dürer: Kunst und Geometrie. Dürers künstlerisches Schaffen aus der Sicht seiner "Underweysung"* (Basel: Birkhäuser, 1980), pp. 64–75.

10. *Melancholia,* Camerarius's 175-word essay devoted wholly to the engraving, was among the ancient and modern pieces the author assembled for the benefit of his students in Tübingen in the *Elementa rhetoricae,* an introduction to the art of rhetoric arranged according to twenty categories; for translation and commentary, see Heckscher, "*Melancholia* (1541)," pp. 31–120.

11. Heinrich Wölfflin, *The Art of Albrecht Dürer*, trans. Alastair Grieve and Heide Grieve (London: Phaidon, 1971), p. 204, who urges the reader to cover up the ladder, an experiment that reveals just how calm the whole *can* look without it: "The lack of a framework, the chaos of the whole, has an unpleasant effect."

12. Heckscher suggests that Camerarius's iconographic frame of reference, and possibly Dürer's as well, was the proverbial wasted effort of those who struggle "to overturn the rock" (*saxum uoluere*), illustrated by Erasmus in the *Adages* by the myth of Sisyphus; see Heckscher, "*Melancholia* (1541)," p. 60.

13. Strauss, *Complete Engravings*, no. 78; Schoch, Mende, and Scherbaum, *Albrecht Dürer*, vol. 1, no. 73.

14. Parshall, "Albrecht Dürer and the Axis of Meaning," p. 21.

15. Panofsky, *Albrecht Dürer*, vol. 1, pp. 160–61; cf. Raymond Klibansky, Erwin Panofsky, and Fritz Saxl, *Saturn and Melancholy: Studies in the History of Natural Philosophy, Religion, and Art* ([London]: Nelson, 1964), pp. 400–402.

16. Terence Lynch, "The Geometric Body in Dürer's Engraving *Melencolia I*," *Journal of the Warburg and Courtauld Institutes* 45 (1982), p. 230.

17. See *ibid.* on this and some of what follows on the polyhedron.

18. Doorly, "Dürer's *Melencolia I*," pp. 269–70, considers the form a deliberately "botched dodecahedron," a form therefore emblematic of Geometry/Melancholy's failure to find a "visual equivalent of the beautiful itself." Cf. the analysis of the polyhedron's deliberate deformation by Ewald Lassnig, "Dürers 'Melencolia-I' und die Erkenntnistheorie bei Ulrich Pinder: Versuch einer Interpretation aus einer Naheliegenden Quelle," *Wiener Jahrbuch für Kunstgeschichte* 57 (2008), pp. 75–82, where it emblematizes a third, still-imperfect stage in the "recognition-process" (*Erkenntnisprozess*) thematized by the picture overall (p. 95).

19. Lynch, "The Geometric Body in Dürer's Engraving *Melencolia I*," p. 228, fig. 5.

20. Bałus, "Dürer's *Melencolia I*," p. 12.

21. Remarked by several earlier writers, the observation is developed furthest by Patrik Reuterswärd, "Sinn und Nebensinn bei Dürer: Randbemerkungen zur 'Melencolia I,'" in Robert Mühler and Johann Fischl (eds.), *Gestalt und Wirklichkeit: Festgabe für Ferdinand Weinhandl* (Berlin: Duncker & Humblot, 1967), pp. 411–36, who interprets *Melencolia* as a *vanitas* image. The present author is among those who can't make out the phantom face.

22. Toccacieli, *Melencolia I di Albrecht Dürer*, pl. 5.

23. Strauss, *Complete Engravings*, no. 37; Schoch, Mende, and Scherbaum, *Albrecht Dürer*, vol. 1, no. 33, pp. 95–99; see also Heckscher, "*Melancholia* (1541)," p. 60. In the woodcut from Charles de Bovelles's *Liber de Sapiente* (Paris, 1510), depicting the confrontation of Fortune and Wisdom (see figure 5.13), Virtue is enthroned upon a sphere (*Sedes fortvne rotvda*) and Wisdom upon a solid rectangular one (*Sedes virtvtis qvadrata*). For this and further aspects of Dürer's Fortuna imagery, see Chapter 5.

24. The German edition of Petrarch was conceived by Sebastian Brant, who evidently worked closely with the pictures' designer (according to the prologue, the work was based on "visierlicher Angebung des Hochgelehrten Doctoris Sebastiani Brant"). For the complete cycle, see Walther Scheidig, *Die Holzschnitte des Petrarca-Meister zu Petrarcas Werk "Von der Artzney bayder Gluck des guten und widerwärtigen"—Augsburg 1532* (Berlin: Henschelverlag, 1955), p. 50; for more recent analyses of the woodcuts, see Karl A. E. Enenkel, "Der Petrarca des 'Petrarca-Meisters': Zum Text-Bild-Verhältnis in illustrierten De Remediis-Ausgaben," in Karl A. E. Enenkel and Jan Papy (eds.), *Petrarch and His Readers in the Renaissance* (Boston: Brill, 2006), pp. 91–170; and Reindert Falkenburg, "Speculative Imagery in Petrarch's *Von der Artzney bayder Glück* (1532)," in *ibid.*, pp. 171–92.

25. Falkenburg, "Speculative Imagery," p. 187.

26. *Ibid.*, p. 188.

27. *Ibid.*, p. 187.

28. *Ibid.*, p. 184.

29. John Dewey, *Art as Experience* (New York: Minton, Balch, and Company, 1934), p. 52.

30. To the extent that human vision itself participates in the malady brought on by the Fall (what Joseph Koerner has called "fallen vision"), it, too, could be a source of misery and stand in need of remedy, though I'm not sure I agree with Falkenburg's closing observation that speculative imagery also provides a "consoling" of the eyes (p. 188).

31. Heckscher, "*Melancholia* (1541)," pp. 53–54, referring to an influential eleventh-century commentary ("rerum dimensio et pondus . . . quantitates sive mensurae rerum"), which in turn reprises Wisdom 11:21: "but thou hast ordered all things in measure, and number, and weight" (*sed omnia in mensura, et numero et pondere disposuisti*).

32. Ernst Cassirer, *The Individual and the Cosmos in Renaissance Philosophy*, trans. Mario Domandi (Oxford: Basil Blackwell, 1963), p. 9.

33. Heckscher, "*Melancholia* (1541)," p. 56. See also Sohm, "Dürer's *Melencolia I*," p. 30.

34. Sohm, "Dürer's *Melencolia I*," p. 30.

35. Heckscher, "*Melancholia* (1541)," p. 57. On the realization of these two directional models in medieval aesthetic experience, see Mary J. Carruthers, *The Experience of Beauty in the Middle Ages* (Oxford: Oxford University Press, 2013), pp. 12–13.

36. On this point, see Doorly, "Dürer's *Melencolia I*," p. 267.

37. Most recently, Michael Stolberg, "Lucas Cranachs 'Melencolia'-Darstellungen und die zeitgenössische Medizin," in Stefan Oehmig (ed.), *Medizin und Sozialwesen in Mitteldeutschland zur Reformationszeit* (Leipzig: Evangelische Verlagsanstalt, 2007), pp. 249–71. Chapter 4 offers a sustained examination of this theme.

38. V. A. Kolve, *Chaucer and the Imagery of Narrative: The First Five Canterbury Tales* (Stanford: Stanford University Press, 1984), p. 30.

39. George W. McClure, *Sorrow and Consolation in Italian Humanism* (Princeton: Princeton University Press, 1991), p. 49.

40. Bałus, "Dürer's *Melencolia I*," p. 16.

41. This model of understanding the communicative function of prints is discussed in Shira Brisman, "The Image That Wants to Be Read: An Invitation to Interpretation in a Drawing by Albrecht Dürer," *Word and Image* 29.3 (2013), pp. 273–303, who describes the exchange as one "in which the image steers the viewer's behavior, and the viewer directs the image's performance."

42. For these two trends respectively, see Falkenburg, "Speculative Imagery"; and Leopoldine van Hogendorp Prosperetti, "Viola Animae: The Art of Jan Brueghel the Elder and the Tradition of Devout Naturalism," *Italian Quarterly* 46.179–182 (Winter–Fall 2009), pp. 107–21. Also my "*Pro remedio animae*: Works of Mercy as Therapeutic Genre," in Birgit Münch and Jürgen Müller (eds.), *Peiraikos' Erben: Die Genese der Genremalerei bis 1500* (Wiesbaden: Reichert, 2015), pp. 97–124.

43. Jeffrey F. Hamburger, "Speculations on Speculation: Vision and Perception in the Theory and Practice of Mystical Devotion," in Walter Haug and Wolfram Schneider-Lastin (eds.), *Deutsche Mystik im abendländischen Zusammenhang: Neu erschlossene Texte, neue methodische Ansätze, neue theoretische Konzepte* (Tübingen: Max Niemeyer, 2000), pp. 353–408; and Herbert L. Kessler, "Speculum," *Speculum* 86 (2011), pp. 1–41.

44. Hamburger, "Speculations on Speculation," p. 359.

45. Boethius, *De Consolatione Philosophiae* 5.6: "qui cum ex alta providentiae specula respexit ... praesentiae infinitaque praeteriti ac futuri spatia complectens omnia." Later, the watchtower metaphor was taken up by Aquinas to describe God's perfect universal foreknowledge: "God's eternity is in present contact with the whole course of time ... much in the way that a person standing on top of a watch-tower embraces in a single glance a whole caravan of passing travelers," *Summa Theologica*, 1aq.14a13, translation from *Compendium theologiae*, trans. Cyril Vollert (St. Louis: Herder, 1947), pp. 142–43. I am grateful to Marius Hauknes for sharing these references with me. His discussion of the *per speculum* and *ad specula* theme appears in Marius Hauknes, "The Painting of Knowledge in Thirteenth-Century Rome," *Gesta* 55.1 (Spring 2016), p. 38.

46. Hamburger, "Speculations on Speculation," p. 394.

47. Carruthers, *The Experience of Beauty in the Middle Ages*, p. 63.

48. I borrow the phrase from Peter Parshall, private correspondence with the author, April 2014.

49. Quoted and discussed in Carruthers, *The Experience of Beauty in the Middle Ages*, p. 155.

50. Jeanneret, *Perpetual Motion*, p. 16, who sees the fallacy of a "compartmented world" as arising from the "fixist variant" of Christian cosmology (p. 26).

51. Quoted in McClure, *Sorrow and Consolation*, p. 47. In the second book of the *Secretum*, we hear the protagonist Franciscus complaining about the temporary effectiveness of the benefits brought by the study of philosophical wisdom, "their effect," McClure explains,

"disappearing soon after his readings were completed" (p. 46). In McClure's view, the response of Augustinus, who urged his partner to employ his memory and craft a personal trove of "salutary maxims," heralds Petrarch's project of compiling a handbook of remedies, which he realized with *De remediis*.

52. Klibansky, Panofsky, and Saxl, *Saturn and Melancholy*, p. 245.

53. *Ibid.*, p. 243.

54. On the Petrarchan paternity of this crisis, see Robert M. Durling, "The Ascent of Mount Ventoux and the Crisis of Allegory," *Italian Quarterly* 18 (1974), pp. 7–28.

CHAPTER THREE: THERAPIES OF THE IMAGE

The epigraph is from the Benjamin Jowett translation of the *Timaeus* and is quoted and discussed in Jacques Derrida, *Dissemination*, trans. Barbara Johnson (Chicago: University of Chicago Press, 1981), pp. 100–101.

1. The medievalist Aron Gurevich usefully defines magic as "a specific mode of human behavior which disregards natural causality and is based on the expectation of results from men's participation in the universe. . . . An ultimate unity and a reciprocal penetration of nature and humankind, organically connected with each other and magically interactive, are taken for granted." Aron Gurevich, *Medieval Popular Culture: Problems of Belief and Perception*, trans. János M. Bak and Paul A. Hollingsworth (New York: Cambridge University Press, 1988), p. 81.

2. On specialization, see Max J. Friedländer, *Landscape, Portrait, Still-Life: Their Origin and Development*, trans. R. F. C. Hull (Oxford: B. Cassirer, 1949); on Italian art theory, E. H. Gombrich, "The Renaissance Theory of Art and the Rise of Landscape," in Gombrich, *Norm and Form: Studies in the Art of the Renaissance* (Oxford: Phaidon, 1966), pp. 107–21; on the effect of cartography, David Summers, *Vision, Reflection, and Desire in Western Painting* (Chapel Hill: University of North Carolina Press, 2007), pp. 82–110.

3. In Ficino's *Commentarium . . . in convivium Platonis de amore* of 1469, chapter 9, he asks, "for what is more agreeable to the spirits of the human body than the voices and faces of men; especially of those who are pleasing not only because of the similarity of nature, but also because of their beauty? Therefore, the choleric and melancholic men pursue, as if the only remedy and solace for their most troublesome complexion of those humors, the pleasures of song and physical form"; *Marsilio Ficino's Commentary on Plato's Symposium*, trans. Sears Reynolds Jayne (Columbia, MO: University of Missouri, 1944), p. 196. On Ficino's music therapy, see Jacomien Prins, "A Philosophic Music Therapy for Melancholy in Marsilio Ficino's 'Timaeus Commentary,'" in Andrea Sieber and Antje Wittstock (eds.), *Melancholie—zwischen Attitüde und Diskurs: Konzepte in Mittelalter und Früher Neuzeit* (Göttingen: V & R Unipress, 2009), pp. 119–43; and my discussion in Chapter 6.

4. Frances Gage, "Exercise for Mind and Body: Giulio Mancini, Collecting, and the Beholding of Landscape Painting in the Seventeenth Century," *Renaissance Quarterly* 61.4

(Winter 2008), p. 1168. A more expansive treatment of this important topic is Frances Gage, *Painting As Medicine in Early Modern Rome: Giulio Mancini and the Efficacy of Art* (University Park: Pennsylvania State University Press, 2016), which appeared after the present chapter was written.

5. Robert Burton, *The Anatomy of Melancholy*, ed. Nicolas K. Kiessling, Thomas C. Faulkner, and Rhonda L Blair, 6 vols. (Oxford: Clarendon Press of Oxford University Press, 1990), vol. 2, p. 85.

6. Gage, "Exercise for Mind and Body," p. 1168.

7. For example, in Melanchthon's effort to detail the interrelation of the soul with the senses, appetites, affects, knowledge, and will through his rereading of Aristotle's *De anima*. Begun in 1533, the *Commentarius de anima* was published in 1540. On this aspect of sixteenth-century natural philosophy, see Sachiko Kusukawa, *The Transformation of Natural Philosophy: The Case of Philip Melanchthon* (Cambridge: Cambridge University Press, 1995), esp. pp. 75–123.

8. Georges Vigarello, "The Upward Training of the Body from the Age of Chivalry to Courtly Civility," in Michel Feher, Ramona Naddaff, and Nadia Tazi (eds.), *Zone 4: Fragments for a History of the Human Body* (New York: Zone Books, 1989), pp. 149–99.

9. Leon Battista Alberti, *Ten Books on Architecture*, bk. 9, ch. 4; quoted and discussed in Gombrich, "The Renaissance Theory of Art and the Rise of Landscape," p. 111. Alberti's ideas about the benefits of viewing water were widely shared by Renaissance physicians; see Gage, *Painting As Medicine in Early Modern Rome*, p. 62.

10. Cited in Gombrich, "The Renaissance Theory of Art and the Rise of Landscape," p. 108.

11. See Reindert L. Falkenburg, *Joachim Patinir: Landscape as an Image of the Pilgrimage of Life*, trans. Michael Hoyle (Amsterdam: Benjamins, 1988), who considers Patinir's landscapes as "meditational images of the pilgrimage of life" (p. 106), but refrains from explicating their therapeutic procedure. For the Antwerp panel illustrated here, see pp. 6, 55, and 65 n.258. On the pilgrimage topos, see Susan K. Hagen, *Allegorical Remembrance: A Study of* The Pilgrimage of the Life of Man *as a Medieval Treatise on Seeing and Remembering* (Athens: University of Georgia Press, 1990); Matthew Botvinick, "The Painting as Pilgrimage: Traces of a Subtext in the Work of Campin and His Contemporaries," *Art History* 15.1 (March 1992), pp. 1–18; Kathryn M. Rudy, "A Guide to Mental Pilgrimage: Paris, Bibliothéque de l'Arsenal ms. 212," *Zeitschrift für Kunstgeschichte* 63.4 (2000), pp. 494–515; and Mitzi Kirkland-Ives, *In the Footsteps of Christ: Hans Memling's Passion Narratives and the Devotional Imagination in the Early Modern Netherlands* (Turnhout: Brepols, 2012).

12. Leopoldine van Hogendorp Prosperetti, *Landscape and Philosophy in the Art of Jan Brueghel the Elder (1568–1625)* (Burlington: Ashgate, 2009), esp. pp. 44–46 on the neo-Stoic "doctrina serena."

13. Similarly, for some medieval writers, the speculative itineraries encountered in or

produced by the process of reading could be occasions for the exercise of mind, soul, and body; see the example of Peter of Celle (d. 1183) in Mary J. Carruthers, *The Experience of Beauty in the Middle Ages* (Oxford: Oxford University Press, 2013), pp. 139–40.

14. Quoted with references in Gage, "Exercise for Mind and Body," pp. 1167–68.

15. For recent contributions across cultures, media, and disciplines, see Dick Houtman and Birgit Meyer (eds.), *Things: Religion and the Question of Materiality* (New York: Fordham University Press, 2012); and Dietrich Boschung and Jan. N. Bremmer (eds.), *The Materiality of Magic* (Paderborn: Wilhelm Fink, 2015).

16. On the implications for medieval visual culture, see Herbert L. Kessler, "Christ the Magic Dragon," *Gesta* 48 (2009), pp. 119–34; and Kessler, "A Sanctifying Serpent: Crucifix as Cure," in Karl F. Morrison and Rudolph M. Bell (eds.), *Studies in Medieval Empathies* (Turnhout: Brepols, 2013), pp. 161–85.

17. For essentials, see Kurt Weitzmann (ed.), *Age of Spirituality: Late Antique and Early Christian Art, Third to Seventh Century*, exhibition catalogue (New York: Metropolitan Museum of Art, 1979), p. 440 (cat. 398); also Jacquelyn Tuerk Stonberg, "An Early Byzantine Inscribed Amulet and its Narratives," *Byzantine and Modern Greek Studies* (1999), pp. 25–42. I thank James Magruder for discussing the New York amulet with me.

18. On this older class of amulets, see Jeffrey Spier, "Medieval Byzantine Magical Amulets and Their Tradition," *Journal of the Warburg and Courtauld Institutes* 56 (1993), pp. 25–62. For the larger family of medical tokens, amulets, rings, armbands, and pilgrimage objects, see Gary Vikan, "Art, Medicine, and Magic in Early Byzantium," *Dumbarton Oaks Papers* 38 (1984), pp. 65–86.

19. See Wikipedia, s.v. "Heliotrope (mineral)," https://en.wikipedia.org/wiki/Heliotrope_(mineral).

20. For Pliny on hematite, see Stonberg, "An Early Byzantine Inscribed Amulet," p. 30; for rust and its medicinal property as the "opposite nature" of iron, see Spike Bucklow, *The Alchemy of Paint: Art, Science and Secrets from the Middle Ages* (London: Marion Boyars, 2009), p. 127.

21. Véronique Dasen, "Probaskani: Amulets and Magic in Antiquity," in Boschung and Bremmer (eds.), *The Materiality of Magic*, p. 184.

22. *Ibid.*, p. 185.

23. Exemplary studies in this vast field include Bernhard Kötting, *Peregrinatio Religiosa: Wallfahrten in der Antike und das Pilgerwesen in der alten Kirche* (Münster: Regensbergsche, 1950); E. D. Hunt, *Holy Land Pilgrimage in the Later Roman Empire, AD 312–460* (Oxford: Clarendon Press of Oxford University Press, 1982); and Peter Brown, "The Rise and Function of the Holy Man in Late Antiquity," in Brown, *Society and the Holy in Late Antiquity* (Berkeley: University of California Press, 1982), pp. 103–52. See also the essays in Robert Ousterhout (ed.), *The Blessings of Pilgrimage* (Urbana: University of Illinois Press, 1990); and David Frankfurter (ed.), *Pilgrimage and Holy Space in Late Antique Egypt* (Leiden: Brill, 1998).

24. See Anna Pawlik, *Das Bildwerk als Reliquiar? Funktionen früher Großplastik im 9. bis 11. Jahrhundert* (Petersberg: Michael Imhoff, 2013), pp. 290–96 (cat. 35). The statue is named for its donor, Bishop Imad, who reigned as bishop of Paderborn from 1051 to 1076.

25. See especially Anton L. Mayer, "Die heilbringende Schau in Sitte und Kult," in Odo Casel (ed.), *Heilige Überlieferung: Ausschnitte aus der Geschichte des Mönchtums und des heiligen Kultes für Ildefons Herwegen* (Münster: Aschendorff, 1938), pp. 234–62. The evolution of these theories is critically traced by Hartmut Kühne, *Ostensio Reliquiarum: Untersuchungen über Entstehung, Ausbreitung, Gestalt und Funktion der Heiltumsweisungen im römische-deutschen Regnum* (Berlin: Walter de Gruyter, 2000), pp. 512–19.

26. Marcia Kupfer, *The Art of Healing: Painting for the Sick and the Sinner in a Medieval Town* (University Park: Pennsylvania State University Press, 2003), p. 1. On "holy matter" as a defining category in pre-Reformation Christianity, see esp. Caroline Walker Bynum, *Christian Materiality: An Essay on Religion in Late Medieval Europe* (New York: Zone Books, 2011).

27. Franz Niehoff (ed.), *Maria allerorten: Die Muttergottes mit dem geneigten Haupt 1699–1999. Das Gnadenbild der Ursulinen zu Landshut—Altbayerische Marienfrömmigkeit im 18. Jahrhundert*, exhibition catalogue (Landshut: Museen der Stadt Landshut, 1999), cat. 1/56b, with further examples discussed and illustrated. Cf. the German nineteenth-century lithographs with the crucified Christ published by A. Hyatt Mayor, *Prints and People: A Social History of Printed Pictures* (Princeton: Princeton University Press, 1971), fig. 12.

28. See my "*Lob und Danck*: On the Social Meaning of Votive Images before the Enlightenment," in Ittai Weinryb (ed.), *Agents of Faith: Material, Place, Memory*, exhibition catalogue (New Haven: Yale University Press, 2018), forthcoming.

29. See Peter Parshall and Rainer Schoch, *Origins of European Printmaking: Fifteenth-Century Woodcuts and Their Public*, exhibition catalogue, National Gallery of Art, Washington (New Haven: Yale University Press, 2005), cat. 93.

30. On the Roman theory of indulgences, see my *Pilgrimage and Pogrom: Violence, Memory, and Visual Culture at the Host-Miracle Shrines of Germany and Austria* (Chicago: University of Chicago Press, 2013), p. 181, with further references; on the *imago pietatis* and its German variants, pp. 83–91.

31. On these changes in the late medieval church's penitential system, see *ibid.*, pp. 4, 160, 179–81, with further references.

32. Christ's healing miracles were extolled as a better form of magic, but were nevertheless only tokens of the greatest power he wielded, aimed at the greatest of human infirmities: sin. The concept of Christ as the divine physician (*Christus medicus*) took shape in the second and third centuries amidst the struggle to displace the cult of Asclepius, and later found its clearest expression in Augustine, who knew from personal experience that the greatest joy was reserved for the recovery of one stricken so ill by sin that "his pulse portends the worst" since "that joy is always greater after greater affliction." Augustine

of Hippo, *Confessions*, trans. Gary Wills (New York: Penguin, 2002), bk. 8, p. 166. On the theme of *Christus medicus*, see Rudolf Arbesmann, "The Concept of 'Christus Medicus' in Augustine," *Traditio* 10 (1954), pp. 1–28; and Johann Anselm Seiger, *Medizinische Theologie: Christus Medicus und Theologia Medicinalis bei Martin Luther und im Luthertum der Barockzeit. Mit Edition dreier Quellentexte* (Leiden: Brill, 2005).

33. See Ruth Slenczka, *Lehrhafte Bildtafeln in spätmittelalterlichen Kirchen* (Cologne: Böhlau, 1998).

34. On the Old Testament sages as guides to wisdom, see John T. McNeill, *A History of the Cure of Souls* (New York: Harper & Brothers, 1951), pp. 1–16.

35. For the suggestion that color vibrations and the dazzling light effects of Grünewald's *Isenheim Altarpiece* were features of its therapeutic use within the setting of the Antonite hospital, see Andrée Hayum, *The Isenheim Altarpiece: God's Medicine and the Painter's Vision* (Princeton: Princeton University Press, 1989), pp. 13–52. For other hospital contexts, see John Henderson, *The Renaissance Hospital: Healing the Body and Healing the Soul* (New Haven: Yale University Press, 1999); Alessandro Orlandini, *Foundlings and Pilgrims: Frescoes in the Sala del Pellegrinaio of the Hospital of Santa Maria della Scala in Siena* (Siena: Nuova Immagine, 2002); Kupfer, *The Art of Healing*; Richard Cork, *The Healing Presence of Art: A History of Western Art in Hospitals* (New Haven: Yale University Press, 2012); and my discussion of Dürer's *Landauer Altar* in Chapter 6.

36. Kupfer, *The Art of Healing*, p. 3.

37. Erwin Panofsky, "*Imago Pietatis*: Ein Beitrag zur Typengeschichte des 'Schmerzensmanns' und der 'Maria Mediatrix'," in *Festschrift für Max J. Friedländer zum 60 Geburtstage* (Leipzig: Seemann, 1927), pp. 261–308.

38. The key account is Hans Belting, *Likeness and Presence: A History of the Image in the Era Before Art*, trans. Edmund Jephcott (Chicago: University of Chicago Press, 1994), esp. pp. 349–408.

39. Jean Wirth, *L'image à la fin du Moyen Âge* (Paris: Cerf, 2011), esp. his chapter 3, "Consolation," pp. 129–46.

40. For the larger altarpiece, see Peter Strieder, *Tafelmalerei in Nürnberg 1350–1550* (Königstein im Taunus: Langewiesche / Hans Köster, 1993), pp. 87–91, figs. 100–103 (cat. 73).

41. For essentials, see F. G. Zehnder (ed.), *Stefan Lochner Meister zu Köln: Herkunft—Werke—Wirkung*, exhibition catalogue (Cologne: Wallraf-Richartz-Museum, 1993), pp. 228–30.

42. On this point, I am embracing Pedro Laín Entralgo's thesis that ancient rhetorical theory, culminating in Aristotle, had already constructed a "fourth type of persuasive word" in addition to the three canonical types (judicial or forensic, deliberative, and apodictic or demonstrative); this he calls the "therapeutic or curative type" and considers it a "speculative form of verbal psychotherapy" that is found "in masked form" (174) in both the *Rhetoric* and, crucially, in Aristotle's theory of *katharsis* (in the *Poetics* and the *Politics*);

Pedro Laín Entralgo, *The Therapy of the Word in Classical Antiquity*, trans. L. J. Rather and John M. Sharp (New Haven: Yale University Press, 1970), pp. 174–79. See also Carruthers, *The Experience of Beauty in the Middle Ages*, pp. 31–35 and 41; and Prologue to Chapters 5 and 6.

43. Thomas Aquinas, *Summa Theologica*, part 1, question 1, article 9: "Est autem naturale homini ut per sensibilia ad intelligibilia veniat, quia omnis nostra cognitio a sensu initium habet" (But it is natural for man to approach intelligible things through sensible things, since all our cognition takes its origin from the senses); *New English Translation of St. Thomas Aquinas's Summa Theologiae (Summa Theologica)*, trans. Alfred J. Freddoso, available at http://www3.nd.edu/~afreddos/summa-translation/Part 1/st1-ques01.pdf, p. 9.

44. See the epigraph for Chapter 4 by Kierkegaard.

45. Religious objects and representations of all kinds thus were held up by churchmen and employed therapeutically by laypeople as *specula* of knowledge, virtue, faith, or love. Rooted in the moral-didactic tradition of *speculum* literature, such metaphorical mirrors exposed the blemishes—sins, lapses, and blindnesses of every conceivable kind—of those who used them with humility. See Herbert Grabes, *Speculum, Mirror und Looking Glass: Kontinuität und Orignalität der Spiegelmetapher in den Buchtiteln des Mittelalters und der englischen Literatur des 13. bis 17. Jahrhunderts* (Tubingen: Max Niemeyer, 1973). For an especially clear-sighted account of these metaphors, see the introduction to Frederick Goldin, *The Mirror of Narcissus in the Courtly Love Lyric* (Ithaca: Cornell University Press, 1967).

46. The following is summarized from my forthcoming essay, "'Return to Your True Self!': Practicing Spiritual Therapy with the *Spiegel der Vernunft* in Munich," in Debra Cashion, Ashley West, and Henry Luttikhuizen (eds.), *The Primacy of the Image in Northern European Art, 1400–1700: Essays in Honor of Larry Silver* (Leiden: Brill, 2017), pp. 362–77. For essential background, see Walter S. Gibson, "Hieronymus Bosch and the Mirror of Man: The Authorship and Iconography of the *Tabletop of the Seven Deadly Sins*," *Oud-Holland* 87 (1973), pp. 223–25 (fig. 15); and Sabine Griese, *Text-Bilder und ihre Kontexte: Medialität und Materialität von Einblatt-Holz- und -Metallschnitten des 15. Jahrhunderts* (Zurich: Chronos, 2011), pp. 99–102.

47. For the Ghisi engraving, see Suzanne Boorsch, Michal Lewis, and R. E. Lewis, *The Engravings of Giorgio Ghisi*, exhibition catalogue (New York: Metropolitan Museum of Art, 1985), pp. 114–20, no. 28.

48. The German art historian and collector Wilhelm Schreiber (1855–1932) gave the woodcut its somewhat misleading title (misleading since it has little to do with the *Speculum humanae salvationis*, known in German as the *Heilsspiegel*); see Richard S. Field, *Fifteenth Century Woodcuts and Metalcuts from the National Gallery of Art, Washington, D.C.* (Washington: National Gallery of Art, n.d. [1965]), cat. 269; Dieter Kuhrmann, *Die Frühzeit des Holzschnitts*, exhibition catalogue (Munich: Staatliche Graphische Sammlung, 1970), cat. 58; Parshall and Schoch, *Origins of European Printmaking*, no. 92 (entry by Sabine Griese); and Griese, *Text-Bilder*, p. 294.

49. See Elizabeth Sears, *The Ages of Man: Medieval Interpretations of the Life Cycle* (Princeton: Princeton University Press, 1986), pp. 146–48.

50. "And God said: We will make man in our image according to our likeness" (*et ait, Faciamus hominem ad imaginem et similtudinem nostrum*). See Dominic Olariu, "Thomas Aquinas' Definition of the *imago Dei* and the Development of Lifelike Portraiture," *Bulletin du centre d'études médiévales Auxerre* 17.2 (2013), available at https://cem.revues.org/13251.

51. Robert Baldwin, "Marriage as a Sacramental Reflection of the Passion: The Mirror in Jan van Eyck's 'Arnolfini Wedding,'" *Oud-Holland* 98.2 (1984), pp. 57–75.

52. Reindert Falkenburg, "Speculative Imagery in Petrarch's *Von der Artzney bayder Glück* (1532)," in Karl A. E. Enenkel and Jan Papy (eds.), *Petrarch and His Readers in the Renaissance* (Boston: Brill, 2006), pp. 174–75. Not coincidentally, this definition fits well the Renaissance understanding of paradoxes; see Mitchell B. Merback, "Nobody Dares: Freedom, Dissent, Self-Knowing and Other Possibilities in Sebald Beham's *Impossible*," *Renaissance Quarterly* 63.4 (Winter 2010), pp. 1037–1105.

53. See in this respect the otherwise fine discussion by Griese, *Text-Bilder*, pp. 99–102.

54. Rainer Schoch, Matthias Mende, and Anna Scherbaum, *Albrecht Dürer: Das druckgraphische Werk*, 3 vols. (Munich: Prestel, 2001–2004), vol. 2, nos. 166–85, pp. 214–79. To date the most complete study is Anna Scherbaum, *Albrecht Dürers Marienleben: Form, Gehalt, Funktion und sozialhistorischer Ort* (Wiesbaden: Harrassowitz, 2004); but see also Junhyoung Michael Shin, *Et in picturam et in sanctitatem: Operating Albrecht Dürer's Marienleben* (Berlin: Verlag für Wissenschaft und Forschung, 2003); and *Albrecht Dürer: Marienleben*, commentary by Anna Scherbaum, trans. Claudia Wiener (Munich: Prestel, 2009). On Chelidonius, see Franz Posset, *Renaissance Monks: Monastic Humanism in Six Biographical Sketches* (Leiden: Brill, 2005), pp. 63–92.

55. Thomas Schauerte, *Albrecht Dürer: Das große Glück. Kunst im Zeichen des geistigen Aufbruchs*, exhibition catalogue (Osnabrück: Kulturgeschichtliches Museum Osnabruck, 2003), cat. 112; Scherbaum, *Albrecht Dürers Marienleben*, pp. 161–64, with further references.

56. "Artifices faber ecce manus ostendit Ioseph. / Aes cudit, cedrum sculpit eburque polit. / Effingit[i]que hominum viuos in marmore vultus. / Alter & egregie daedalus aedificat. / Hoc studio victum domui quaesivit. & vna / Traxit cum Maria laetius exilium." (Joseph the craftsman displays his skillful hands. / He carves in bronze, sculpts in cedar wood, and polishes ivory. / And depicts the vivid faces of men in marble / Spendidly he builds as a second Daedalus / With this trade he sought the means of living / And along with Mary he spent more joyously the time of exile); from the 1511 edition, with original typographic deviations. Translation by Joaquin Dominguez Arduengo; cf. Shin, *Et in picturam et in sanctitatem*, p. 109 n.55. On the Daedalus theme, see Erwin Panofsky, *Albrecht Dürer*, 2 vols. (Princeton: Princeton University Press, 1943), vol. 1, pp. 98–99; and Hartmut Krohm, "Alter Daedalus: Zum Begriff künstlerischer Tätigkeit in Dürers 'Marienleben,'" in Bodo Brinkmann, Hartmut Krohm, and Michael

Roth (eds.), *Aus Dürers Welt: Festschrift für Fedja Anzelewsky* (Turnhout: Brepols, 2001), pp. 77–90.

57. Cynthia Hahn, "Joseph as Ambrose's 'Artisan of the Soul' in the *Holy Family in Egypt* by Albrecht Dürer," *Zeitschrift für Kunstgeschichte* 47.4 (1984), p. 517. Dürer's conception reprises an iconography that blossomed in late medieval narratives of Mary's life (*Marien-vita*) and Christ's early life by authors such as Ludolph of Saxony and Michael de Massa, books that were extensively illustrated in both manuscript versions and printed editions.

58. Walter S. Melion, *The Meditative Art: Studies in the Northern Devotional Print, 1550–1625* (Philadelphia: Saint Joseph's University Press, 2009), p. 5.

59. Explored in Ralph Dekoninck, "*Ad vivum*: Pictorial and Spiritual Imitation in the Allegory of the Pictura Sacra by Frans Francken II," in Walter S. Melion, Ralph Dekoninck, and Agnès Guiderdoni-Bruslé (eds.), *Ut Pictura Meditatio: The Meditative Image in Northern Art, 1500–1700* (Turnhout: Brepols, 2012), pp. 318–36.

60. Andrea Catellani, "Before the Preludes: Some Semiotic Observations on Vision, Meditation, and the 'Fifth Space' in Early Jesuit Spiritual Illustrated Literature," in Melion, Dekoninck, and Guiderdoni-Bruslé (eds.), *Ut Pictura Meditatio*, pp. 157–202, esp. pp. 194–202.

61. Melion, *The Meditative Art*, p. 3.

62. Shin, *Et in picturam et in sanctitatem*, pp. 75–80.

63. Pierre Hadot, *Philosophy as a Way of Life: Spiritual Exercises from Socrates to Foucault*, ed. Arnold I. Davidson, trans. Michael Chase (Oxford: Blackwell, 1995), pp. 126–44.

64. Karin Leonhard, "Pictura's Fertile Field: Otto Marseus van Schrieck and the Genre of *Sottobosco* Painting," *Simiolus* 34.2 (2009–2010), pp. 95–118; and Leonhard, "Painted Poison: Venomous Beasts, Herbs, Gems, and Baroque Color Theory," *Nederlands Kunsthistorisch Jaarboek* 61 (2011), p. 137 (same language on p. 139).

65. Leonhard, "Painted Poison," p. 129.

66. *Ibid.*, p. 135.

67. Hans Ulrich Gumbrecht, *Production of Presence: What Meaning Cannot Convey* (Stanford: Stanford University Press, 2004).

68. Leonhard, "Painted Poison," p. 135.

69. Derrida, *Dissemination*, pp. 90–120; discussed in Leonhard, "Painted Poison," pp. 119–20, who already wants to add *artist* to Derrida's composite healing deity.

70. Pamela H. Smith, *The Body of the Artisan: Art and Experience in the Scientific Revolution* (Chicago: University of Chicago Press, 2004), pp. 129–49, with an emphasis on alchemy.

71. For the corporate identification of painters with St. Luke, and further references, see the Prologue to Chapters 5 and 6.

72. The notes for Chapter 4 offer a sampling of the enormous literature on melancholia as a temperament, condition, and pathology. The indispensible overviews, each with extensive bibliographies, are Raymond Klibansky, Erwin Panofsky, and Fritz Saxl, *Saturn and Melancholy: Studies in the History of Natural Philosophy, Religion, and Art* ([London]:

Nelson, 1964); Stanley W. Jackson, *Melancholia and Depression: From Hippocratic Times to Modern Times* (New Haven: Yale University Press, 1986); and Matthew Bell, *Melancholia: The Western Malady* (Cambridge: Cambridge University Press, 2014).

CHAPTER FOUR: THE NARRATIVE QUALITY OF MELANCHOLIA

The epigraph is from Søren Kierkegaard, "At a Graveside," in *Three Discourses on Imagined Occasions*, ed. and trans. Howard V. Hong and Edna H. Hong (Princeton: Princeton University Press, 1993), p. 78.

1. For example, in the *Nemesis* of 1502 (see figure 2.8); the *Fall of Man* of 1504 (Walter Strauss, *The Complete Engravings, Etchings and Drypoints of Albrecht Dürer* [New York: Dover, 1973], no. 42); and several other engravings and etchings.

2. Erwin Panofsky, *Albrecht Dürer*, 2 vols. (Princeton: Princeton University Press, 1943), vol. 1, p. 160. In a later comment on the contrast, Panofsky ventures that the figuration of inner cognitive action in Melancholy, which typifies "Theoretical Insight" (that is, thinking without acting), is contrasted with the figuration of "Practical Skill" (acting without thinking) in the putto. "Theory and practice are . . . thoroughly disunited; and the result is impotence and gloom" (vol. 1, p. 163). Dissent from the view that the putto is a countermodel to Melancholy's paralysis is the starting point of Rainer Hoffmann, *Im Zwielicht: Zu Albrecht Dürers Meisterstich* Melencolia I (Cologne: Böhlau, 2014), for whom putto and goddess are locked in a common inactivity.

3. In early desert monasticism, the Greek *akēdeia* (Latinized as *acedia*) referred not to simple laziness, but to a kind of spiritual boredom and disgust; like the Latin *taedium*, which replaced it (along with *tristitia*, or spiritual sadness), it was considered a fundamental vice and the monk's gravest adversary, for the *taedium animi* undermined every practical activity of the religious life, especially prayer and contemplation of God. For the early development of these terms, see Siegfried Wenzel, *The Sin of Sloth: Acedia in Medieval Thought and Literature* (Chapel Hill: University of North Carolina Press, 1967); and for their aesthetic implications, Mary J. Carruthers, *The Experience of Beauty in the Middle Ages* (Oxford: Oxford University Press, 2013), pp. 30–31 and 146–47.

4. See Raymond Klibansky, Erwin Panofsky, and Fritz Saxl, *Saturn and Melancholy: Studies in the History of Natural Philosophy, Religion, and Art* (London: Nelson, 1964), pp. 299–300 and fig. 89b; and Gerlinde Lütke Notarp, *Von Heiterkeit, Zorn, Schwermut und Lethargie: Studien zur Ikonographie der vier Temperamente in der niederländischen Serien- und Genregraphik des 16. und 17. Jahrhunderts* (Münster: Waxmann, 1998), pp. 61–65, 176–77, and figs. 18–21.

5. On "vigilant repose" in late medieval devotional imagery, see Mitchell B. Merback, "The Man of Sorrows in Northern Europe: Ritual Metaphor and Therapeutic Exchange," in Catherine R. Puglisi and William L. Barcham (eds.), *New Perspectives on the Man of Sorrows* (Kalamazoo: Medieval Institute Publications, 2013), pp. 77–116.

6. Panofsky, *Albrecht Dürer*, vol. 1, p. 163; his remarks about the "superior being" are on p. 160.

7. *Ibid.*, p. 171. Repeatedly throughout his career, Panofsky defined the greatness of artworks in terms of their capacity to synthesize multiple concerns into single, expressive unities; thus in the brilliant conclusion to his study of *Melencolia I* did he find the engraving to be "at the same time the objective statement of a general philosophy and the subjective confession of an individual man" (*ibid.*).

8. For a closer reading of this panel than I am able to give here, see my "Man of Sorrows in Northern Europe," with further references. For fundamental work on the metaphors and typologies operating through the *sessio Christi* theme, see F. P. Pickering, *Literature and Art in the Middle Ages* (Coral Gables: University of Miami Press, 1970); for the "Christus in Elend" theme specifically, see Sabine Fehlemann, "Christus im Elend: Vom Andachtsbild zum realistischen Bilddokument," in Bazon Brock and Achim Preiß (eds.), *Ikonographia: Anleitung zum Lesen von Bildern (Festschrift Donat de Chapeaurouge)* (Munich: Klinkhardt & Biermann, 1990), pp. 79–96.

9. See Drew Daniel, *Melancholy Assemblage: Affect and Epistemology in the English Renaissance* (New York: Fordham University Press, 2013), who argues that the "visual experience of looking at a melancholy portrait . . . 'relocates' the phenomenon of melancholy itself, shifting its terrain from the inaccessibly private interiority of a lone sufferer . . . to the social field in place between the sufferer and the observer(s)" (p. 55).

10. Philip L. Sohm, "Dürer's *Melencolia I*: The Limits of Knowledge," *Studies in the History of Art* 9 (1980), p. 29.

11. *Ibid.*, pp. 16–17.

12. Significantly, Beham replicated the spelling of Dürer's title in his version; see Jeffrey Chipps Smith, *Nuremberg: A Renaissance City, 1500–1618*, exhibition catalogue (Austin: University of Texas Press, 1983), no. 86; Stephen Goddard (ed.), *The World in Miniature: Engravings by the German Little Masters, 1500–1550*, exhibition catalogue (Lawrence: Spencer Museum of Art, The University of Kansas, 1988), cat. 11; and Rainer Schoch, Matthias Mende, and Anna Scherbaum, *Albrecht Dürer: Das druckgraphische Werk*, 3 vols. (Munich: Prestel, 2001–2004), vol. 1, no. 71, p. 182.

13. On subversion in the work of Beham and other artists in Dürer's circle, see the essays in Jürgen Müller and Thomas Schauerte (eds.), *Die gottlosen Maler von Nürnberg: Konvention und Subversion in der Druckgrafik der Beham-Brüder* exhibition catalogue (Nuremberg: Museen de Stadt Nürnberg, 2011); Thomas Schauerte, Jürgen Müller and Bertram Kaschek (eds.), *Von der Freiheit der Bilder: Spott, Kritik und Subversion in der Kunst der Dürerzeit* (Petersberg: Michael Imhoff, 2013); and my "Nobody Dares: Freedom, Dissent, Self-Knowing and Other Possibilities in Sebald Beham's *Impossible*," *Renaissance Quarterly* 63.4 (Winter 2010), pp. 1037–1105.

14. Cf. Sohm, "Dürer's *Melencolia I*," p. 22 (for the scales), p. 29 (for the other objects).

On the scales as symbols of justice, see Elfreide Scheil, "Albrecht Dürer's *Melencholia I* und die Gerechtigkeit," *Zeitschrift für Kunstgeschichte* 70.2 (2007), pp. 201–14.

15. Hoffman, *Im Zwielicht*, p. 10.

16. "Indeed the significance of Melancholy's depression," Sohm concludes, "is conveyed primarily by means of temporal imagery." Sohm, "Dürer's *Melencolia I*," p. 29.

17. Stephen Crites, "The Narrative Quality of Experience," *Journal of the American Academy of Religion* 39.3 (September 1971), pp. 291–311.

18. Stanley W. Jackson, *Melancholia and Depression: From Hippocratic Times to Modern Times* (New Haven: Yale University Press, 1986), pp. 10–11, and see below.

19. Panofsky, *Albrecht Dürer*, vol. 1, pp. 160–61.

20. Jackson, *Melancholia and Depression*, p. 6.

21. See Klibansky, Panofsky, and Saxl, *Saturn and Melancholy*, pp. 382–84, fig. 128; Dieter Koepplin and Tilman Falk, *Lukas Cranach: Gemälde, Zeichnungen, Druckgraphik*, 2 vols., exhibition catalogue (Basel: Birkhäuser, 1974), vol. 1, no. 171; cf. Charles Zika, *Exorcising Our Demons: Magic, Witchcraft and Visual Culture in Early Modern Europe* (Leiden: Brill, 2003), pp. 333–74, with discussion of Cranach's other versions.

22. On Graf's image, which depicts Mars and Bellona fomenting chaos while the demonic horde takes to the battlefield below, see Christian Müller, *Urs Graf: Die Zeichnungen im Kupferstichkabinett Basel* (Basel: Schwabe, 2001), pp. 362–64.

23. See Bodo Brinkmann and Berthold Hinz, *Hexenlust und Sündenfall: Die seltsamen Phantasien des Hans Baldung Grien / Witches' Lust and the Fall of Man: The Strange Fantasies of Hans Baldung Grien*, exhibition catalogue (Petersberg: Michael Imhof, 2007), cat. 6; the best interpretation of Baldung's witches remains Joseph Leo Koerner, *The Moment of Self-Portraiture in German Renaissance Art* (Chicago: University of Chicago Press, 1993), pp. 323–44.

24. Charles Zika, "Wild Riders, Popular Folklore and Moral Disorder," in Zika, *The Appearance of Witchcraft: Print and Visual Culture in Sixteenth-Century Europe* (London: Routledge, 2007), pp. 99 and 102.

25. On Goya's witches as both cause and effect of melancholic disturbance, see the excellent study by Guy Tal, "An 'Enlightened' View of Witches: Melancholy and Delusionary Experience in Goya's *Spell*," *Zeitschrift für Kunstgeschichte* 75.1 (2012), pp. 33–50. Tal cites the ideas of the Dutch physician Johann Weyer (1515–88), who argued that melancholy, especially in women, weakens the mind's defenses against the Devil, who enters them and provokes them to delusion. See also the essays collected in Roy Porter (ed.), *Medicine in the Enlightenment* (Amsterdam: Rodopi, 1994), especially by Johanna Geyer-Kordesch, "Whose Enlightenment? Medicine, Witchcraft, Melancholia, and Pathology," pp. 113–27.

26. See Chapter 1.

27. The literature on melancholia's appearance in Greek nosological and therapeutic medicine is vast, and the topic far exceeds my competence. Recent studies make clear that melancholia as a peculiar form of mental aberration based in organic imbalance was

unthinkable before the rise of a realist tradition of "scientific medicine" as founded by the Greeks; see Jacques Jouanna, "At the Roots of Melancholy: Is Greek Medicine Melancholic?" in Jouanna, *Greek Medicine from Hippocrates to Galen: Selected Papers*, ed. Philip van der Eijk, trans. Neil Allies (Leiden: Brill, 2012), pp. 229–58; and Matthew Bell, *Melancholia: The Western Malady* (Cambridge: Cambridge University Press, 2014), esp. pp. 23–32, who emphasizes the necessity of "culturally specific notions of the self" (p. 18) for any working definition of melancholia or depression.

28. Jackson, *Melancholia and Depression*, pp. 30–31, with quote from the Hippocratic corpus on p. 30.

29. *Hippocrates*, vol. 4, trans. W. H. S. Jones (London: Heinemann, 1931), pp. 184–85, quoted and discussed in Angus Gowland, "Melancholy, Imagination, and Dreaming in Renaissance Learning," in Yasmin A. Haskell (ed.), *Diseases of the Imagination and Imaginary Disease in the Early Modern Period* (Turnhout: Brepols, 2011), p. 56.

30. Angus Gowland, "Medicine, Psychology, and the Melancholic Subject in the Renaissance," in Elena Carrera (ed.), *Emotions and Health, 1200–1700* (Leiden: Brill, 2013), pp. 191–92. For the humors and the systematization of the temperaments in ancient and medieval medicine, consult Klibansky, Panofsky, and Saxl, *Saturn and Melancholy*, pp. 3–15 and 97–123; Notarp, *Von Heiterkeit, Zorn, Schwermut und Lethargie*; and Noga Arikha, *Passions and Tempers: A History of the Humours* (New York: Ecco, 2007).

31. Gowland, "Medicine, Psychology, and the Melancholic Subject," p. 192.

32. See the Epilogue.

33. The modern notion of melancholy as a special brand of inwardness, a distinctive inner "mood," is anticipated in certain aspects of medieval poetry; see Klibansky, Panofsky, and Saxl, *Saturn and Melancholy*, pp. 217–40.

34. Quoted in Jackson, *Melancholia and Depression*, p. 32, from [Pseudo-Aristotle], *Problemata*, in *The Works of Aristotle*, 11 vols. ed. J. A. Smith and W. D. Ross (Oxford: Clarendon Press of Oxford University Press, 1908–31), p. 7, 953a–955a. Cf. Klibansky, Panofsky, and Saxl, *Saturn and Melancholy*, pp. 18–29 (Greek text and translation) and pp. 29–41 (discussion). In this model, thermal imbalance can be caused by many factors, even external situations affecting mood; see Winfried Schleiner, *Melancholy, Genius and Utopia in the Renaissance* (Wiesbaden: Otto Harrassowitz, 1991), pp. 20–25; Eckart Schütrumpf, "Black Bile as the Cause of Human Accomplishments and Behaviors in *Pr.* 30.1: Is the Concept Aristotelian?," in Robert Mayhew (ed.), *The Aristotelian Problemata Physica: Philosophical and Scientific Investigations* (Leiden: Brill, 2015), p. 359, who also points out (p. 357 and n.4), contra Klibansky, Panofsky, and Saxl (*Saturn and Melancholy*, p. 29), that in the *Problemata* "mixture" refers to temperatures, not black bile's relationship to other humors. The latter idea was introduced by Ficino.

35. Klibansky, Panofsky, and Saxl, *Saturn and Melancholy*, p. 4; also see the valuable discussion in Alina N. Feld, *Melancholy and the Otherness of God: A Study in the Hermeneutics of Depression* (Lanham: Lexington, 2011), pp. 11–13.

36. Hippocratic doctors, recognizing a commonality of symptoms (depressive fear, paralysis, troubles in speech, mental disturbance), established for melancholia "a clear conceptual position between epilepsy and madness"; Jouanna, "At the Roots of Melancholy," p. 236.

37. Here I rely on the clear-sighted discussion in Jackson, *Melancholia and Depression*, pp. 41–45. Without adding anything fundamentally new to existing humoral theory, Galen's diagnostic framing of melancholia remained authoritative until the eighteenth century.

38. In the broad rehabilitation of Aristotle in the Middle Ages, efforts to address the *Problemata*'s validation of melancholy's "gifts" were halfhearted; see Klibansky, Panofsky, and Saxl, *Saturn and Melancholy*, pp. 67–74. For the phrase "eucrasia within an anomaly," see p. 40.

39. On Constantinus Africanus, the most prominent figure of the Salernan school of medicine (ninth century onward), see Klibansky, Panofsky, and Saxl, *Saturn and Melancholy*, pp. 82–86, with the older literature; for Rufus's treatise, see the essays in Rufus of Ephesus, *On Melancholy*, ed. and trans. Peter E. Pormann (Tübingen: Mohr Siebeck, 2008).

40. Quoted in Klibansky, Panofsky, and Saxl, *Saturn and Melancholy*, p. 83.

41. Quoted and discussed in *ibid.*, pp. 83–84.

42. Quoted in translation in *ibid.*, p. 84.

43. Quoted by Peter-Klaus Schuster and Jörg Völlnagel, "Dürer and Rufus: *Melencolia I* in the Medical Tradition," in Rufus of Ephesus, *On Melancholy*, p. 212, who strain the historical connections between Rufus's doctrines and *Melencolia I*.

44. Rufus, discussed in Jackson, *Melancholia and Depression*, p. 37.

45. Klibansky, Panofsky, and Saxl, *Saturn and Melancholy*, p. 88.

46. Jason Pratensis, *De tuenda sanitate libri quatuor* (Antwerp, 1538), p. 263; cited and discussed in Michael Stolberg, "Lucas Cranachs 'Melencolia'-Darstellungen und die zeitgenössische Medizin," in Stefan Oehmig (ed.), *Medizin und Sozialwesen in Mitteldeutschland zur Reformationszeit* (Leipzig: Evangelische Verlagsanstalt, 2007), pp. 255–56.

47. Klibansky, Panofsky, and Saxl, *Saturn and Melancholy*, p. 87.

48. Gowland, "Melancholy, Imagination, and Dreaming," p. 57.

49. Quoted and discussed in Jackson, *Melancholia and Depression*, p. 44. Similar processes involving the inflammation of the hypochondriacal tissues surrounding the stomach, resulting in "noxious vapors or aurae," are described by Byzantine physicians, for example Paul of Aegina (625–690); see *ibid.*, p. 55.

50. Quoted in Jackson, *Melancholia and Depression*, p. 42.

51. Stolberg, "Lucas Cranachs 'Melencolia'-Darstellungen," p. 266.

52. Luther's repeated insistence that the melancholic constitution was "the devil's well-prepared bath" (*Melancholicum caput est paratum balneum Diaboli*) left unresolved the question whether the mind's derangement was the direct result of demonic manipulation of the soul or an effect of the soul's tortured response to carnal temptations; see H. Günter

Schmitz, "Das Melancholieproblem in Wissenschaft und Kunst der frühen Neuzeit," *Sud-hoffs Archiv* 60.2 (1976), pp. 143 and 152–54; and Noel L. Brann, *The Debate over the Origin of Genius during the Italian Renaissance: The Theories of Supernatural Frenzy and Natural Melancholy in Accord and in Conflict on the Threshold of the Scientific Revolution* (Leiden: Brill, 2002), pp. 6–7. For Luther's statements, recorded with variations in the "Table Talk," see Koepplin and Falk, *Lucas Cranach*, vol. 1, p. 292; Schleiner, *Melancholy, Genius and Utopia*, p. 67 and n.72 (citing all the variations found in the *Tischreden*); also Stuart Clark, *Vanities of the Eye: Vision in Early Modern European Culture* (Oxford: Oxford University Press, 2007), ch. 2.

53. Stolberg, "Lucas Cranachs 'Melencolia'-Darstellungen," p. 269. On Melanchthon's treatise, see Schleiner, *Melancholy, Genius and Utopia*, pp. 56–66; and Sachiko Kusukawa, *The Transformation of Natural Philosophy: The Case of Philip Melanchthon* (Cambridge: Cambridge University Press, 1995), pp. 100–14.

54. This is how Aretaeus of Cappadocia (ca. first century CE) described the condition; see Jackson, *Melancholia and Depression*, p. 39.

55. A valuable overview that explores how ancient practitioners negotiated this divide is Jean Starobinski, *Geschichte der Melancholiebehandlung von den Anfängen bis 1900* (Basel: J. R. Geigy, 1960).

56. For the remedies of Soranus, I follow Jackson, *Melancholia and Depression*, p. 35.

57. In Christian ascetic perspective, melancholia was a sign of grace, a test by which God demonstrated his love for his children; reason therefore dictated bearing it with humility. See Klibansky, Panofsky, and Saxl, *Saturn and Melancholy*, pp. 75–78, who note the genre of the "Anti-melancholy hortations" (pp. 77–78 n.25); see also Feld, *Melancholy and the Otherness of God*, pp. 15–42.

58. For the following remedies of Rufus, see Jackson, *Melancholia and Depression*, pp. 38–39; for Galen's views, pp. 44–45. On the enduring importance of bloodletting in pre-modern medicine, see Shigehisa Kuriyama, "Interpreting the History of Bloodletting," *Journal of the History of Medicine and Allied Sciences* 50 (1995), pp. 11–46.

59. C. J. S. Thompson, *The Mystery and Art of the Apothecary* (London: John Lane, Bodley Head, 1929), pp. 35–43; and Jackson, *Melancholia and Depression*, p. 53.

60. Quoted in Jackson, *Melancholia and Depression*, p. 45.

61. These are Jackson's words, *Melancholia and Depression*, p. 51.

62. Quoted and discussed in *ibid.*, p. 56.

63. "Coitus, inquit, pacificat, austeriorem superbiam refrenat, melancholicos adiuvat"; quoted and discussed in Klibansky, Panofsky, and Saxl, *Saturn and Melancholy*, p. 84. For Constantinus's overall therapeutic methodology, see Starobinski, *Geschichte der Melancholiebehandlung*, pp. 40–41.

64. Overexertion and excessive animal heat during intercourse also threatened the male seed, which contained *pneuma* (spirit); see Aline Rousselle, *Porneia: On Desire and the Body in Antiquity*, trans. Felicia Pheasant (Oxford: Basil Blackwell, 1988), pp. 13–23.

65. Quoted in Jackson, *Melancholia and Depression*, p. 41. For Aretaeus's alleviative methods, see Starobinski, *Geschichte der Melancholiebehandlung*, pp. 24-26.

66. Brann, *The Debate over the Origin of Genius during the Italian Renaissance*, p. 19.

67. For Albertus Magnus (d. 1280), the "natural" melancholic represented the "complexio sicca et frigida" and was thus incompatible with genuine intellectual ability, which required the qualities of warmth and moisture; he therefore had to create a special category—"melancholicus de melancholia adusta calida"—when reconciling his views with the claims of the Aristotelian *Problemata*; see Klibansky, Panofsky, and Saxl, *Saturn and Melancholy*, p. 71.

68. Leon Golden, "The Clarification Theory of *Katharsis*," *Hermes* 104.4 (1976), pp. 437-452; for the therapeutic implications in Aristotle, see especially Pedro Láin Entralgo, *The Therapy of the Word in Classical Antiquity*, trans. L. J. Rather and John M. Sharp (New Haven: Yale University Press, 1970), pp. 183-204.

69. Karl Giehlow, "Dürers Stich Melencolia I und der maximilianische Humanistenkreis," *Mitteilungen der Gesellschaft für vervielfältigende Künste* 26.2 (1903), pp. 29—41; 27.3 (1904), pp. 6—18; and 27.4 (1904), pp. 57—78.

70. The text of the *Picatrix* is an eleventh-century compilation of older traditions; first entitled *Ghayat al-Hakim* (Goal of the Sage), translated into Spanish under Alfonso the Wise of Castile in the thirteenth century and later translated into Latin, it is largely given over to instructions for making magical images that mobilize and harness astral spirits to affect sublunary objects; see Henry Kahane, Renée Kahane, and Angelina Pietrangeli, "'Picatrix' and the Talismans," *Romance Philology* 19.4 (May 1966), pp. 574-93; and for recent studies, Jean-Patrice Boudet, Anna Caiozzo, and Nicolas Weill-Parot (eds.), *Images et magie: Picatrix entre Orient et Occident* (Paris: Honoré Champion, 2011).

71. Klibansky, Panofsky, and Saxl, *Saturn and Melancholy*, p. 94.

72. *Ibid.*, p. 97.

73. *Ibid.*, p. 277, with references to the editions.

74. Aby Warburg, "Pagan-Antique Prophecy in Words and Images in the Age of Luther," in Warburg, *The Renewal of Pagan Antiquity: Contributions to the Cultural History of the European Renaissance*, trans. David Britt (Los Angeles: Getty Research Institute for the History of Art and the Humanities, 1999), p. 636. This reprises the conclusion of Karl Giehlow; see Chapter 1.

75. Gowland, "Melancholy, Imagination, and Dreaming," pp. 53-102, esp. pp. 54-60.

76. Klibansky, Panofsky, and Saxl, *Saturn and Melancholy*, p. 278.

77. *Ibid.*, pp. 279-80; Schoch, Mende, and Scherbaum, *Albrecht Dürer*, vol. 3, no. 269.2 (with full bibliography); Thomas Schauerte, *Albrecht Dürer: Das große Glück. Kunst im Zeichen des geistigen Aufbruchs* (Bramsche: Kulturgeschichtliches Museum Osnabruck, 2003), cat. 102; and Schauerte, "Von der 'Philosophia' zur 'Melencolia I': Anmerkungen zu Dürers Philosophie-Holzschnitt für Konrad Celtis," in Franz Fuchs (ed.), *Konrad Celtis*

und Nürnberg: Akten des interdisziplinären Symposions vom 8. und 9. November 2002 im Caritas-Pirckheimer-Haus in Nürnberg (Wiesbaden: Harrassowitz, 2004), pp. 117–139. A few years later, the block was reused in Augsburg to illustrate the so-called *Ligirinus* (Erhard Oeglin, April 1507), the twelfth-century poem "discovered" by Celtis around 1500 in the Cistercian monastery at Ebrach.

78. "Quicquid habet Coelum quid Terra quid Aer & aequor / Quicquid in humanis rebus & esse potest / Et deus in toto quicquid facit igneus orbe / Philosophia meo pectore cuncta gero" (Whatever heaven contains, what earth, the air, and the water, / Whatever can exist among all things that are human, / Whatever the fire-god makes in the whole circle of earth, / All that I, Philosophy, carry within my own breast); translation from Smith, *Nuremberg: A Renaissance City*, p. 103 (cat. 10). See also Charles Talbot (ed.), *Dürer in America: His Graphic Work*, exhibition catalogue (New York: MacMillan, 1971), cat. 212; and Lewis W. Spitz, *The Religious Renaissance of the German Humanists* (Cambridge, MA: Harvard University Press, 1963), p. 87.

79. Schauerte, *Albrecht Dürer*, p. 161. The obelisk's coding of learning's "ascent" is basically modeled after Boethius (*De consolatione Philosophiae*, 1.1), who said the scale should rise from *pi* to *theta* (practice to theory), but Dürer has the *phi* at the bottom (for philosophy) and *theta* at the top (presumably for theology); see Gerd Unverfehrt (ed.), *Dürers Dinge: Einblattgraphik und Buchillustrationen Albrecht Dürers aus dem Besitz der Georg-August-Universität Göttingen*, exhibition catalogue (Göttingen: Kunstsammlung der Universität Göttingen, 1997), cat. 34; and Klibansky, Panofsky, and Saxl, p. 279 n.11.

80. For further discussion with references, see the Epilogue.

81. See Chapter 5 for my discussion of Dürer's metalpoint self-portrait of 1522 (figure 5.8). The quote is from Klibansky, Panofsky, and Saxl, *Saturn and Melancholy*, p. 280.

82. Marsilio Ficino, *Three Books On Life*, ed. and trans. Carol V. Kaske and John R. Clark (Binghamton, NY: Medieval and Renaissance Texts and Studies, in conjunction with the Renaissance Society of America, 1989), bk. 3, ch. 22, pp. 363–65.

83. Warburg, "Pagan-Antique Prophecy," p. 641.

84. For the most recent—and ambitious—effort to use the "key" of the magic square to "unlock" the encoded meanings of the engraving, see Leonhard G. Richter, *Dürer-Code: Albrecht Dürers entschlüsselte Meisterstiche* (Dettelbach: J. H. Röll, 2014).

85. These patterns are usefully laid out by Jill Britton in "Melancholia Magic Square," online at http://britton.disted.camosun.bc.ca/jbmelancholia.html.

86. Michael H. Shank, "The Faces of Saturn: Images and Texts from Augustus through Dürer and Galileo," in Marvin Bolt and Stephen Case (eds.), *Engaging the Heavens: Inspiration of Astronomical Phenomena 5* (San Francisco: Astronomical Society of the Pacific, 2012), p. 112.

87. I. R. F. Calder, "A Note on Magic Squares in the Philosophy of Agrippa of Nettisheim," *Journal of the Warburg and Courtauld Institutes* 12 (1949), p. 197.

88. For example, Shank, "The Faces of Saturn," p. 118. Panofsky, in *Albrecht Dürer*, vol. 1, pp. 170-71, discounts the likelihood that the engraving originated from the merely personal circumstances of Dürer's grieving, as well as the insinuation that the square's numerology refers to his mother's death date.

89. Klibansky, Panofsky, and Saxl, *Saturn and Melancholy*, p. 256. Furthermore, the horoscope showed the malign planet in the sign of Aquarius, Saturn's "night abode."

90. Panofsky, *Albrecht Dürer*, vol. 1, p. 165; see also Heinrich Wölfflin, *The Art of Albrecht Dürer*, trans. Alastair Grieve and Heide Grieve (London: Phaidon, 1971), p. 203; and Sohm, "Dürer's *Melencolia I*," p. 16.

91. Ficino, *Three Books On Life*, bk. 2, ch. 15, an important passage quoted in full in Klibansky, Panofsky, and Saxl, *Saturn and Melancholy*, pp. 271-73 (quoted material on 272).

92. Warburg, "Pagan-Antique Prophecy," pp. 645-47, with my emphasis. Johannes Lichtenberger (d. 1503) was an astrologer well known for his *Prognosticatio in latino* (1488), which went through numerous editions.

93. For Warburg, the liberating message of the work "can be understood only if we recognize that the artist has taken a magical and mythical logic and made it spiritual and intellectual" ("Pagan-Antique Prophecy," p. 644). Cf. the original statement: "Der recht eigentlich schöpferische Akt, der Dürers 'Melencolia I' zum humanistischen Trostblatt wider Saturnfürchtigkeit macht, kann erst begriffen werden, wenn man dies magische Mythologik als eigentliches Objekt der künstlerisch-vergeistigenden Umformung erkennt." Aby Warburg, "Heidnisch-antike Weissagung in Wort und Bild zu Luthers Zeiten," in *Sitzungsberichte der Heidelberger Akademie der Wissenschaften, Philosophisch-Historische Klasse*, 26 (1919) (Heidelberg, 1920), p. 61.

94. Cf. Eisler's shrewd remarks: "The great print is at once descriptive and diagnostic, the objective characterization of a state. For all the mysterious depths of reference the engraving is the most enlightened of Dürer's works, rooted in recognition as a prelude to healing—salvation." See Colin Eisler, "Maximilian and Dürer's Major Engravings," in Juliusz A. Chrościcki and Jan Białostocki (eds.), *Ars auro prior: Studia Ioanni Białostocki sexagenario dicata* (Warsaw: Państwowe Wydawnictwo Naukowe, 1981), p. 299.

95. Frank Ankersmit, *Sublime Historical Experience* (Stanford: Stanford University Press, 2005), p. 145.

96. Adapted from Günter Grass, "On Stasis in Progress: Variations on Albrecht Dürer's Engraving *Melencolia I*," in Giulia Bartrum et al., *Albrecht Dürer and His Legacy: The Graphic Work of a Renaissance Artist*, exhibition catalogue (Princeton: Princeton University Press, 2002), pp. 76 and 69.

PROLOGUE TO CHAPTERS FIVE AND SIX

The epigraph is from Paracelsus, *Sämtliche Werke*, ed. Karl Sudhoff, 14 vols. (Munich: Oldenburg, 1922-33), vol. 8, p. 71: "ein arzt ein menschen also lauter durchsehe, als durchzusehen ist ein distillirter tau, in dem sich kein fünklin verbergen mag, das nit gesehen werd. und also durchsichtig sol er hinein sehen als durch einen quellenden brunnen, wie viel stein und sandkörner, mit was farben, formen . . . sie sind"; quoted in translation in Lilla Vekerdy, "Paracelsus's *Great Wound Surgery*," in Elizabeth Lane Furdell (ed.), *Textual Healing: Essays On Medieval and Early Modern Medicine* (Leiden: Brill, 2005), p. 90.

1. Friedrich Winkler, *Die Zeichnungen Albrecht Dürers*, 4 vols. (Berlin: Deutscher Verein für Kunstwissenschaft, 1936–39), vol. 2, no. 272; John Rowlands, *The Age of Dürer and Holbein: German Drawings 1400–1550*, exhibition catalogue (Cambridge: Cambridge University Press, 1988), no. 50; John Rowlands, with assistance of Giulia Bartrum, *Drawings by German Artists and Artists from German-Speaking Regions of Europe: The Fifteenth Century and the Sixteenth Century by Artists Born before 1530*, 2 vols. (London: British Museum, 1993), vol. 1, no. 154; Giulia Bartrum et al., *Albrecht Dürer and His Legacy: The Graphic Work of a Renaissance Artist*, exhibition catalogue (Princeton: Princeton University Press, 2002), cat. 82; and Daniel Hess and Thomas Eser (eds.), *The Early Dürer*, exhibition catalogue (Nuremberg: Germanisches National Museum; New York: Thames and Hudson, 2012), cat. 191, with full references. The German inscription is variously rendered: "Die 2 angsicht hab ich vch erl . . . [probably *erlich*] gemacht jn meiner Kranckheit."

2. Since this and the *Head of Christ* are almost always exhibited together, see the above sources as follows: Winkler, *Die Zeichnungen Albrecht Dürers*, vol. 2, no. 271; Rowlands, *The Age of Dürer and Holbein*, cat. 49; Rowlands and Bartrum, *Drawings by German Artists and Artists from German-Speaking Regions of Europe*, cat. 153; Bartrum et al., *Albrecht Dürer and His Legacy*, cat. 81; and Hess and Eser (eds.), *The Early Dürer*, cat. 190.

3. Francis Ames-Lewis, *The Intellectual Life of the Early Renaissance Artist* (New Haven: Yale University Press, 2000), p. 8. Essential reading on this sprawling topic in Dürer studies includes Erwin Panofsky, *Albrecht Dürer*, 2 vols. (Princeton: Princeton University Press, 1943); Joseph Leo Koerner, *The Moment of Self-Portraiture in German Renaissance Art* (Chicago: University of Chicago Press, 1993); Philipp P. Fehl, "Dürer's Literal Presence in His Pictures: Reflections on His Signatures in the Small Woodcut Passion," in Matthias Winner (ed.), *Künstler über sich in seinem Werk: Internationales Symposium der Bibliotheca Hertziana, Rom 1989* (Weinheim: VCH, Acta Humaniora, 1992), pp. 191–244; Ernst Ullmann, *Albrecht Dürer-Selbstbildnisse und autobiographische Schriften als Zeugnisse der Entwicklung seiner Persönlichkeit* (Berlin: Akademie, 1994); Erika Boeckeler, "Painting Writing in Albrecht Dürer's *Self-Portrait* of 1500," *Word and Image* 28.1 (May 2012), pp. 30–56; and Shira Brisman, "The Image That Wants to Be Read: An Invitation to Interpretation in a Drawing by Albrecht Dürer," *Word and Image* 2.3 (2013), pp. 273–303.

4. Rensselaer W. Lee, "*Ut Pictura Poesis*: The Humanistic Theory of Painting," *Art Bulletin* 22.4 (December 1940), pp. 197–269.

5. Petrarch, *Trionfo della fama* (after 1348), and Fazio, *De viris illustribus* (1456); for both quotations and discussion, see Ames-Lewis, *The Intellectual Life of the Early Renaissance*

Artist, p. 164. Attributed by Plutarch to Simonides, the pendant clichés, "painting is mute poetry" and "poetry a speaking picture," were beloved by humanists; Lee, "*Ut Pictura Poesis*," p. 197.

6. When Chelidonius composed his thirty-seven poems on the history of salvation to complement Dürer's woodcuts for the *Small Passion* (1508–1511), he made explicit reference to specific poetic modes, designations that signaled either their metrical structure or the principal motifs they employed; see Franz Posset, *Renaissance Monks: Monastic Humanism in Six Biographical Sketches* (Leiden: Brill, 2005), pp. 72–73. See also above, Chapter 3, for the collaboration on Dürer's *Marienleben*.

7. Less a grammar school in the standard sense, the *Poetenschule* was more an academy for interested laymen and thus rightly has been compared to what is today called "continuing education." Jane Campbell Hutchison, *Albrecht Dürer: A Biography* (Princeton: Princeton University Press, 1990), p. 55 (with founding date incorrectly given as 1498). First proposed in 1492 by Celtis, the school was not inaugurated until 1496, with Dr. Johann Pirckheimer as its "spiritus rector"; it was located in the old city Weighing House in the Winklerstrasse, only a few doors away from Dürer's birthplace. See also Thomas Schauerte, "*Peripeteia*: Konrad Celtis, the Nuremberg School of Poets, and Dürer's 'Ercules,'" trans. Randall Herz, in Hess and Eser (eds.), *The Early Dürer*, pp. 208–20.

8. See Catherine King, "National Gallery 3902 and the Theme of Luke the Evangelist as Artist and Physician," *Zeitschrift für Kunstgeschichte* 48.2 (1985), pp. 250–52; and Till H. Borchert, "Rogier's *St. Luke*: The Case for Corporate Identification," in Carol J. Purtle (ed.), *Rogier van der Weyden: St. Luke Drawing the Virgin. Selected Essays in Context* (Turnhout: Brepols, 1997), p. 65. On the tradition of St. Luke Madonnas, see Rona Goffen, "Icon and Vision: Giovanni Bellini's Half-Length Madonnas," *Art Bulletin* 57.4 (December 1975), pp. 505–509.

9. See King, "National Gallery 3902."

10. In 1520, Cranach acquired the apothecary shop and house of Martin Polich of Mellrichstadt (d. 1513) in Wittenberg, and in the same year was reassigned Mellrichstadt's apothecary privileges by his patron, Friedrich the Wise; see Werner Schade, *Cranach: A Family of Master Painters*, trans. Helen Sebba (New York: G. P. Putnam's Sons, 1980), p. 43.

11. David Summers uses the term in discussing the intercourse of optics, perspective, geometry, architecture, and painting during the Quattrocento; see Summers, *Vision, Reflection, and Desire in Western Painting* (Chapel Hill: University of North Carolina Press, 2007), p. 78, but the term may be extended to other areas of multidisciplinary practice.

12. Leon Battista Alberti, *On Painting*, trans. John R. Spencer (New Haven: Yale University Press, 1970), p. 77.

13. From a letter of 1452, quoted and discussed in John R. Spencer, "Ut Rhetorica Pictura: A Study in Quattrocento Theory of Painting," *Journal of the Warburg and Courtauld Institutes* 20.1–2 (1957), p. 27.

14. The key transformation of Plato's view by Aristotle is captured by the Spanish

philologist Antonio Tovar in his edition of the *Rhetoric* (which I have been unable to consult), when he states that for Aristotle, "rhetoric does not endeavor merely to *déloun* [to cause to see]" but "it is legitimate for it also to *psychagôgein* [to lead souls] to which end one must study character and the passions"; quoted in Pedro Laín Entralgo, *The Therapy of the Word in Classical Antiquity*, trans. L. J. Rather and John M. Sharp (New Haven: Yale University Press, 1970), p. 175; see also Mary J. Carruthers, *The Experience of Beauty in the Middle Ages* (Oxford: Oxford University Press, 2013), pp. 41-44. Pre-Socratic ideas concerning the effect of speech on the condition of the soul likened that effect to "the power of drugs over the nature of bodies" (Gorgias's *Encomium of Helen*); see Jacques Derrida, *Dissemination*, trans. Barbara Johnson (Chicago: University of Chicago Press, 1981), pp. 115-17.

15. Laín Entralgo, *The Therapy of the Word in Classical Antiquity*. In chapter 5 ("The Power of the Word in Aristotle"), the author argues forcefully for "a fourth type of persuasive word, the therapeutic or curative type," whose construction was begun by the pre-Aristotelian rhetoricians (Gorgias and Antiphon) and Plato (particularly in the *Phaedrus*); much of what Aristotle says about the three types of persuasion he does distinguish—deliberative, judicial, and demonstrative—can be recast, Laín Entralgo suggests, in therapeutic terms. Closest in purpose is the "deliberative" mode, whose principal aim is "the useful" (*to sympheron*), a technical term that recurs in the Hippocratic corpus to denote "the supreme criterion of therapeutic action." The analysis is worth quoting in full here: "Deliberative persuasion has as its object the possible, but not that which is possible by nature (*physei*), such as the fact that the oak grows from the acorn or that a bath is refreshing, nor that which is possible as a result of chance (*apo tychês*), such as meeting a friend whom one does not expect to see, but 'the things that can depend upon us and whose reason for occurrence consists in us' (I, 4, 1359, a 38). And is not this also the object of medicine? . . . [Rudolf] Virchow once wrote that 'politics is medicine on a large scale.' From the point of view of the relationship between therapeutic persuasion and deliberative or political persuasion it could also be said, in the Aristotelian manner, that medicine is politics on a small scale. Health, too, is found among the goods that for Aristotle make up 'the useful' (I, 6, 1362, b14)" (p. 177).

16. Martha C. Nussbaum, *The Therapy of Desire: Theory and Practice in Hellenistic Ethics* (Princeton: Princeton University Press, 1994), chs. 1–3.

17. Rita Copeland and Ineke Sluiter, "General Introduction," in Rita Copeland and Ineke Sluiter (eds.), *Medieval Grammar and Rhetoric: Language Arts and Literary Theory, AD 300–1475* (Oxford: Oxford University Press, 2009), p. 23.

18. Aristotle, *The "Art" of Rhetoric*, trans. John Henry Freese (Cambridge, MA: Harvard University Press, 1975), pp. 17–18.

19. Laín Entralgo, *The Therapy of the Word in Classical Antiquity*, p. 179.

20. *Ibid.*, p. 176, citing the *Rhetoric*, 1.1.1355, b10–15.

21. Laín Entralgo, *The Therapy of the Word in Classical Antiquity*, p. 179.

22. Aristotle, *Rhetoric* 1.8; in *The "Art" of Rhetoric*, p. 89.

23. Laín Entralgo, *The Therapy of the Word in Classical Antiquity*, p. 178.

24. George W. McClure, *Sorrow and Consolation in Italian Humanism* (Princeton: Princeton University Press, 1991), p. 4.

25. Marcus Tullius Cicero, *Tusculan Disputations*, rev. ed., trans. J. E. King (Cambridge: Harvard University Press, 1971), pp. 230–31, a book that McClure, in *Sorrow and Consolation*, calls "the single most comprehensive and influential source for Renaissance psychological theory" (p. 7). For Petrarch's medical terminology in the *Letters of Old Age*, see *ibid.*, p. 31.

26. For Petrarch's dispute with the doctors, see McClure, *Sorrow and Consolation*, pp. 49–54 (quote on p. 50).

27. The full title is *Epistolarum mearum ad diversos liber* (A book of my letters to different people); Petrarch apparently settled on the idea of collecting his own after discovering Cicero's letters in 1345. For Petrarch as a "public" consoler, see McClure, *Sorrow and Consolation*, pp. 30–45.

28. McClure, *Sorrow and Consolation*, pp. 46 and 51, who also locates the term *medici animorum* at the end of chapter 93, "On Misery and Sadness" (p. 214 n.102). Whereas in the earlier *De otio religioso* (On religious leisure), Petrarch speaks of consolations for the soul (*anima*), *De remediis* he regarded as therapy for the mind (*animus*); *ibid.*, p. 48. The threefold division of Petrarch's self-identification as a rhetorical healer and the corresponding division of his works by genre employed here I owe to McClure's study.

CHAPTER FIVE: THE ARTIST AS MEDICUS, PART ONE

The epigraph is from Jacob Burckhardt, *Weltgeschichtliche Betrachtungen*, translated and discussed in Frank Ankersmit, *Sublime Historical Experience* (Stanford: Stanford University Press, 2005), pp. 163–64; cf. the translation by M. D. Hottinger (1943), republished as *Reflections On History* (Indianapolis: Liberty Classics, 1979), p. 34.

1. Franz Posset, *Renaissance Monks: Monastic Humanism in Six Biographical Sketches* (Leiden: Brill, 2005), p. 83. Kress's bronze epitaph by Peter Vischer the Younger is still in the Lorenzkirche (130 cm H). See Rainer Kahsnitz and William D. Wixom (eds.), *Gothic and Renaissance Art in Nuremberg, 1300–1550*, exhibition catalogue, Metropolitan Museum of Art and Germanisches Nationalmuseum (Munich: Prestel, 1986), cat. 54 (on the Kress Missal).

2. In 1506, Dürer left Barbara in charge of selling his prints during the annual *Heiltumsfest* in Nuremberg, which occurred annually on the second Friday after Easter; Jane Campbell Hutchison, *Albrecht Dürer: A Biography* (Princeton: Princeton University Press, 1990), p. 83, notes that, in Nuremberg, it was customary for women to handle retail sales.

3. Preserved in Berlin (Kupferstichkabinett, Sign. Clm. 32), the single surviving leaf from Dürer's *Gedenckbuch* features on its reverse his report of the portentous "rain of crucifixes" he claims to have witnessed in Nuremberg in 1503, "the greatest marvel I have seen

in all my days" (*Daz grost wunderwerck, daz jch all mein dag gesehen hab*); it is accompanied by a nebulous three-figure Crucifixion rendered in wash. See Michael Roth (ed.), *Dürers Mutter: Schönheit, Alter und Tod im Bild der Renaissance* (Berlin: Staatliche Museen zu Berlin / Nicolaische Verlagsbuchhandlung, 2006), cat. 2 (M. Roth); Peter Parshall, "Albrecht Dürer's *Gedenckbuch* and the Rain of Crosses," *Word and Image* 22.3 (2006), pp. 202–10; and Helmut Puff, "Memento Mori, Memento Mei: Albrecht Dürer and the Art of Dying," in Lynne Tatlock (ed.), *Enduring Loss in Early Modern Germany: Cross Disciplinary Perspectives* (Leiden: Brill, 2010), 103–32, esp. pp. 103–11. The reverse side also features Dürer's summary of his financial situation around 1506–1507.

4. Translation from Hutchison, *Albrecht Dürer*, p. 122.

5. See Roth (ed.), *Dürers Mutter*, no. 1 (Michael Roth).

6. Translation from Hutchison, *Albrecht Dürer*, p. 122. The authors in *Dürers Mutter* rightly highlight the "staged quality" of the portrait (p. 131).

7. Hutchison, *Albrecht Dürer*, p. 122.

8. In addition to confirming Dürer's mastery of the eye's anatomy, Wolfgang Pirsig usefully points out that the clearly described divergence of the right eye's axis of vision (strabismus) is a feature that recurs in Dürer's portrait heads of family, friends, and others, including himself; see Wolfgang Pirsig, "'Dürers Mutter'—aus ärztlicher Sicht," in *Dürers Mutter*, pp. 17–22.

9. Otto Benesch, *The Art of the Northern Renaissance: Its Relation to the Contemporary Spiritual and Intellectual Movements*, rev. ed. (London: Phaidon, 1965), p. 8.

10. *Portrait Diptych of Barbara Dürer*, née Holper (left), and *Albrecht Dürer the Elder* (right), ca. 1490; oil on fir panels, 47 cm x 35.8 cm (Barbara), and 47.5 cm x 39.5 cm (Albrecht), Nuremberg, Germanisches Nationalmuseum (no. 1160; Barbara) and Florence, Galleria degli Uffizi (no. 1086; Albrecht). Separated since at least 1628, the two panels were reunited for the exhibition *The Early Dürer* in 2012. See Daniel Hess and Thomas Eser (eds.), *The Early Dürer*, exhibition catalogue (Nuremberg: Germanisches National Museum; New York: Thames and Hudson, 2012), nos. 7 and 8.

11. Maureen Carroll, "*Memoria* and *Damnatio Memoriae*: Preserving and Erasing Identities in Roman Funerary Commemoration," in Maureen Carroll and Jane Rempel (eds.), *Living Through the Dead: Burial and Commemoration in the Classical World* (Oxford: Oxbow, 2011), pp. 66–67.

12. Cf. the sensitive commentary by Jeffrey Chipps Smith, "Dürer's Losses and the Dilemmas of Being," in Tatlock (ed.), *Enduring Loss in Early Modern Germany*, pp. 71–101, esp. p. 74.

13. For graphic industry as release, see Andrew Robison et al., *Albrecht Dürer: Master Drawings, Watercolors, and Prints from the Albertina*, exhibition catalogue (Washington, D.C.: National Gallery of Art / Munich: Delmonico Books, Prestel, 2013), p. 201 (cat. 80, by Matthias Mende).

14. *Ibid.*

15. Erwin Panofsky, *Albrecht Dürer*, 2 vols. (Princeton: Princeton University Press, 1943), vol. 1, p. 171.

16. Matthias Mende, in Robison et al., *Albrecht Dürer*, p. 201, translation modified.

17. See the discussion in Chapter 4. For the variegated history of the term, see s.v. "Trostbrief," *Deutsches Wörterbuch von Jacob und Wilhelm Grimm*, 16 vols. (Leipzig, 1854–1961; Quellenverzeichnis, 1971).

18. *Ibid.*

19. See Ronald K. Rittgers, "Christianization through Consolation: Urban Rhegius' Soul Medicine for the Healthy and the Sick in These Dangerous Times (1529)," in Anna Marie Johnson and John A. Maxfield (eds.), *Reformation as Christianization: Essays on Scott Hendrix's Christianization Thesis* (Tübingen: Mohr Siebeck, 2012), pp. 321–48.

20. Ioan P. Couliano, *Eros and Magic in the Renaissance*, trans. Margaret Cook (Chicago: University of Chicago Press, 1987), p. 50. On 21 May 1991, Couliano was murdered in a bathroom at the University of Chicago's Divinity School, possibly by Romanian intelligence agents in retaliation for his criticisms of the Communist regime of Nicolae Ceaușescu.

21. Friedrich Winkler, *Die Zeichnungen Albrecht Dürers*, 4 vols. (Berlin: Deutscher Verein für Kunstwissenschaft, 1936–39), vol. 1, no. 26; Winkler, *Albrecht Dürer: Leben und Werk* (Berlin: Gebr. Mann, 1957), pp. 36–37, with the identification of the headgear as a bandage and the perception of physical rather than spiritual pain; *Albrecht Dürer 1471–1971*, exhibition catalogue (Nuremberg: Prestel, 1971), cat. 65 (where it is labeled "Selbstbildnis mit Binde," self-portrait with bandage); Joseph Leo Koerner, *The Moment of Self-Portraiture in German Renaissance Art* (Chicago: University of Chicago Press, 1993), pp. 3–5, 4–17, 21 (with doubts about Winkler's identification of the bandage); Rainer Schoch, *100 Meister-Zeichnungen aus der Graphischen Sammlung der Universität Erlangen-Nürnberg*, exhibition catalogue (Nuremberg: Germanisches Nationalmuseum, 2008), cat. 38; Christiane Andersson and Larry Silver, "Dürer's Drawings," in Larry Silver and Jeffrey Chipps Smith (eds.), *The Essential Dürer* (Philadelphia: University of Pennsylvania Press, 2010), pp. 18–20; and Hans Dickel (ed.), *Zeichnen seit Dürer: Die süddeutschen und schweizerischen Zeichnungen der Renaissance in der Universitätsbibliothek Erlangen*, exhibition catalogue (Petersberg: Michael Imhof, 2014), cat. 78v. Dürer set out on his *Wanderjahre* in 1490, around Eastertide, and traveled for four years, but it is not certain where he made this drawing.

22. Joanna Woods-Marsden, *Renaissance Self-Portraiture: The Visual Construction of Identity and the Social Status of the Artist* (New Haven: Yale University Press, 1998), pp. 35–36.

23. Trevor Anderson, "Dental Treatment in Medieval England," *British Journal of Dentistry* 197.7 (October 2004), pp. 419–25.

24. See especially David Kunzle, "The Art of Pulling Teeth in the Seventeenth and Nineteenth Centuries: From Public Martyrdom to Private Nightmare and Political Struggle?," in Michel Feher, Ramona Naddaff, and Nadia Tazi (eds.), *Zone 5: Fragments for a History of the Human Body* (New York: Zone Books, 1989), pp. 29–89, who coined the phrase

"dental martyrdom"; and John Gash, "The Caravaggesque Toothpuller," in Tom Nichols (ed.), *Others and Outcasts in Early Modern Europe: Picturing the Social Margins* (Aldershot: Ashgate, 2007), pp. 133–55.

25. If real, we may also ask whether it is not pain mixed with the anxious anticipation of worse pain, the pain of surgery; if we are to understand the depiction as postsurgical, what we see mixed with pain may be, rather, humiliation.

26. All of the commentators cited above have adduced the connection. However, here it is the cheekbone that anchors the supporting hand, rather than the chin, suggestive of a pained weariness, rather than afflicted thought.

27. Dürer treated this theme in the so-called *Jabach Altarpiece*; see Chapter 6.

28. See Jean Starobinski, *Geschichte der Melancholiebehandlung von den Anfängen bis 1900* (Basel: J. R. Geigy, 1960), p. 42.

29. Winkler, *Die Zeichnungen Albrecht Dürers*, vol. 2, no. 482, who favors an earlier date, accepting Flechsig's argument that Dürer's relative age here places the self-portrait closer to those embedded in the *Feast of the Rose Garlands* (1506) and the *Heller Altar* (ca. 1510); and Anne Röver-Kann, with Manu von Miller, *Dürer-Zeit: Die Geschichte der Dürer-Sammlung in der Kunsthalle Bremen*, exhibition catalogue (Munich: Hirmer, 2012), pp. 110–15 (no. 32), with complete references to the older literature.

30. Panofsky, *Albrecht Dürer*, vol. 1, p. 171. On the question of whether Dürer himself was a melancholic in any clinical sense, which will not be decided here, see also Raymond Klibansky, Erwin Panofsky, and Fritz Saxl, *Saturn and Melancholy: Studies in the History of Natural Philosophy, Religion, and Art* (London: Nelson, 1964), p. 363 n.271; and Friedbert Ficker, "Albrecht Dürer und die Medizin seiner Zeit," *Münchener medizinische Wochenschrift* 113 (21 May 1971), pp. 814–18, who likewise connects the drawing to the artist's commitment to humoral pathology.

31. Accordng to Johanna Geyer-Kordesch, patient narratives in the early eighteenth century were transmitted along a familiar course: first the patient tells "a relative or local doctor about [an] illness, who writes it down, often with a wonderful sense of drama.... This was sent to a consultant, after, probably, reading it over to the client, for a written medical opinion. The recipient, usually a medical faculty professor, writes a response, in which he draws together salient points and reaches both a diagnostic conclusion and recommendations for medication and therapy"; see Geyer-Kordesch, "Whose Enlightenment? Medicine, Witchcraft, Melancholia, and Pathology," in Roy Porter (ed.), *Medicine in the Enlightenment* (Amsterdam: Rodopi, 1994), p. 114. In Dürer studies, the consultation theory is accepted by Winkler, *Die Zeichnungen Albrecht Dürers*, vol. 2, no. 141; Panofsky, *Albrecht Dürer*, vol. 1, p. 171; and Ficker, "Albrecht Dürer und die Medizin seiner Zeit" among others. Röver-Kann, *Dürer-Zeit*, p, 111, regards it as a consensus among researchers.

32. On the significance of letters and distant communication in Dürer's oeuvre, see

Shira Brisman, *Albrecht Dürer and the Epistolary Mode of Address* (Chicago: University of Chicago Press, 2017).

33. Koerner, *The Moment of Self-Portraiture in German Renaissance Art*, p. 177. As the comparisons assembled by Koerner also make clear, the self-pointing gesture has a conventional and performative character.

34. The strongest case for the persistence of premodern collective perceptions in responses to images remains David Freedberg, *The Power of Images: Studies in the History and Theory of Response* (Chicago: University of Chicago Press, 1989).

35. See Hutchison, *Albrecht Dürer: A Biography*, p. 149.

36. See Jan Białostocki, *Dürer and His Critics 1500–1971: Chapters in the History of Ideas Including a Collection of Texts* (Baden-Baden: Valentin Koerner, 1986), pp. 105–14 and fig. 43 (a drawing of 1829 by Johann Philipp Walther, after Fellner's painting).

37. "Vnd am mondag frühe fuhren wir zu schiff wieder aus und führen für die Fahr und für Zürchse. Wolt den grosen fisch gesehen haben, da hett in die Fortuna wieder weg geführt," entry for 10 December 1520 in Hans Rupprich (ed.), *Dürer: Schriftlicher Nachlass*, 3 vols. (Berlin: Deutscher Verein für Kunstwissenschaft, 1956–69), vol I, p. 163, translation from Hutchison, *Albrecht Dürer: A Biography*, p. 156.

38. Journal entry for April 11, 1521, in Jan-Albert Goris and George Marlier (eds.), *Albrecht Dürer's Diary of His Journey to the Netherlands, 1520–1521* (Greenwich: New York Graphic Society, 1971), p. 88; for the original German, see Rupprich (ed.), *Dürer: Schriftlicher Nachlass*, vol. 1, pp. 168–69; also discussed in Smith, "Dürer's Losses and the Dilemmas of Being," p. 88.

39. Hanns M. Seitz, "'Do der gelb fleck ist...': Dürers Malaria, eine Fehldiagnos," *Wiener klinische Wochenschrift* 122, supplement 3 (October 2010), pp. 10–13, rejects the diagnosis of the natural course of a *Plasmodium vivax* infection as the cause of Dürer's recurring fevers or his eventual death at age fifty-seven. See the case for malaria in Rupprich (ed.), *Dürer: Schriftlicher Nachlass*, vol. 1, p. 195 n.585; Hutchison, *Albrecht Dürer: A Biography*, pp. 153–54 and 162–63; and Smith, "Dürer's Losses and the Dilemmas of Being," p. 87. If not properly treated, malarial infections generally recur for years after onset, with somewhat milder symptoms. For the possibility that Dürer had contracted syphilis, see R. F. Timken-Zinkann, "Medical Aspects of the Art and Life of Albrecht Dürer (1471–1528)," *Proceedings of the XXIII International Congress of the History of Medicine, London 2–9 September 1972*, vol. 2 (London: Wellcome Institute for the History of Medicine, 1974), pp. 870–75.

40. Hutchison, *Albrecht Dürer: A Biography*, p. 163 (for payments to doctors) and p. 158 (for myrobolans).

41. Albrecht Dürer, *The Writings of Albrecht Dürer*, ed. and trans. William Martin Conway (New York: Philosophical Library, 1958), pp. 89–90; discussed in Hutchison, *Albrecht Dürer: A Biography*, p. 127; and Smith, "Dürer's Losses and the Dilemmas of Being," p. 87. Notable in this connection are the corrective glasses Dürer mentions buying during his

travels in the Netherlands; see Goris and Marlier (eds.), *Albrecht Dürer's Diary*, p. 71; also cited in Smith, "Dürer's Losses and the Dilemmas of Being," p. 87.

42. Letter dated 18 January 1519; quoted in Hutchison, *Albrecht Dürer A Biography*, p. 127.

43. Winkler, *Die Zeichnungen Albrecht Dürers*, vol. 4, no. 886; Walter Strauss, *The Complete Drawings of Albrecht Dürer*, 6 vols. (New York: Abaris, 1974), vol. 4, no. 1522/8; T. A. Ilatovskaya, *West European Drawing of XVI–XX Centuries: Kunsthalle Collection in Bremen — Catalogue* (Moscow: Kultura, 1992), cat. 40; and Röver-Kann, *Dürer-Zeit*, pp. 156–61 (cat. no. 46), with the most comprehensive bibliography.

44. Anne Röver-Kann, "Dürer Zeit — Schöne Zeit: Die Bremer Sammler Klugkist, Lahmann und Schwarting," in *Dürer-Zeit*, pp. 18–23.

45. The return of this drawing, along with important paintings by Masolino, Altdorfer, and Toulouse-Lautrec, was secured by Günter Busch (director of the Kunsthalle until 1984) in the early 1950s; see Röver-Kann, "Dürer Zeit," p. 20.

46. In 2003, the objects were collectively declared the property of the Russian state. For current information, see the Deutsches Zentrum Kulturgutverluste at http://www.lostart.de/Webs/DE/Provenienz/Auslagerungsorte/Index.html?cms_param=AUSLORT_ID=14944%26ORT_ID=318. The collection is now divided between two museums. A useful table of the location of the drawings is in Röver-Kann, *Dürer-Zeit*, pp. 242–45. On the absconding by Baldin and legal efforts to repatriate what remains, see also Konstantin Akinsha, Grigoriĭ Kozlov, and Sylvia Hochfield, *Beautiful Loot: The Soviet Plunder of Europe's Art Treasures* (New York: Random House, 1995), pp. 243–50.

47. Panofsky, *Albrecht Dürer*, vol. 1, p. 241; Koerner, *The Moment of Self-Portraiture in German Renaissance Art*, pp. 179, 191, 241–43; and Ernst Ullmann, *Albrecht Dürer-Selbstbildnisse und autobiographische Schriften als Zeugnisse der Entwicklung seiner Persönlichkeit* (Berlin: Akademie, 1994).

48. In 1924, Emmy Voigtländer, following a suggestion by Friedrich Schneider, declared the figure to be a self-portrait; see Friedrich Schneider, "Albrecht Dürers Tafelgemälde 'Barmherzigkeit' 1523, ehemals im Dom zu Mainz," *Mainzer Zeitschrift* 2 (1907), p. 83; and Emmy Voigtländer, "Ein Selbstbildnis aus Dürers Spätzeit," *Repertorium für Kunstwissenschaft* 44 (1924), pp. 282–87.

49. Gustav Pauli (ed.), *Die Kunst Albrecht Dürers: Seine Werke in Originalen und Reproduktionen geordnet nach der Zeitfolge ihrer Entstehung*, exhibition catalogue (Bremen: Kunsthalle, 1911), no. 1127 (which I have not been able to consult); cited in Röver Kann, *Dürer-Zeit*, p. 158.

50. On "Christomorphic" self-portraiture, see above all Koerner, *The Moment of Self-Portraiture in German Renaissance Art*, p. 179. For a critique, see Margaret A. Sullivan, "*Alter Apelles*: Dürer's 1500 *Self-Portrait*," *Renaissance Quarterly* 68.4 (Winter 2016), pp. 1161–91, with brief comment on the Bremen drawing on 1186.

51. Panofsky, *Albrecht Dürer*, vol. 1, p. 241. Noteworthy is the fact that Princeton Uni-

versity Press selected the Bremen drawing as the frontispiece to its fourth edition of Panofsky's book. See also Roland H. Bainton, "Dürer and Luther as the Man of Sorrows," *Art Bulletin* 29.4 (December 1947), pp. 269–72, who amplifies the *imitatio Christi* theme and traces parallels in representations of Luther's persecution at the hands of his political enemies.

52. Also relevant here is Dürer's pen-and-ink Man of Sorrows of ca. 1510 in the British Museum in London; see Koerner, *The Moment of Self-Portraiture in German Renaissance Art*, p. 178 (fig. 93).

53. *Ibid.*, p. 179.

54. *Ibid.*

55. Hans Belting's term, "Passionsbildnis Jesu" (Passion portrait of Christ), coined for the icon type that came to be known as the *imago pietatis*, remains broadly useful for images that refer across the categories of "cultic," "devotional," and "narrative"; see Belting, *Das Bild und sein Publikum in Mittelalter: Form und Funktion früher Bildtafeln der Passion* (Berlin: Gebr. Mann, 1981), available as *The Image and Its Public in the Middle Ages: Form and Function of Early Paintings of the Passion*, trans. Mark Bartusis and Raymond Meyer (New Rochelle: Aristotle D. Caratzas, 1990).

56. Mitchell B. Merback, "The Man of Sorrows in Northern Europe: Ritual Metaphor and Therapeutic Exchange," in Catherine R. Puglisi and William L. Barcham (eds.), *New Perspectives on the Man of Sorrows* (Kalamazoo: Medieval Institute Publications, 2013), pp. 77–116, esp. pp. 110–12.

57. Michel Foucault, "Technologies of the Self," in *Ethics: Subjectivity and Truth*, ed. Paul Rabinow, trans. Robert Hurley and others (New York: New Press, 1997), pp. 223–51; Pierre Hadot, *Philosophy as a Way of Life: Spiritual Exercises from Socrates to Foucault*, ed. Arnold I. Davidson, trans. Michael Chase (Oxford: Blackwell, 1995), pp. 206–13; and for a critique of Foucault, see Roland Boer, "Foucault's Care," *Political Theology Today*, 20 February 2014, http://www.politicaltheology.com/blog/foucaults-care.

58. The cardinal may have ordered the work in person during a visit to Nuremberg for the Reichstag, between 10 April 1522 and 8 February 1523. The first to identify the Pommersfelden panel with the Bremen drawing was Eduard Flechsig, *Albrecht Dürer: Sein Leben und seine künstlerische Entwickelung*, 2 vols. (Berlin: G. Grote'sche, 1928–31), vol. 1, p. 428, and vol. 2, pp. 254–55, 262, 263, 601 n.1224. See also Fedja Anzelewsky, *Albrecht Dürer: Das Malerische Werk*, ed. Deutschen Verein für Kunstwissenschaft (Berlin: Deutscher Verlag für Kunstwissenschaft, 1971), pp. 267–68 (no. 170K); Herman Maué and Sonja Brink (eds.), *Die Grafen von Schönborn: Kirchenfürsten, Sammler, Mäzene*, exhibition catalogue (Nuremberg: Germanisches Nationalmuseum, 1989), cat. 275; and Röver Kann, *Dürer-Zeit*, p. 161 and p. 194 n.5.

59. Rainer Schoch, Matthias Mende, and Anna Scherbaum, *Albrecht Dürer: Das druckgraphische Werk*, 3 vols. (Munich: Prestel, 2001–2004), vol. 1, no. 78.

60. Cf. Voigtländer, "Ein Selbstbildnis aus Dürers Spätzeit," p. 284, who believes the decision to convert a sitting-figure study into a *Schmerzensmann* was made only subsequently. The same author points out that the Pommersfelden copy switches the left-right placement of the flail and birch (p. 283).

61. Röver-Kann, *Dürer-Zeit*, p. 156, describes it simply as "wehenden Haaren," windblown hair, with no further comment.

62. Strauss, *The Complete Engravings, Etchings and Drypoints*, no. 53.

63. *Ibid.*, no. 29, with "D" in monogram reversed; Schoch, Mende, and Scherbaum, *Albrecht Dürer*, vol. 1, no. 28, pp. 86–87.

64. Leon Battista Alberti, *On Painting*, from Aby Warburg, "Sandro Botticelli's *Birth of Venus* and *Spring:* An Examination of Concepts of Antiquity in the Italian Early Renaissance," in Warburg, *The Renewal of Pagan Antiquity: Contributions to the Cultural History of the European Renaissance*, trans. David Britt (Los Angeles: Getty Research Institute for the History of Art and the Humanities, 1999), p. 96. Cf. the more restrained translation in Alberti, *Leon Battista Alberti: A New Translation and Critical Edition*, ed. and trans. Rocco Sinisgalli (Cambridge: Cambridge University Press, 2011), p. 21.

65. Warburg, "Sandro Botticelli's *Birth of Venus* and *Spring*," p. 96. As Warburg mentions, the connection was first drawn by Anton Springer in 1883.

66. Alberti, *On Painting*, as quoted in Warburg, "Sandro Botticelli's *Birth of Venus* and *Spring*," p. 96.

67. Discussed in Chapter 4, with references.

68. Strauss, *The Complete Engravings, Etchings and Drypoints*, no. 7; Schoch, Mende, and Scherbaum, *Albrecht Dürer*, vol. 1, no. 5, p. 36.

69. Joseph Leo Koerner, "The Fortune of Dürer's 'Nemesis'," in Walter Haug and Burghart Wachinger (eds.), *Fortuna* (Tübingen: Max Niemeyer, 1995), pp. 239–94.

70. In addition to the catalogues cited above (in Chapter 2), see Koerner, "The Fortune of Dürer's 'Nemesis'," pp. 257–64; Thomas Schauerte, *Albrecht Dürer*, pp. 154–56 (no. 98).

71. Koerner, "The Fortune of Dürer's 'Nemesis'," pp. 250–51.

72. On the connections between Charles de Bovelle's *Liber de sapiente* and German humanism, likewise the relevance of the Fortune/Wisdom woodcut to Dürer's *Melencolia*, see Peter-Klaus Schuster, *Melencolia I: Dürers Denkbild*, 2 vols. (Berlin: Gebr. Mann, 1991), vol. 1, pp. 307–22; and Peter-Klaus Schuster and Jörg Völlnagel, "Dürer and Rufus: *Melencolia I* in the Medical Tradition," in Rufus of Ephesus, *On Melancholy*, ed. Peter E. Pormann (Tübingen: Mohr Siebeck, 2008), pp. 204–205 and 209–11. Key iconographic studies of Fortuna and her allegorical counterparts are Alfred Doren, "Fortuna im Mittelalter und in der Renaissance," *Vorträge der Bibliothek Warburg* 1 (1922–23), pp. 71–144; F. P. Pickering, *Literature and Art in the Middle Ages* (Coral Gables: University of Miami Press, 1970), pp. 168–222; and Simona Cohen, *Transformations of Time and Temporality in Medieval and Renaissance Art* (Leiden: Brill, 2014), pp. 73–79.

73. Aby Warburg, "Francesco Sassetti's Last Injunctions to His Sons," in *The Renewal of Pagan Antiquity*, pp. 223–62.

74. Quoted in *ibid.*, p. 237 (with Italian original on p. 235).

75. Quoted and discussed in *ibid.*, p. 241 and p. 258 n.49.

76. *Ibid.*, p. 242.

77. *Ibid.*, pp. 244–45.

78. *Ibid.*, p. 249.

79. For all three references, see *ibid.*, p. 258 n.50, which cites Oskar Brenner (ed.), *Ein altes italienisch-deutsches Sprachbuch: Ein Beitrag zur Mundartenkunde des 15. Jahrhunderts*, vol. 2 (Munich: Christian Kaiser, 1895), p. 2.

80. Warburg, "Sassetti's Last Injunctions to His Sons," p. 241; cf. Koerner, "The Fortune of Dürer's 'Nemesis',￼" p. 256.

81. Winkler, *Die Zeichnungen Albrecht Dürers*, vol. 4, no. 944; Rupprich (ed.), *Dürer: Schriftlicher Nachlass*, vol. 1, pp. 214–15; translation from Jean Michel Massing, "Dürer's Dreams," *Journal of the Warburg and Courtauld Institutes* 49 (1986), p. 241. See also Karl Möseneder, *Paracelsus und die Bilder: Über Glauben, Magie und Astrologie im Reformationszeitalter* (Tübingen: Max Niemeyer, 2009), p. 114, emphasizing its place in contemporary discussions of a "second flood"; and Smith, "Dürer's Losses and the Dilemmas of Being," p. 89.

82. Letter to Giovanni Barrili, in Francesco Petrarch, *Letters on Familiar Matters*, trans. Aldo S. Bernardo, 3 vols. (Albany: State University of New York Press, 1975–85), vol. 2, p. 162; see the Introduction for further references.

CHAPTER SIX: THE ARTIST AS MEDICUS, PART TWO

The epigraph is from Wolfgang Stechow, "Alberti Dureri Praecepta," *Studies in the History of Art* 4 (1971–72), p. 91. These words are from Stechow's invitational address at the Germanisches National Museum on the occasion of the landmark Dürer exhibition, May 21, 1971.

1. For essentials on the altarpiece, see Fedja Anzelewsky, *Albrecht Dürer: Das Malerische Werk*, ed. Deutschen Verein für Kunstwissenschaft (Berlin: Deutscher Verlag für Kunstwissenschaft, 1971), pp. 175–79 (nos. 72–75); Peter Strieder, *Tafelmalerei in Nürnberg 1350–1550* (Königstein im Taunus: K. Robert, 1993), p. 103; Doris Kutschbach, *Albrecht Dürer: Die Altäre* (Stuttgart: Belser, 1995), pp. 49–64; Bodo Brinkmann and Stephan Kemperdick, *Deutsche Gemälde im Städel 1500–50* (Mainz am Rhein: Philipp von Zabern, 2005), pp. 257–69; and Daniel Hess and Thomas Eser (eds.), *The Early Dürer*, exhibition catalogue (Nuremberg: Germanisches National Museum; New York: Thames & Hudson, 2012), nos. 109 and 110.

2. Munich, Alte Pinakothek, inv. WAF 228 and WAF 229. Early in the nineteenth century, when the panels were in the possession of the Cologne painter Joseph Hoffmann, they were split for more profitable sale; see Gisela Goldberg, Bruno Heimberg, and Martin Schawe, *Albrecht Dürer: Die Gemälde der Alten Pinakothek*, ed. Bayerische Staatsgemäldesammlungen München (Heidelberg: Edition Braus, 1998), pp. 385–415, no. 9.

3. Günter Bandmann, *Melancholie und Musik: Ikonographische Studien* (Cologne: Westdeutscher, 1960), p. 56; and Tobias Leuker, *Dürer als ikonographischer Neuerer* (Freiburg: Rombach, 2001), pp. 22–23. The evidence for the Wittenberg provenance is reviewed critically by Joachim Jacoby, "A Note on Dürer's So-Called Jabach Altarpiece," *Bibliothèque d'Humanisme et Renaissance* 63.1 (2001), pp. 58–59.

4. Jacoby, "A Note on Dürer's So-Called Jabach Altarpiece," p. 61. In addition to the commission for the chapel's decoration, Dürer had multiple contacts with the Fuggers. He made a portrait in chalk (now lost) of Georg, who lived in Nuremberg for a time, while his portrait of Jakob Fugger ("the Rich") is preserved in the Staatsgalerie Augsburg (no. 717); see Sebastian Gulden, "An Ideal Neighborhood: The Physical Environment of the Early Dürer as a Space of Experience," in Hess and Eser (eds.), *The Early Dürer*, p. 37.

5. Anzelewsky, *Albrecht Dürer*, p. 149.

6. See the discussion in Brinkmann and Kemperdick, *Deutsche Gemälde im Städel 1500–50*, pp. 267–68.

7. Jerome interpreted Job as a prophet of the Resurrection in his exegesis of Job 19:25–26 ("For I know that my Redeemer liveth, and in the last day I shall rise out of the earth. And I shall be clothed again with my skin, and in my flesh I will see my God"); discussed in Marguerite L. Brown, "The Subject Matter of Duerer's *Jabach Altar*," *Marsyas* 1 (1941), p. 56; and Kathi Meyer, "St. Job as a Patron of Music," *Art Bulletin* 35.1 (March 1954), pp. 30–31.

8. Jacoby, "A Note on Dürer's So-Called Jabach Altarpiece," p. 61.

9. Erwin Panofsky, *Albrecht Dürer*, 2 vols. (Princeton: Princeton University Press, 1943), vol. 1, p. 94.

10. Fedja Anzelewsky, *Dürer-Studien: Untersuchungen zu den ikonographischen und geistesgeschichtlichen Grundlagen seiner Werke zwischen den beiden Italienreisen* (Berlin: Deutscher Verlag für Kunstwissenschaft, 1983), p. 161.

11. Recent technical examination has revealed that Dürer distressed the painted surface, using the ball of his hand to create texture in areas of shading and then, across the open expanses of Job's skin, sprayed or splashed solvents onto the freshly applied glazes, creating small craters that simulate the blistering of skin lesions; see Daniel Hess and Oliver Mack, "Dürer as Painter: The Early Work up to 1505," in Hess and Eser (eds.), *The Early Dürer*, p. 185.

12. Jacoby, "A Note on Dürer's So-Called Jabach Altarpiece," p. 49, with further references. Jacoby is preceded in this theory by Samuel Terrien, *The Iconography of Job through the Centuries: Artists as Biblical Interpreters* (University Park: Pennsylvania State University Press, 1996), pp. 139–45.

13. Jacoby, "A Note on Dürer's So-Called Jabach Altarpiece," p. 50, with further references.

14. See especially Gert von der Osten, "Job and Christ: The Development of a Devotional Image," *Journal of the Warburg and Courtauld Institutes* 16.1–2 (January–June 1953), pp.

153–58; Bandmann, *Melancholie und Musik*, pp. 55–62; and F. P. Pickering, *Literature and Art in the Middle Ages* (Coral Gables: University of Miami Press, 1970), pp. 92–114, esp. figs. 9a–d.

15. Rainer Schoch, Matthias Mende, and Anna Scherbaum, *Albrecht Dürer: Das druckgraphische Werk*, 3 vols. (Munich: Prestel, 2001–2004), vol. 2, no. 186.

16. Thomas Aquinas, *Expositio super Iob ad litteram:* Commentary on the Book of Job, ed. Joseph Kenny, O.P., trans. Brian Mulladay, available online at http://dhspriory.org/thomas/SSJob.htm. I owe the identification of this source to Leuker, *Dürer als ikonographischer Neuerer*, pp. 25–27.

17. Aquinas, *Expositio super Iob ad litteram*, ch. 30. Here I have used the English translation of Job provided by Aquinas's translators to avoid confusions in the commentary's biblical quotes.

18. Jacoby, "A Note on Dürer's So-Called Jabach Altarpiece," p. 51: "The evidence gained from medical sources quite clearly demonstrates that the pouring of water in Dürer's painting represents a medical procedure."

19. Now in the Wallraf-Richartz Museum in Cologne; for a review of examples, see Brown, "The Subject Matter of Duerer's *Jabach Altar*," pp. 57–58.

20. Hans Kauffmann, "Der sogennante Jabasche Altar und die Dichtung des Buches Hiob," *Kunstwissenschaftliche Beiträge, August Schmarsow gewidmet zum fünfzigsten Semester* (1907), pp. 153–62; cited in Leuker, *Dürer als ikonographischer Neuerer*, p. 27.

21. Rudolf Preimesberger, "Albrecht Dürers Jabachaltar—'Trommler und Pfeifer,'" in Ekkehard Mai (ed.), *Die Zukunft der Alten Meister: Perspektiven und Konzepte für das Kunstmuseum von heute* (Cologne: Böhlau, 2001), pp. 175–76.

22. Meyer, "St. Job as a Patron of Music."

23. For the biblical themes, see Bandmann, *Melancholie und Musik*, pp. 11–30.

24. Marsilio Ficino, letter to Antonio Canisiano (*De musica*); quoted and discussed in D. P. Walker, *Spiritual and Demonic Magic from Ficino to Campanella* (1958; University Park: Pennsylvania State University Press, 2000), p. 6.

25. Penelope Gouk, "Music and Spirit in Early Modern Thought," in Elena Carrera (ed.), *Emotions and Health, 1200-1700* (Leiden: Brill, 2013), pp. 233–34.

26. On Ficino's astrological music, see Walker, *Spiritual and Demonic Magic*, pp. 18–24; and more recently, Hyun-Ah Kim, *The Renaissance Ethics of Music* (New York: Routledge, 2015), ch. 4, "Divine Music: The Platonic-Humanist Tradition."

27. "Daz sext, ob sich der jung zw fill vbte do fan jm dy Melecoley vber hant mocht nemen, daz er durch kurtzwelich seiten spill zw leren do von gezogen werd zw ergetzlikeit seins geplütz," in Hans Rupprich (ed.), *Dürer: Schriftlicher Nachlass*, 3 vols. (Berlin: Deutscher Verein für Kunstwissenschaft, 1956–69), vol. 2, p. 92 (with Rupprich's useful overview on pp. 83–90). My translation is adapted from Albrecht Dürer, *The Writings of Albrecht Dürer*, ed. and trans. William Martin Conway (New York: Philosophical Library, 1958), p. 171, with another rendition of the original German on p. 189. Cf. Heinrich Wölfflin, *The Art of Albrecht Dürer*,

trans. Alastair Grieve and Heide Grieve (London: Phaidon, 1971), p. 202, where the phrase about melancholia's onset is translated as "[getting] out of hand"; see also Raymond Klibansky, Erwin Panofsky, and Fritz Saxl, *Saturn and Melancholy: Studies in the History of Natural Philosophy, Religion, and Art* (London: Nelson, 1964), who translate the article as follows: "Sixthly, see that the youth does not practise too much, whereby melancholy might get the upper hand of him; see that he learns to distract himself by pleasant airs on the lute, to delight his blood" (p. 282). The semantic range of *ergetzlikeit* in Dürer's Early New High German (*Frühneuhochdeutsch*) extends to notions of delighting, pleasuring, cheering, and refreshment; see Peter O. Müller, *Substantiv-Derivation in den Schriften Albrecht Dürers: Ein Beitrag zur Methodik historisch-synchroner Wortbildungsanalysen* (Berlin: Walter de Gruyter, 1993), p. 303.

28. Hjalmar G. Sandar, "Beiträge zur Biographie Hugos van der Goes und zur Chronologie seiner Werke," *Repertorium für Kunstwissenschaft* 35 (1912), pp. 519-45.

29. On the close connection between Job and syphilis, see Terrien, *The Iconography of Job*, pp. 140-42 (who unfortunately refers to Saint Job as "the intercessor for sexual reprobates"); and Jacoby, "A Note on Dürer's So-Called Jabach Altarpiece," pp. 52-55, who treats the issue more prudently.

30. Brown, "Subject Matter of Duerer's *Jabach Altar*," p. 61.

31. See Chapter 3 for a discussion of delegate figures, a term I have borrowed from Andrea Catellani.

32. My thanks to Lorenzo Pericolo for discussing this and related terms with me (personal correspondence, May 2016).

33. A magnificent overview is Christoph Stiegemann (ed.), *Caritas: Nächstenliebe von den frühen Christen bis zur Gegenwart*, exhibition catalogue, Erzbischöflichen Diözesansmuseum Paderborn (Petersberg: Michael Imhoff, 2015).

34. From Augustine, *De trinitate*, book 8, discussed in Timothy Verdon, "Masaccio's Trinity: Theological, Social, and Civic Meanings," in Diane Cole Ahl (ed.), *The Cambridge Companion to Masaccio* (Cambridge: Cambridge University Press, 2002), p. 165.

35. See *ibid*.

36. Preface to "Jesus Maria 1509"; original German in Moritz Thausing, *Dürers Briefe, Tagebücher und Reime, nebst einem Anhange von Zuschriften an und für Dürer* (Vienna: Wilhelm Braumüller, 1872), pp. 143-45; translation in Dürer, *The Writings of Albrecht Dürer*, where the editor credits Mrs. Charles Heaton, *The History of the Life of Albrecht Dürer of Nürnberg, with a Translation of His Letters and Journal & Some Account of His Works* (London: Macmillan, 1870).

37. Reproduced in Thausing, *Dürers Briefe, Tagebücher und Reime*, pp. 145-46; edited text with commentary in Berndt Hamm and Wolfgang Huber (eds.), *Lazarus Spengler: Schriften*, vol. 1, *Schriften der Jahre 1509 bis Juni 1525* (Gütersloh: Gütersloher Verlagshaus, 1995), pp. 3-5 (no. 1).

38. Dürer, *The Writings of Albrecht Dürer*, p. 282 (Heaton translation as cited above). Dürer's verses are difficult here: "Dass mir desgleichen nicht wiederfahr' / Thut's Noth, das ich

nicht mit Lernen spar' / Und dass ich Fleiss auch daran wende, Es ist noch Zeit zu gutem Ende"; in Thausing, *Dürers Briefe, Tagebücher und Reime*, p. 148. For Vitruvius, the architect "should be lettered, so that he may leave a lasting memorial in his treatises; know how to draw; be instructed in geometry; and now history, philosophy, music, medicine, law, and astrology" (*De architectura* 1.1.3); quoted and discussed in Patrick Doorly, "Dürer's *Melencolia I*: Plato's Abandoned Search for the Beautiful," *Art Bulletin* 86.2 (June 2004), p. 258.

39. Dürer, *The Writings of Albrecht Dürer*, p. 282 (Heaton translation as cited above); original in Thausing, *Dürers Briefe, Tagebücher und Reime*, pp. 147-49, corrected and edited, including the addition of line breaks, as follows: "Doch will ich nicht nur Reime schreiben, / Sondern auch Arzneikunde treiben. / Denn wunderlich ist es zu merken, / Wie die Arznei'n des Malers stärken. / D'rum hört, was solch' ein Arzt euch lehrt, / Viel gut' Ding', der Geseundheit werth: / Ein kleines Tröpflein reiner Laugen / Ist gut zu träufeln in die Augen. / Und wer scharf hören will und schnell, / Der thu' in die Ohren Mandelöl. / Wer das Zipperlein los will sein, / Der trinke Wasser, nicht starken Wein; / Und wer will gesunde Beine behalten, / Der Soll einen Block nich stehend spalten. / Wer darnach alt wird hundert Jahr, / Bezeugt, wie gut mein Ratschlag war." Cf. the version in Rupprich (ed.), *Dürer: Schriftlicher Nachlass*, vol. 1, pp. 130-31.

40. "Gleich wie Dürer indr molerei, / also dieser inn der ercznerei, / vor in vnd nach in niemand drad / in irer kuns gegleichet hat, / mvst es darvm vom tevfel sein / das sei ferne, och nein och nein"; from the engraving published by Balthasar Jenichen, 1572 (Nuremberg, Germanisches Nationalmuseum); reproduced and discussed in Karl Möseneder, *Paracelsus und die Bilder: Über Glauben, Magie und Astrologie im Reformationszeitalter* (Tübingen: Max Niemeyer, 2009), pp. 13-14 and fig. 5. The text was reused in the *Paracelsus-Flugblatt* by Matthis Quad of Kinckelbach (1606), which includes the same Agrippan "magic square" Dürer used in the *Melencolia* (see Chapter 4), but rotated 45 degrees counterclockwise; see Rupprich (ed.), *Dürer: Schriftlicher Nachlass*, vol. 1, p. 319 (no. 28); Möseneder, *Paracelsus und die Bilder*, p. 143 and fig. 7; and Carlos Gilly, "Der Paracelsus-Einblattdruck des Matthis Quad von 1606: Kritische Überlegungen über die sogenannten Rosenkreuzer-Bildnisse des Paracelsus," online at http://www.ritmanlibrary.com/collection/424-2. I am grateful to Peter Starenko for collaborating with me on the translation.

41. Friedrich Winkler, *Die Zeichnungen Albrecht Dürers*, 4 vols. (Berlin: Deutscher Verein für Kunstwissenschaft, 1936-39), vol. 1, no. 58; and Peter Prange, *Deutsche Zeichnungen, 1450-1800: Die Sammlungen der Hamburger Kunsthalle, Kupferstichkabinett. Bestandkatalog*, ed. Hubertus Gaßner and Andreas Stolzenburg, 2 vols. (Cologne: Böhlau, 2007), no. 290 (by Petra Roettig), with full bibliography.

42. Jane Campbell Hutchison, *Albrecht Dürer: A Biography* (Princeton: Princeton University Press, 1990), p. 56, referring to Erika Simon, "Das Werk: Die Rezeption der Antike," in *Albrecht Dürer 1471-1971*, exhibition catalogue (Nuremberg: Prestel, 1971), pp. 263-64 and cat. 506; and Anzelewsky, *Dürer-Studien*, pp. 45-56.

43. Hutchison, *Albrecht Dürer: A Biography*, p. 50. For Pirckheimer's role and influence on city culture, see Franz Xaver Pröll (ed.), *Willibald Pirckheimer, 1470-1970: Eine Dokumentation in der Stadtbibliothek Nürnberg*, exhibition catalogue (Nuremberg: Stadtbibliothek, 1970).

44. Hutchison, *Albrecht Dürer: A Biography*, p. 107. Of course, the period encompassed by the *Poetenschule* also saw the production of several brilliant reinterpretations of "religious" themes in the medium of engraving: the *Prodigal Son* (1496), the *Saint Eustace* (1501), Dürer's largest engraving, and the *Adam and Eve* (1504), to mention only the finest.

45. Lorraine Smith Pangle, *Aristotle and the Philosophy of Friendship* (Cambridge: Cambridge University Press, 2003), p. 39.

46. *Ibid.*, p. 196.

47. See James McEvoy, "The Theory of Friendship in Erasmus and Thomas More," *American Catholic Philosophical Quarterly* 80.2 (2006), pp. 227-52, with quote on p. 230 n.8.

48. Glenn Lesses, "Austere Friends: The Stoics and Friendship," *Apeiron* 26.1 (March 1, 1993), pp. 57-75; the quoted passage is Lesses's words, p. 68.

49. Cicero, *De finibus bonorum et malorum* 3.70, discussed in Lesses, "Austere Friends," p. 74. For Aristotle, "The excellent person is related to his friend in the same way as he is related to himself, since a friend is another himself"; Aristotle, *Nicomachean Ethics*, trans. Terence Irwin (Indianapolis: Hackett, 1985), p. 260 (1170b6).

50. Marcus Tullius Cicero, *Tusculan Disputations*, rev. ed., trans. J. E. King (Cambridge, MA: Harvard University Press, 1971), p. 225.

51. I am borrowing the phrase from Ronald K. Rittgers, *The Reformation of Suffering: Pastoral Theology and Lay Piety in Late Medieval and Early Modern Germany* (Oxford: Oxford University Press, 2012), p. 47.

52. Willibald Pirckheimer, *De his qui tarde a numine corripiuntur libellus* [Plutarch's *On the Delays of the Divine Vengeance*] (Nuremberg: F. Peypus, 1513), quoted in Lewis W. Spitz, *The Religious Renaissance of the German Humanists* (Cambridge, MA: Harvard University Press, 1963), p. 165.

53. Letter 8, Nuremberg Stadtbibliothek, Pirckheimer-Papiere 396; translation in Hutchison, *Albrecht Dürer: A Biography*, p. 93.

54. Hutchison, *Albrecht Dürer: A Biography*, p. 85. Ten of Dürer's letters survive from the Italian sojourn—eight of these were fortuitously preserved in a wall in the Pirckheimer family home on Egidienplatz and discovered during remodeling in 1748.

55. Beate Bockem, "The Young Dürer and Italy: Contact with Italy and the Mobility of Art and Artists around 1500," in Hess and Eser (eds.), *The Early Dürer*, p. 61.

56. "Vnd als jr schreibt, jch soll pald kumen oder jr wolt mirs weib kristiren, jst ewch vnerlawbt, jr prawt sy den zw thott"; Letter 10, from Venice, circa 13 October 1506, London, British Library, Sloane Collection, Harl. 4935, fol. 41; Rupprich (ed.), *Dürer: Schriftlicher Nachlass*, vol. 1, pp. 58-60. Cf. the more genteel translation in Hutchison, *Albrecht Dürer: A Biography*, p. 95: "Don't try it, you'll kill her." As Corine Schleif points out, the verb

klistieren (alt: *klysieren*) can refer to the administration of rectal or vaginal enemas and clearly has a smutty intent here; likewise the verb *brauten*, a transitive verb for "male-initiated coitus"; Corinne Schleif, "Albrecht Dürer between Agnes Frey and Willibald Pirckheimer," in Larry Silver and Jeffrey Chipps Smith (eds.), *The Essential Dürer* (Philadelphia: University of Pennsylvania Press, 2010), pp. 185–86.

57. Colin Eisler, "Review of *Albrecht Dürer: A Biography*, by Jane Campbell Hutchison," *Renaissance Quarterly* 45.1 (Spring, 1992), p. 165.

58. Quote from Willehad Paul Eckert and Christoph von Imhoff, *Willibald Pirckheimer Dürers Freund im Spiegel seines Lebens, seiner Werke und seiner Umwelt*, 2nd. ed. (Cologne: Wienand, 1982), p. iv, with an otherwise excellent treatment of the men's relationship on pp. 69–122 (by Eckert); see also Schleif, "Albrecht Dürer," esp. pp. 195–201 on "the ever-expanding myths of the evil wife Agnes" (p. 196).

59. Eisler, "Review of *Albrecht Dürer: A Biography*," pp. 165–66.

60. Pirckheimer to Johann Tschertte, Nuremberg, November 1530, quoted and discussed in Schleif, "Albrecht Dürer," p. 191. For the original document, see Rupprich, *Dürer: Schriftlicher Nachlass*, vol. 1, pp. 283–88 (no. 137).

61. Eisler, "Review of *Albrecht Dürer: A Biography*," p. 165

62. Friedrich Winkler, *Albrecht Dürer: Leben und Werk* (Berlin: Gebr. Mann, 1957), p. 179; Winkler, *Die Zeichnungen Albrecht Dürers*, vol. 2, no. 268; Michael Roth (ed.), *Dürers Mutter: Schönheit, Alter und Tod im Bild der Renaissance* (Berlin: Staatliche Museen zu Berlin / Nicolaische Verlagsbuchhandlung, 2006), cat. 88; also discussed in Schleif, "Albrecht Dürer," p. 203 (with further references in n.47), from which this translation comes.

63. Scurrilous rumor and innuendo appear in the letters of Lorenz Behaim (ca. 1457–1521), the Bamberg canon, humanist, astrologer, and alchemist who corresponded often with Pirckheimer. Having made Dürer's beard an object of ongoing ridicule, he once interjected (in Italian) the rumor that Dürer's "boy" (*gerzone*) couldn't stand the beard; quoted and discussed in Schleif, "Albrecht Dürer," p. 189 with further references. In addition to the references above, Eisler's assertions about Dürer's bisexuality appear in "Who Is Dürer's 'Syphilitic Man'?," *Perspectives in Biology and Medicine* 52.1 (Winter 2009), pp. 48–60. Also see Robert Smith, "Dürer, Sexuality, Reformation," in Bernard Smith (ed.), *Culture and History: Essays Presented to Jack Lindsay* (Sydney: Hale & Iremonger, 1984), pp. 304–34.

64. The phrase is from Schleif, "Albrecht Dürer," p. 189, who inclines toward this conclusion, too.

65. Hutchison, *Albrecht Dürer: A Biography*, p. 86.

66. Winkler, *Die Zeichnungen Albrecht Dürers*, vol. 2, no. 270; Roth (ed.), *Dürers Mutter*, cat. 89. Preserved in Berlin is also an even larger charcoal portrait of Crescentia, dated 1503 (314 x 242 mm; Staatliche Museen, Kupferstichkabinett); Winkler, *Die Zeichnungen Albrecht Dürers*, vol. 2, no. 269.

67. Schoch, Mende, and Scherbaum, *Albrecht Dürer*, vol. 1, no. 199; and Jeffrey Chipps Smith, *Nuremberg: A Renaissance City, 1500-1618*, exhibition catalogue (Austin: University of Texas Press, 1983), cat. 30. On the portraitist's ambition to capture invisible qualities of "mind," see especially Frank Zöllner, "The 'Motions of the Mind' in Renaissance Portraits: The Spiritual Dimension of Portraiture," *Zeitschrift für Kunstgeschichte* 68.1 (2005), pp. 23-40

68. By contrast, Dürer did paint Spengler's portrait, though the panel has not survived and is known only through an eighteenth-century print; see Anzelewsky, *Albrecht Dürer*, pp. 248-49 (nos. 140K-141K); the portrait of a man Dürer did in charcoal and brown chalk, now in the British Museum (inv. SL, 5218.52), has been connected with the lost panel.

69. Roth (ed.), *Dürers Mutter*, cat. 31.

70. MVLIERI INCOM[PARABILI]: CONIVGIQUE CHAR[ISSIMAE]: CRESSENCI[A]E / M[O]ES[TISSIMVS]: BILIBALDVS PIRCKHEYMER MARITVS QVEM NU[M]Q[UAM]: / NISI MORTE SVA TVUBAVIT MONVMENTVM POSVIT. and in the middle field: MIGRAVIT EX [A]ERVMNIS IN DOMIN[I] XVI. K[A]L[ENDAS] IVNII ANNO SALVTIS N[OST]R[A]E / 1504.

71. Pliny the Elder, *Naturalis historia*, bk. 35; translation from Liana De Girolami Cheney, *The Homes of Giorgio Vasari* (New York: Peter Lang, 2006), p. 152.

72. Winkler, *Die Zeichnungen Albrecht Dürers*, vol. 4, nos. 925 and 926; John Rowlands, with assistance of Giulia Bartrum, *Drawings by German Artists and Artists from German-Speaking Regions of Europe: The Fifteenth Century and the Sixteenth Century by Artists Born before 1530*, 2 vols. (London: British Museum, 1993), cat. 245 and 246; also discussed in Schuster, *Melencolia I*, vol. 1, pp. 206-207.

73. For the Weimar sheet and the dating of each group, see Winkler, *Die Zeichnungen Albrecht Dürers*, vol. 4, nos. 93-94 (discussing nos. 924-26). The reversal of tinctures on the London sheet was noted by Campbell Dodgson, as mentioned by Rowlands, *Drawings by German Artists*, p. 110 (cat. 246).

74. Hutchison, *Albrecht Dürer: A Biography*, p. 119. On the evolving attitude toward the Reformation among Dürer, Pirckheimer, and Spengler, see Gerhard Pfeiffer, "Albrecht Dürer und Lazarus Spengler," in Dieter Albrecht, Andreas Kraus, and Kurt Reindel (eds.), *Festschrift für Max Spindler, zum 75. Geburtstag* (Munich: C. H. Beck, 1969), pp. 379-400. More recently, Berndt Hamm, *Lazarus Spengler (1479-1534)* (Tübingen: Mohr Siebeck, 2004).

75. Hutchison, *Albrecht Dürer: A Biography*, pp. 123-24.

76. See Harold J. Grimm, *Lazarus Spengler: A Lay Leader of the Reformation* (Columbus: Ohio State University Press, 1978), pp. 36-38. In a letter of circa 1520 to Georg Spalatin, chaplain to Friedrich the Wise, Dürer mentions the hot water Spengler's *Defense* landed him in, but does not render an opinion on its contents; for the letter, see Dürer, *The Writings of Albrecht Dürer*, pp. 89-90.

77. Hutchison, *Albrecht Dürer: A Biography*, p. 126. Eck considered Spengler's *Defense*

a personal attack; likewise the anonymously published satire of February 1520, *The Corner [Ecke] Planed Smooth (Eccius dedolatus)*, which many assumed had been written by
Pirckheimer.

78. Alfred Wendehorst, "Nuremberg, the Imperial City: From Its Beginnings to the
End of Its Glory," in Rainer Kahsnitz and William D. Wixom (eds.), *Gothic and Renaissance
Art in Nuremberg, 1300–1550*, exhibition catalogue (Munich: Prestel, 1986), p. 17; Hutchison,
Albrecht Dürer: A Biography, p. 120.

79. Grimm, *Lazarus Spengler*, p. 20; also Hutchison, *Albrecht Dürer: A Biography*, p. 119.

80. Winkler, *Die Zeichnungen Albrecht Dürers*, vol. 3, no. 623; Walter Strauss, *The Complete Drawings of Albrecht Dürer*, 6 vols. (New York: Abaris, 1974), vol. 3, p. 1290. Translation
adapted from Hutchison, *Albrecht Dürer: A Biography*, pp. 120–21. See also Grimm, *Lazarus Spengler*, p. 28; Pfeiffer, "Albrecht Dürer und Lazarus Spengler"; and Shira Brisman,
Albrecht Dürer and the Epistolary Mode of Address (Chicago: University of Chicago Press,
2017), p. 10 (fig. 0.7).

81. Lazarus Spengler, *Ermanung und Undterwaysung zu einem tugendhaften Wandel*
(Nuremberg: Friedrich Peypus, 1520[?]); edited text with commentary in Rupprich, *Dürer:
Schriftlicher Nachlass*, vol. 1, pp. 74–75 (no. 21) and p. 221 (no. 2, Dürer's entry in his own copy
of Spengler's *Ermanung*, received as a gift from the author); also Hamm and Huber (eds.),
Schriften der Jahre 1509 bis Juni 1525, pp. 4–55 (no. 2); also discussed in Grimm, *Lazarus
Spengler*, p. 28.

82. As Winkler pointed out, the decorative treatment of the banderoles in the lower
zones (twisting scrollwork and little duck-billed faces in the corner finials) shows up in
Dürer's repertoire soon after 1520; see Winkler, *Die Zeichnungen Albrecht Dürers*, vol. 4, no.
93, who credits Eduard Flechsig with the founding observation.

83. "Wer zu mir reich well kömenn / der sol sein kreücz auf sich nemen / Vnd sol
trewlich das nach mir tragenn / Vnd der weltt pey czeyt wider sagen." See Peter Parshall
and Rainer Schoch, *Origins of European Printmaking: Fifteenth-Century Woodcuts and their
Public*, exhibition catalogue (New Haven: Yale University Press, 2005), cat. 87 (entry by
Sabine Griese).

84. See Rittgers, *The Reformation of Suffering*.

85. Moritz Thausing, *Dürer: Geschichte seines Lebens und seiner Kunst* (Leipzig: E. A.
Seemann, 1876), p. 309 ("ein wahres Juwel der Kunst"). Among the many studies, see
Erwin Panofsky, *Albrecht Dürer*, 2 vols. (Princeton: Princeton University Press, 1943), vol.
1, pp. 125–31; Anzelewsky, *Albrecht Dürer*, no. 118; Strieder, *Tafelmalerei in Nürnberg*, no. 416;
and Karl Schütz, *Albrecht Dürer im Kunsthistorischen Museum* (Vienna: Kunsthistorisches
Museum Wien / Milan: Electra, 1994), pp. 13–39.

86. According to a dedicatory letter by Christoph Scheurl, Dürer's unusual use of the
imperfect form of the verb *facere* (rather than the imperfect indicative *fecit*) was urged on

him by Pirckheimer, who wanted his friend to follow the example of Apelles. Pliny had explained that the imperfect form designated a work that was still in process, never thoroughly complete; see Joan Stack, "Albrecht Dürer's Curls: Melchior Lorck's 1550 Engraved Portrait and Its Relationship to Dürer's Self-Fashioned Public Image," *MUSE* 42 (2009), pp. 57–59; for Scheurl's dedicatory letter, see Rupprich, *Dürer: Schriftlicher Nachlass*, vol. 1, pp. 292–93.

87. Black chalk drawing, 27.2 x 18.9 cm, dated 1511 with monogram and inscription: "landawer styfter" (Frankfurt, Städel Museum, inv. 6951); Winkler, *Die Zeichnungen Albrecht Dürers*, vol. 2, no. 511; Strauss, *Complete Drawings*, vol. 3, no. 1511/17; and Edmund Schilling and Kurt Schwarzweller (eds.), *Katalog der Deutschen Zeichnungen: Alte Meister*, 3 vols. (Munich: Prestel, 1973), vol. 2, no. 93. Dürer translated the sketch into the painting's embedded *Stifterbild* with virtually no changes.

88. See Winkler, *Die Zeichnungen Albrecht Dürers*, vol. 2, no. 445; Strieder, *Tafelmalerei in Nürnberg*, no. 414; Strauss, *Complete Drawings*, vol. 2, no. 1508/23; David Mandrella (ed.), *Dessins allemands et flamands du musée Condé à Chantilly: De Dürer à Rubens* (Paris: Éditions de la Réunion des musées nationaux, 1999), no. 7.

89. The original reads: *mathes landauer hat entlich vollbracht / das gottes haus der tzwelf brüder / samt der stiftnus und dieser thafell / nach xps gepurd mccccxj jor.* Linden wood with remnants of gilding, 284 x 213 cm (Nuremberg, Germanisches Nationalmuseum); see Strieder, *Tafelmalerei in Nürnberg*, no. 415.

90. For the windows, destroyed in the Second World War, see Hermann Schmitz, *Die Glasgemälde des Königlichen Kunstgewerbe-museums zu Berlin*, 2 vols. (Berlin: Julius Bard, 1913), vol. 2, nos. 236–41. The east windows were designed as a triple lancet flanked by double lancets, and a cartoon for the Rebel Angels panel, probably by Dürer's own hand, survives in Boston; see Barbara Butts, "Albrecht Dürer and the Stained Glass for the All Saints Chapel of the House of the Twelve Brethren: The Boston Cartoon Reconsidered," *Journal of the Museum of Fine Arts, Boston* 2 (1990), pp. 65–79.

91. Schmitz, *Die Glasgemälde*, vol. 1, p. 129; as cited in Butts, "Albrecht Dürer and the Stained Glass," p. 65.

92. For Beaune, see Barbara G. Lane, "'Requiem aeternam dona eis': The Beaune 'Last Judgment' and the Mass of the Dead," *Simiolus* 19.3 (1989), pp. 166–80; for Isenheim, see Andrée Hayum, *The Isenheim Altarpiece: God's Medicine and the Painter's Vision* (Princeton: Princeton University Press, 1989); for Laatsch, see Rainer Kahsnitz, *Carved Splendor: Late Gothic Altarpieces in Southern Germany, Austria, and South Tirol*, trans. Russell Stockman (Los Angeles: J. Paul Getty Museum, 2006), no. 19.

93. Panofsky, *Albrecht Dürer*, vol. 1, pp. 129–30, where the doctrinal concept announced in the title of Augustine's last chapter ("The eternal bliss of the City of God and the perpetual Sabbath") is proposed as the "precise and exhaustive appellation" for Dürer's painting.

94. Panofsky, *Albrecht Dürer*, vol. 1, p. 129.

95. Carolyn M. Carty, "Albrecht Dürer's *Adoration of the Trinity*: A Reinterpretation," *Art Bulletin* 67.1 (March 1985), p. 152.

96. See Ann Eljenholm Nichols, "The Bread of Heaven: Foretaste or Foresight?," in Clifford Davidson (ed.), *The Iconography of Heaven* (Kalamazoo, MI: Medieval Institute Publications, 1994), pp. 40–68.

97. A distinction worked out by Alexander of Hales in his *Sentences* of ca. 1222, at a time when scholastic theology maintained a general insistence that "eating by sight" was not properly sacramental, but only an aid to devotion; see Miri Rubin, *Corpus Christi: The Eucharist in Late Medieval Culture* (Cambridge: Cambridge University Press, 1991), p. 64.

98. Schoch, Mende, and Scherbaum, *Albrecht Dürer*, vol. 2, no. 231; and Giulia Bartrum et al., *Albrecht Dürer and His Legacy: The Graphic Work of a Renaissance Artist*, exhibition catalogue, British Museum (Princeton: Princeton University Press, 2002), no. 120. Also see Smith, "Dürer, Sexuality, Reformation," pp. 319–20, for evident borrowings from the Laocoön and Michelangelo's *Pietà*.

EPILOGUE

1. The original reads: "Auch sein noch in diser eren porten vill annder getzerden, dauon vil zuschreiben were, die ein yeder beseher selbs auslegen vnnd interpretieren mag, die ich vonn kurz wegen ytz vnnderlasse"; see Eduard Chmelaz (ed.), *Maximilian's Triumphal Arch: Woodcuts by Albrecht Dürer and Others* (New York: Dover, 1972), plate 36. The exhaustive study is Thomas Ulrich Schauerte, *Die Ehrenpforte für Kaiser Maximilian I: Dürer und Altdorfer im Dienst des Herrschers* (Munich: Deutscher Kunstverlag, 2001); also see Rainer Schoch, Matthias Mende, and Anna Scherbaum, *Albrecht Dürer: Das druckgraphische Werk*, 3 vols. (Munich: Prestel, 2001–2004), vol. 2, no. 238; Thomas Ulrich Schauerte, *Albrecht Dürer: Das große Glück. Kunst im Zeichen des geistigen Aufbruchs* (Bramsche: Kulturgeschichtliches Museum Osnabruck, 2003), p. 158 (cat. 99); Schauerte "Von der 'Philosophia' zur 'Melencolia I': Anmerkungen zu Dürers Philosophie-Holzschnitt für Konrad Celtis," in Franz Fuchs (ed.), *Konrad Celtis und Nürnberg: Akten des interdisziplinären Symposions vom 8. und 9. November 2002 im Caritas-Pirckheimer-Haus in Nürnberg* (Wiesbaden: Harrassowitz, 2004), pp. 129–30; Larry Silver, *Marketing Maximilian: The Visual Ideology of a Holy Roman Emperor* (Princeton: Princeton University Press, 2008); and Karl Möseneder, *Paracelsus und die Bilder: Über Glauben, Magie und Astrologie im Reformationszeitalter* (Tübingen: Max Niemeyer, 2009), pp. 106–107.

2. For this portion of Stabius's text, see Peter-Klaus Schuster, *Melencolia I: Dürers Denkbild*, 2 vols. (Berlin: Gebr. Mann, 1991), vol. 1, pp. 274–75; Schauerte, *Die Ehrenpforte Kaiser Maximilian I*, pp. 400–402 (Clavis II) and p. 248 (summary). For the allegorical transpositions between the *Ehrenpforte* and Pirckheimer's *Hieroglyphica*, see especially Karl

Giehlow, *The Humanist Interpretation of Hieroglyphs in the Allegorical Studies of the Renaissance*, trans. Robin Raybould (Leiden: Brill, 2015), pp. 11–23.

3. As Schuster has remarked, summing up nearly a century of research, "the interest of the humanists in Hercules is inseparable from humanistic interest in melancholia"; Schuster, *Melencolia I*, vol. 1, p. 275.

4. *Ibid.*

5. Schoch, Mende, and Scherbaum, *Albrecht Dürer*, vol. 2, no. 105, pp. 45–48. Erwin Panofsky, in *Hercules am Scheidewege, und andere antike Bildstoffe in der neueren Kunst*, new edition (Berlin: Gebr. Mann, 1997), pp. 181–86, first reinterpreted the scene as Hercules punishing Cacus. More recently, Thomas Schauerte has connected the scene with the theme of Hercules's "madness" and Seneca's tragedy, *Hercules furens*; see his *"Peripeteia*: Konrad Celtis, the Nuremberg School of Poets, and Dürer's 'Ercules,'" trans. Randall Herz, in Daniel Hess and Thomas Eser (eds.), *The Early Dürer*, exhibition catalogue (Nuremberg: Germanisches National Museum; New York: Thames and Hudson, 2012), pp. 210–12.

6. [Pseudo-] Aristotle, *Problemata physica*, book 30, lines 1–3, in *The Works of Aristotle*, vol. 7: *Problemata*, trans. E. S. Foster (Oxford: Clarendon Press of Oxford University Press, 1927), available online at https://archive.org/stream/worksofaristotle07arisuoft/worksofaristotle07arisuoft_djvu.txt.

7. Karl Giehlow, "Dürers Stich *Melencolia I* und der maximilianische Humanistenkreis," *Mitteilungen der Gesellschaft für vervielfältigende Künste* 26.2 (1903), pp. 29–34. Raymond Klibansky, Erwin Panofsky, and Fritz Saxl, *Saturn and Melancholy: Studies in the History of Natural Philosophy, Religion, and Art* (London: Nelson, 1964), p. 278 n.5, note that Peutinger's statement also betrays a knowledge of Ficino's *De triplici vita*. See also Hermann Wiesflecker, *Kaiser Maximilian I: Das Reich, Österreich und Europa an der Wende der Neuzeit*, 5 vols. (Vienna: Verlag für Geschichte und Politik, 1971–85), vol. 5, pp. 336–38, who points out that Maximilian was actually born under the sign of Mercury; Schuster, *Melencolia I*, vol. 1, p. 276; and Schauerte, *Albrecht Dürer*, p. 158 (no. 99).

8. This according to Aby Warburg, "Pagan-Antique Prophecy in Words and Images in the Age of Luther," in *The Renewal of Pagan Antiquity: Contributions to the Cultural History of the European Renaissance*, trans. David Britt (Los Angeles: Getty Research Institute for the History of Art and the Humanities, 1999), p. 641, who cites the letter from Melanchthon to Camerarius dated 13 January 1532: "My brother has lost his son, a very fine boy.... The father has Saturn in the fifth locus—just like Maximilian, and you know what his domestic fate was" (pp. 690–91 n.108). See also Colin Eisler, "Maximilian and Dürer's Major Engravings," in Juliusz A. Chrościcki and Jan Białostocki (eds.), *Ars auro prior: Studia Ioanni Białostocki sexagenario dicata* (Warsaw: Państwowe Wydawnictwo Naukowe, 1981), p. 299. It remains unclear to what extent Tannstetter actually served as Maximilian's personal physician, but he is recorded after the emperor's death in the service of the young prince,

Ferdinand I; see Franz Graf-Stuhlhofer, *Humanismus zwischen Hof und Universität: Georg Tannstetter (Collimitius) und sein wissenschaftliches Umfeld im Wien des frühen 16. Jahrhunderts* (Vienna: WUV-Universitätsverlag, 1996), pp. 75–78, and p. 131 for Tannstetter's linkage of the solar eclipse of 1518 with an escalation of black bile in the emperor's body.

9. Wiesflecker, *Kaiser Maximilian*, vol. 4, p. 421. In the weeks following the Augsburger Reichstag of 1518 until the time of his death in January 1519, Maximilian suffered from a "secret illness" historians now assume to be syphilis and the actual cause of his death; see *ibid.*, vol. 4, p. 492; also vol. 5, p. 338.

10. See Chapter 1 for my discussion with references.

11. Schuster, *Melencolia I*, pp. 276–77. Eisler, "Maximilian and Dürer's Major Engravings," places *Melencolia* on his short list of engravings Dürer produced "with an eye toward Maximilian's special appreciation"—the others being the *Vision of St. Eustace* of ca. 1500, the *Nemesis* (see figure 2.8), and the *Knight, Death, and the Devil* of ca. 1513 (see figure I.7). Eisler insists (p. 299): "How can one question the relevance of *Melencolia I* to Maximilian, Dürer's major art patron at the time of its engraving and the best-known melancholic of his day?" Yet Panofsky and Saxl had done just that; see Erwin Panofsky and Fritz Saxl, *Dürers Melencolia I: Eine quellen- und typengeschichtliche Untersuchung* (Leipzig: B. G. Teubner, 1923), p. 54 n.1, an opinion repeated in Klibansky, Panofsky, and Saxl, *Saturn and Melancholy*, p. 327 n.148, claiming the connection can not be proved.

12. Schauerte, *Albrecht Dürer*, p. 158 (no. 99).

13. Frances A. Yates, *The Occult Philosophy in the Elizabethan Age* (London: Routledge & Kegan Paul, 1979), p. 58; a similar proposal was advanced in 1967 by Patrik Reuterswärd, "Sinn und Nebensinn bei Dürer: Randbemerkungen zur 'Melencolia I,'" in Robert Mühler and Johann Fischl (eds.), *Gestalt und Wirklichkeit: Festgabe für Ferdinand Weinhandl* (Berlin: Duncker & Humblot, 1967), p. 429, where the author confidently assigned Dürer's *Knight, Death, and the Devil* (see figure I.7) the role of a "Melencolia II." For discussion of the *St. Jerome* engraving (figure 2.1), see Chapter 2 above. The literature holds no shortage of claims to "explain precisely" the "I" in the engraving's title; see Peter-Klaus Schuster and Jörg Völlnagel, "Dürer and Rufus: *Melencolia I* in the Medical Tradition," in Rufus of Ephesus, *On Melancholy*, ed. Peter E. Pormann (Tübingen: Mohr Siebeck, 2008), p. 210.

14. Schauerte, "Von der 'Philosophia' zur 'Melencolia I,'" p. 133.

15. I. R. F. Calder, "A Note on Magic Squares in the Philosophy of Agrippa of Nettisheim," *Journal of the Warburg and Courtauld Institutes* 12 (1949), p. 198 n.4.

16. Erwin Panofsky, *Albrecht Dürer*, 2 vols. (Princeton: Princeton University Press, 1943), vol. 1, p. 167.

17. *Ibid.*, vol. 1, p. 168. Panofsky considered Agrippa the most important literary source for the concept behind *Melencolia I*. Also see Klibansky, Panofsky, and Fritz Saxl, *Saturn and Melancholy*, pp. 351–64: "There is no work of art which corresponds more nearly to

Agrippa's notion of melancholy than Dürer's engraving, and there is no text with which Dürer's engraving accords more nearly than Agrippa's chapters on melancholy" (p. 360).

18. Giehlow, "Dürers Stich Melencolia I," p. 75 ("Zinn oder Silber"); and Heinrich Wölfflin, *The Art of Albrecht Dürer*, trans. Alastair Grieve and Heide Grieve (London: Phaidon, 1971), p. 203.

19. Lisolotte Hansmann and Lenz Kriss-Rettenbeck, *Amulett — Magie — Talisman* (Hamburg: Nikol, 1977), p. 197.

20. For a sparkling discussion, see Spike Bucklow, *The Alchemy of Paint: Art, Science and Secrets from the Middle Ages* (London: Marion Boyars, 2009), pp. 118–26 (quoted material on p. 119).

Bibliography

SOURCES BEFORE 1800

Alberti, Leon Battista, *On Painting*, trans. John R. Spencer (New Haven: Yale University Press, 1970).

———, *Leon Battista Alberti: A New Translation and Critical Edition*, ed. and trans. Rocco Sinisgalli (Cambridge: Cambridge University Press, 2011).

Aquinas, Thomas, *Expositio super Iob ad litteram* (Commentary on the Book of Job), trans. Brian Mulladay, ed. Joseph Kenny, O.P., available at http://dhspriory.org/thomas/SSJob.htm.

Aristotle, *The "Art" of Rhetoric*, trans. John Henry Freese (Cambridge: Harvard University Press; London: William Heinemann, 1975).

———, *Nicomachean Ethics,* trans. Terence Irwin (Indianapolis: Hackett, 1985).

[Pseudo-] Aristotle, *Problemata physica*, in *The Works of Aristotle*, vol. 7: *Problemata*, trans. E. S. Foster (Oxford: Clarendon Press of Oxford University Press, 1927).

Augustine of Hippo, *Confessions*, trans. Gary Wills (New York: Penguin, 2002).

Burton, Robert, *The Anatomy of Melancholy*, eds. Nicolas K. Kiessling, Thomas C. Faulkner, and Rhonda L Blair, 6 vols. (Oxford: Clarendon Press of Oxford University Press, 1989–2001).

Cicero, Marcus Tullius, *Tusculan Disputations*, rev. ed., trans. J. E. King (Cambridge, MA: Harvard University Press, 1971).

Dürer, Albrecht, *The Writings of Albrecht Dürer*, ed. and trans. William Martin Conway (New York: Philosophical Library, 1958).

Erasmus, Desiderius, *Manual of a Christian Knight* (*Enchiridion milites Christiani*), available at http://oll.libertyfund.org/index.php?option=com_staticxt&staticfile=show.php%3Ftitle=191&layout=html - toc_list.

Ficino, Marsilio, *Marsilio Ficino's Commentary on Plato's* Symposium, trans. Sears Reynolds Jayne (Columbia: University of Missouri Press, 1944).

———, *Three Books On Life*, ed. and trans. Carol V. Kaske and John R. Clark (Binghamton, NY: Medieval and Renaissance Texts and Studies, in conjunction with the Renaissance Society of America, 1989).

Goris, Jan-Albert, and George Marlier (eds.), *Albrecht Dürer's Diary of His Journey to the Netherlands, 1520–1521* (Greenwich: New York Graphic Society, 1971).

Hamm, Berndt, and Wolfgang Huber (eds.), *Lazarus Spengler: Schriften*, vol. 1, *Schriften der Jahre 1509 bis Juni 1525* (Gütersloh: Gütersloher Verlagshaus, 1995).

Paracelsus [Theophrast von Hohenheim], *Sämtliche Werke*, ed. Karl Sudhoff, 14 vols. (Munich: Otto Wilhelm Barth, 1922–33).

Petrarch, Francesco, *Letters on Familiar Matters*, trans. Aldo S. Bernardo, 3 vols. (Albany: State University of New York Press, 1975–85).

——, *Petrarch's Remedies for Fortune Fair and Foul: A Modern English Translation of De Remediis Utriusque Fortune, with a Commentary*, trans. Conrad H. Rawski, 5 vols. (Bloomington: Indiana University Press, 1991).

——, *Letters of Old Age — Rerum senilium libri I–XVIII*, trans. Aldo S. Bernardo, Saul Levin, and Reta S. Bernardo, 2 vols. (Baltimore: Johns Hopkins University Press, 1992).

Rufus of Ephesus, *On Melancholy*, ed. Peter E. Pormann (Tübingen: Mohr Siebeck, 2008).

Rupprich, Hans (ed.), *Dürer: Schriftlicher Nachlass*, 3 vols. (Berlin: Deutscher Verein für Kunstwissenschaft, 1956–69).

Thausing, Moritz (ed.), *Dürers Briefe, Tagebücher und Reime, nebst einem Anhange von Zuschriften an und für Dürer* (1872; Osnabrück: Otto Zeller, 1970).

SECONDARY LITERATURE

Albrecht Dürer 1471–1971, exhibition catalogue (Nuremberg: Prestel, 1971).

Albrecht Dürer: Marienleben, commentary by Anna Scherbaum, trans. Claudia Wiener, and introduction by Rainer Schoch (Munich: Prestel, 2009).

Akinsha, Konstantin, Grigoriĭ Kozlov, and Sylvia Hochfield, *Beautiful Loot: The Soviet Plunder of Europe's Art Treasures* (New York: Random House, 1995).

Ames-Lewis, Francis, *The Intellectual Life of the Early Renaissance Artist* (New Haven: Yale University Press, 2000).

Anderson, Trevor, "Dental Treatment in Medieval England," *British Journal of Dentistry* 197.7 (October 2004), pp. 419–25.

Andersson, Christiane, and Larry Silver, "Dürer's Drawings," in Larry Silver and Jeffrey Chipps Smith (eds.), *The Essential Dürer* (Philadelphia: University of Pennsylvania Press, 2010), pp. 12–34.

Ankersmit, Frank, *Sublime Historical Experience* (Stanford: Stanford University Press, 2005).

Anzelewsky, Fedja, *Albrecht Dürer: Das Malerische Werk*, ed. Deutschen Verein für Kunstwissenschaft (Berlin: Deutscher Verlag für Kunstwissenschaft, 1971).

——, *Dürer-Studien: Untersuchungen zu den ikonographischen und geistesgeschichtlichen Grundlagen seiner Werke zwischen den beiden Italienreisen* (Berlin: Deutscher Verlag für Kunstwissenschaft, 1983).

Arbesmann, Rudolf, "The Concept of 'Christus Medicus' in Augustine," *Traditio* 10 (1954), pp. 1–28.

Arikha, Noga, *Passions and Tempers: A History of the Humours* (New York: Ecco, 2007).

Bainton, Roland H., "Dürer and Luther as the Man of Sorrows," *Art Bulletin* 29.4 (December 1947), pp. 269–72.

Baldwin, Robert, "Marriage as a Sacramental Reflection of the Passion: The Mirror in Jan van Eyck's 'Arnolfini Wedding,'" *Oud-Holland* 98.2 (1984), pp. 57–75.

Bałus, Wojciech, "Dürer's *Melencolia I:* Melancholy and the Undecidable," *Artibus et historiae* 15.30 (1994), pp. 9–21.

Bandmann, Günter, *Melancholie und Musik. Ikonographische Studien* (Cologne: Westdeutscher, 1960).

Bartrum, Giulia et al., *Albrecht Dürer and His Legacy: The Graphic Work of a Renaissance Artist,* exhibition catalogue, British Museum (Princeton: Princeton University Press, 2002).

Bell, Matthew, *Melancholia: The Western Malady* (Cambridge: Cambridge University Press, 2014).

Belting, Hans, *Das Bild und sein Publikum in Mittelalter: Form und Funktion früher Bildtafeln der Passion* (Berlin: Gebr. Mann, 1981).

——, *The Image and Its Public in the Middle Ages: Form and Function of Early Paintings of the Passion,* trans. Mark Bartusis and Raymond Meyer (New Rochelle: Aristotle D. Caratzas, 1990).

——, *Likeness and Presence: A History of the Image in the Era Before Art,* trans. Edmund Jephcott (Chicago: University of Chicago Press, 1994).

Benesch, Otto, *The Art of the Northern Renaissance: Its Relation to the Contemporary Spiritual and Intellectual Movements,* rev. ed. (London: Phaidon, 1965).

Benjamin, Walter, *The Origin of German Tragic Drama,* trans. John Osbourne (London: Verso, 1977).

Białostocki, Jan, *Dürer and His Critics 1500–1971: Chapters in the History of Ideas Including a Collection of Texts* (Baden-Baden: Valentin Koerner, 1986).

Bock, Wolfgang, *Walter Benjamin—Die Rettung der Nacht: Sterne, Melancholie und Messianismus* (Bielefeld: Aisthesis, 2000).

Bockem, Beate, "The Young Dürer and Italy: Contact with Italy and the Mobility of Art and Artists around 1500," in Daniel Hess and Thomas Eser, (eds.), *The Early Dürer,* exhibition catalogue (Nuremberg: Germanisches National Museum; New York: Thames and Hudson, 2012), pp. 52–64.

Boeckeler, Erika, "Painting Writing in Albrecht Dürer's *Self-Portrait* of 1500," *Word and Image* 28.1 (May 2012), pp. 30–56.

Boer, Roland, "Foucault's Care," *Political Theology Today* (20 February 2014), available at http://www.politicaltheology.com/blog/foucaults-care.

Böhme, Hartmut, *Albrecht Dürer, Melencolia I: Im Labyrinth der Deutung* (Frankfurt am Main: Fischer Tachenbuch, 1987).

Boorsch, Suzanne, Michal Lewis, and R. E. Lewis, *The Engravings of Giorgio Ghisi*, exhibition catalogue (New York: Metropolitan Museum of Art, 1985).

Boschung, Dietrich, and Jan. N. Bremmer (eds.), *The Materiality of Magic* (Paderborn: Wilhelm Fink, 2015).

Botvinick, Matthew, "The Painting as Pilgrimage: Traces of a Subtext in the Work of Campin and His Contemporaries," *Art History* 15.1 (March 1992), pp. 1–18.

Boudet, Jean-Patrice, Anna Caiozzo, and Nicolas Weill-Parot (eds.), *Images et magie: Picatrix entre Orient et Occident* (Paris: Honoré Champion, 2011).

Bouwsma, William J., "The Two Faces of Humanism: Stoicism and Augustinianism in Renaissance Thought," in Bouwsma, *A Usable Past: Essays in European Cultural History* (Berkeley: University of California Press, 1990), pp. 19–64.

——, "The Renaissance Discovery of Human Creativity," in John W. O'Malley, Thomas M. Izbicki, and Gerald Christianson (eds.), *Humanity and Divinity in Renaissance and Reformation: Essays in Honor of Charles Trinkhaus* (Leiden: Brill, 1993), pp. 17–34.

Bredekamp, Horst, "A Neglected Tradition? Art History as *Bildwissenschaft*," *Critical Inquiry* 29 (Spring 2003), pp. 418–28.

Brann, Noel L., *The Debate over the Origin of Genius during the Italian Renaissance: The Theories of Supernatural Frenzy and Natural Melancholy in Accord and in Conflict on the Threshold of the Scientific Revolution* (Leiden: Brill, 2002).

Brenner, Oskar (ed.), *Ein altes italienisch-deutsches Sprachbuch. Ein Beitrag zur Mundartenkunde des 15. Jahrhunderts* (Munich: Christian Kaiser, 1895).

Brinkmann, Bodo, and Stephan Kemperdick, *Deutsche Gemälde im Städel 1500–50* (Mainz am Rhein: Philipp von Zabern, 2005).

——, and Berthold Hinz, *Hexenlust und Sündenfall: Die seltsamen Phantasien des Hans Baldung Grien / Witches' Lust and the Fall of Man: The Strange Fantasies of Hans Baldung Grien*, exhibition catalogue (Petersberg: Michael Imhof, 2007).

Brisman, Shira, "The Image That Wants to Be Read: An Invitation to Interpretation in a Drawing by Albrecht Dürer," *Word and Image* 29.3 (2013), pp. 273–303.

——, *Albrecht Dürer and the Epistolary Mode of Address* (Chicago: University of Chicago Press, 2017).

Brown, Marguerite L., "The Subject Matter of Duerer's *Jabach Altar*," *Marsyas* 1 (1941), pp. 55–68.

Brown, Peter, "The Rise and Function of the Holy Man in Late Antiquity," in Brown, *Society and the Holy in Late Antiquity* (Berkeley: University of California Press, 1982), pp. 103–52.

Büchsel, Martin, "Die gescheiterte 'Melancholia generosa': *Melencolia I*," *Städel-Jahrbuch*, new series 9 (1983), pp. 84–119.

——, *Albrecht Dürers Stich* Melencolia, I: *Zeichen und Emotion—Logik einer Kunsthistorischen Debatte* (Munich: Wilhelm Fink, 2010).

Bucklow, Spike, *The Alchemy of Paint: Art, Science and Secrets from the Middle Ages* (London: Marion Boyars, 2009).

Burckhardt, Jacob, *Reflections On History*, trans. M. D. Hottinger (Indianapolis: Liberty Classics, 1979).

Butts, Barbara, "Albrecht Dürer and the Stained Glass for the All Saints Chapel of the House of the Twelve Brethren: The Boston Cartoon Reconsidered," *Journal of the Museum of Fine Arts, Boston* 2 (1990), pp. 65–79.

Bynum, Caroline Walker, *Christian Materiality: An Essay on Religion in Late Medieval Europe* (New York: Zone Books, 2011).

Calder, I. R. F., "A Note on Magic Squares in the Philosophy of Agrippa of Nettisheim," *Journal of the Warburg and Courtauld Institutes* 12 (1949), pp. 196–99.

Camille, Michael, "Walter Benjamin and Dürer's *Melencolia I*: The Dialectics of Allegory and the Limits of Iconology," *Ideas and Production: A Journal in the History of Ideas* 5 (1986), pp. 58–79.

Carroll, Maureen, "*Memoria* and *Damnatio Memoriae*: Preserving and Erasing Identities in Roman Funerary Commemoration," in Maureen Carroll and Jane Rempel (eds.), *Living Through the Dead: Burial and Commemoration in the Classical World* (Oxford: Oxbow, 2011), pp. 65–90.

Carruthers, Mary J., *The Experience of Beauty in the Middle Ages* (Oxford: Oxford University Press, 2013).

Carty, Carolyn M., "Albrecht Dürer's *Adoration of the Trinity*: A Reinterpretation," *Art Bulletin* 67.1 (March 1985), pp. 146–53.

Cassirer, Ernst, *The Individual and the Cosmos in Renaissance Philosophy*, trans. Mario Domandi (Oxford: Basil Blackwell, 1963).

Catellani, Andrea, "Before the Preludes: Some Semiotic Observations on Vision, Meditation, and the 'Fifth Space' in Early Jesuit Spiritual Illustrated Literature," in Walter S. Melion, Ralph Dekoninck, and Agnès Guiderdoni-Bruslé (eds.), *Ut Pictura Meditatio: The Meditative Image in Northern Art, 1500–1700* (Turnhout: Brepols, 2012), pp. 157–202.

Cheney, Liana De Girolami, *The Homes of Giorgio Vasari* (New York: Peter Lang, 2006).

Chmelaz, Eduard (ed.), *Maximilian's Triumphal Arch: Woodcuts by Albrecht Dürer and Others* (New York: Dover, 1972).

Clark, Stuart, *Vanities of the Eye: Vision in Early Modern European Culture* (Oxford: University Press, 2007).

Cohen, Simona, *Transformations of Time and Temporality in Medieval and Renaissance Art* (Leiden: Brill, 2014).

Copeland, Rita, and Ineke Sluiter (eds.), *Medieval Grammar and Rhetoric: Language Arts and Literary Theory, AD 300–1475* (Oxford: Oxford University Press, 2009).

Cork, Richard, *The Healing Presence of Art: A History of Western Art in Hospitals* (New Haven: Yale University Press, 2012).

Couliano, Ioan P., *Eros and Magic in the Renaissance*, trans. Margaret Cook (Chicago: University of Chicago Press, 1987).

Crites, Stephen, "The Narrative Quality of Experience," *Journal of the American Academy of Religion* 39.3 (September 1971), pp. 291–311.

Daniel, Drew, *Melancholy Assemblage: Affect and Epistemology in the English Renaissance* (New York: Fordham University Press, 2013).

Dasen, Véronique, "Probaskani: Amulets and Magic in Antiquity," in Dietrich Boschung and Jan. N. Bremmer (eds.), *The Materiality of Magic* (Paderborn: Wilhelm Fink, 2015), pp. 177–203.

Dekoninck, Ralph, "*Ad vivum:* Pictorial and Spiritual Imitation in the Allegory of the Pictura Sacra by Frans Francken II," in Walter S. Melion, Ralph Dekoninck, and Agnès Guiderdoni-Bruslé (eds.), *Ut Pictura Meditatio: The Meditative Image in Northern Art, 1500–1700* (Turnhout: Brepols, 2012), pp. 318–36.

Derrida, Jacques, *Dissemination*, trans. Barbara Johnson (Chicago: University of Chicago Press, 1981).

Dewey, John, *Art as Experience* (New York: Minton, Balch, and Company, 1934).

Dickel, Hans (ed.), *Zeichnen seit Dürer: Die süddeutschen und schweizerischen Zeichnungen der Renaissance in der Universitätsbibliothek Erlangen*, exhibition catalogue (Petersberg: Michael Imhof, 2014).

Doorly, Patrick, "Dürer's *Melencolia I*: Plato's Abandoned Search for the Beautiful," *Art Bulletin* 86.2 (June 2004), pp. 255–76.

Doren, Alfred, "Fortuna im Mittelalter und in der Renaissance," *Vorträge der Bibliothek Warburg* 1 (1922–23), pp. 71–144.

Durling, Robert M., "The Ascent of Mount Ventoux and the Crisis of Allegory," *Italian Quarterly* 18 (1974), pp. 7–28.

Eckert, Willehad Paul, and Christoph von Imhoff, *Willibald Pirckheimer: Dürers Freund im Spiegel seines Lebens, seiner Werke und seiner Umwelt*, 2nd. ed. (Cologne: Wienand, 1982).

Eisler, Colin, "Maximilian and Dürer's Major Engravings," in Juliusz A. Chrościcki and Jan Białostocki (eds.), *Ars auro prior: Studia Ioanni Białostocki sexagenario dicata* (Warsaw: Państwowe Wydawnictwo Naukowe, 1981), pp. 297–99.

——, "Review of *Albrecht Dürer: A Biography*, by Jane Campbell Hutchison," *Renaissance Quarterly* 45.1 (Spring, 1992), pp. 163–66.

——, "Who Is Dürer's 'Syphilitic Man?,'" *Perspectives in Biology and Medicine* 52.1 (Winter 2009), pp. 48–60.

Enenkel, Karl A. E., "Der Petrarca des 'Petrarca-Meisters': Zum Text-Bild-Verhältnis in illustrierten De Remediis-Ausgaben," in Karl A. E. Enenkel and Jan Papy (eds.), *Petrarch and His Readers in the Renaissance* (Boston: Brill, 2006), pp. 91–170.

Falkenburg, Reindert, *Joachim Patinir: Landscape as an Image of the Pilgrimage of Life*, trans. Michael Hoyle (Amsterdam: Benjamins, 1988).

————, "Speculative Imagery in Petrarch's *Von der Artzney bayder Glück* (1532)," in Karl A. E. Enenkel and Jan Papy (eds.), *Petrarch and His Readers in the Renaissance* (Boston: Brill, 2006), pp. 171–92

Fehl, Philipp P., "Dürer's Literal Presence in His Pictures: Reflections on His Signatures in the Small Woodcut Passion," in Matthias Winner (ed.), *Künstler über sich in seinem Werk: Internationales Symposium der Bibliotheca Hertziana, Rom 1989* (Weinheim: VCH, Acta Humaniora, 1992), pp. 191–244.

Fehlemann, Sabine, "Christus im Elend: Vom Andachtsbild zum realistischen Bilddokument," in Bazon Brock and Achim Preiß (eds.), *Ikonographia: Anleitung zum Lesen von Bildern (Festschrift Donat de Chapeaurouge)* (Munich: Klinkhardt and Biermann, 1990), pp. 79–96.

Feld, Alina N., *Melancholy and the Otherness of God: A Study in the Hermeneutics of Depression* (Lanham, MD: Lexington, 2011).

Ficker, Friedbert, "Albrecht Dürer und die Medizin seiner Zeit," *Münchener medizinische Wochenschrift* 113 (21 May 1971), pp. 814–18.

Field, Richard S., *Fifteenth Century Woodcuts and Metalcuts from the National Gallery of Art, Washington, D.C.* (Washington: National Gallery of Art, n.d. [1965]).

Flechsig, Eduard, *Albrecht Dürer: Sein Leben und seine künstlerische Entwicklung*, 2 vols. (Berlin: G. Grote'sche, 1928–31).

Foucault, Michel, "Technologies of the Self," in *Ethics: Subjectivity and Truth*, ed. Paul Rabinow, trans. Robert Hurley and others (New York: The New Press, 1997), pp. 223–51.

Frankfurter, David (ed.), *Pilgrimage and Holy Space in Late Antique Egypt* (Leiden: Brill, 1998).

Freedberg, David, *The Power of Images: Studies in the History and Theory of Response* (Chicago: University of Chicago Press, 1989).

Freud, Sigmund, *Beyond the Pleasure Principle* (1920), in *The Standard Edition of the Complete Psychological Works of Sigmund Freud*, trans. James Strachey et al., vol. 18 (London: The Hogarth Press and the Institute of Psycho-Analysis, 1953–74).

Friedländer, Max J., *Landscape, Portrait, Still-Life: Their Origin and Development*, trans. R. F. C. Hull (Oxford: B. Cassirer, 1949).

Gash, John, "The Caravaggesque Toothpuller," in Tom Nichols (ed.), *Others and Outcasts in Early Modern Europe: Picturing the Social Margins* (Aldershot: Ashgate, 2007), pp. 133–55.

Gay, Peter, "Weimar Culture: The Outsider as Insider," in Donald Fleming and Bernard Bailyn (eds.), *The Intellectual Migration: Europe and America, 1930–1960* (Cambridge, MA: Belknap Press of Harvard University Press, 1969), pp. 11–93.

Gage, Frances, "Exercise for Mind and Body: Giulio Mancini, Collecting, and the Beholding of Landscape Painting in the Seventeenth Century," *Renaissance Quarterly* 61.4 (Winter 2008), pp. 1167–1207.

————, *Painting as Medicine in Early Modern Rome: Giulio Mancini and the Efficacy of Art* (University Park: Pennsylvania State University Press, 2016).

Geyer-Kordesch, Johanna, "Whose Enlightenment? Medicine, Witchcraft, Melancholia, and Pathology," in Roy Porter (ed.), *Medicine in the Enlightenment* (Amsterdam: Rodopi, 1994), pp. 113–27.

Gibson, Walter S., "Hieronymus Bosch and the Mirror of Man: The Authorship and Iconography of the *Tabletop of the Seven Deadly Sins*," *Oud-Holland* 87 (1973), pp. 205–26.

Giehlow, Karl, "Dürers Stich *Melencolia I* und der maximilianische Humanistenkreis," *Mitteilungen der Gesellschaft für vervielfältigende Künste* 26.2 (1903), pp. 29–41; 27.3 (1904), pp. 6–18; and 27.4 (1904), pp. 57–78.

——, *The Humanist Interpretation of Hieroglyphs in the Allegorical Studies of the Renaissance*, trans. Robin Raybould (Leiden: Brill, 2015).

Gilly, Carlos, "Der Paracelsus-Einblattdruck des Matthis Quad von 1606: Kritische Überlegungen über die sogenannten Rosenkreuzer-Bildnisse des Paracelsus," available at http://www.ritmanlibrary.com/collection/424-2.

Goddard, Stephen (ed.), *The World in Miniature: Engravings by the German Little Masters, 1500–1550*, exhibition catalogue (Lawrence: Spencer Museum of Art, University of Kansas, 1988).

Goffen, Rona, "Icon and Vision: Giovanni Bellini's Half-Length Madonnas," *Art Bulletin* 57.4 (December 1975), pp. 505–509.

Goldberg, Gisela, Bruno Heimberg, and Martin Schawe, *Albrecht Dürer: Die Gemälde der Alten Pinakothek*, ed. Bayerische Staatsgemäldesammlungen München (Heidelberg: Edition Braus, 1998).

Golden, Leon, "The Clarification Theory of *Katharsis*," *Hermes* 104 (1976), pp. 437–52.

Goldin, Frederick, *The Mirror of Narcissus in the Courtly Love Lyric* (Ithaca: Cornell University Press, 1967).

Gombrich, E. H., "The Renaissance Theory of Art and the Rise of Landscape," in Gombrich, *Norm and Form: Studies in the Art of the Renaissance* (Oxford: Phaidon, 1966), pp. 107–21.

Gouk, Penelope, "Music and Spirit in Early Modern Thought," in Elena Carrera (ed.), *Emotions and Health, 1200–1700* (Leiden: Brill, 2013), pp. 221–39.

Gowland, Angus, "Melancholy, Imagination, and Dreaming in Renaissance Learning," in Yasmin A. Haskell (ed.), *Diseases of the Imagination and Imaginary Disease in the Early Modern Period* (Turnhout: Brepols, 2011), pp. 53–102.

——, "Medicine, Psychology, and the Melancholic Subject in the Renaissance," in Elena Carrera (ed.), *Emotions and Health, 1200–1700* (Leiden: Brill, 2013), pp. 185–219.

Grabes, Herbert, *Speculum, Mirror und Looking Glass: Kontinuität und Orignalität der Spiegelmetapher in den Buchtiteln des Mittelalters und der englischen Literatur des 13. bis 17. Jahrhunderts* (Tubingen: Max Niemeyer, 1973).

Graf-Stuhlhofer, Franz, *Humanismus zwischen Hof und Universität: Georg Tannstetter (Collimitius) und sein wissenschaftliches Umfeld im Wien des frühen 16. Jahrhunderts* (Vienna: WUV-Universitätsverlag, 1996).

Grass, Günter, "On Stasis in Progress: Variations on Albrecht Dürer's Engraving *Melencolia I*," in Giulia Bartrum et al., *Albrecht Dürer and His Legacy: The Graphic Work of a Renaissance Artist*, exhibition catalogue (Princeton: Princeton University Press, 2002), pp. 61–76.

Griese, Sabine, *Text-Bilder und ihre Kontexte. Medialität und Materialität von Einblatt-Holz- und -Metallschnitten des 15. Jahrhunderts* (Zurich: Chronos, 2011).

Grigg, Robert, "Studies on Dürer's Diary of His Journey to the Netherlands: The Distribution of the 'Melencolia I,'" *Zeitschrift für Kunstgeschichte* 49.3 (1986), pp. 398–409.

Grimm, Harold J., *Lazarus Spengler: A Lay Leader of the Reformation* (Columbus: Ohio State University Press, 1978).

Gulden, Sebastian, "An Ideal Neighborhood: The Physical Environment of the Early Dürer as a Space of Experience," in Daniel Hess and Thomas Eser (eds.), *The Early Dürer*, exhibition catalogue (Nuremberg: Germanisches National Museum; New York: Thames and Hudson, 2012), pp. 29–38.

Gumbrecht, Hans Ulrich, *Production of Presence: What Meaning Cannot Convey* (Stanford: Stanford University Press, 2004).

Gurevich, Aron, *Medieval Popular Culture: Problems of Belief and Perception*, trans. János M. Bak and Paul A. Hollingsworth (New York: Cambridge University Press, 1988).

Hadot, Pierre, *Philosophy as a Way of Life: Spiritual Exercises from Socrates to Foucault*, ed. Arnold I. Davidson, trans. Michael Chase (Oxford: Blackwell, 1995).

Hagen, Susan K., *Allegorical Remembrance: A Study of* The Pilgrimage of the Life of Man *as a Medieval Treatise on Seeing and Remembering* (Athens: University of Georgia Press, 1990).

Hahn, Cynthia, "Joseph as Ambrose's 'Artisan of the Soul' in the *Holy Family in Egypt* by Albrecht Dürer," *Zeitschrift für Kunstgeschichte* 47.4 (1984), pp. 515–22.

Hamburger, Jeffrey F., "Speculations on Speculation: Vision and Perception in the Theory and Practice of Mystical Devotion," in Walter Haug and Wolfram Schneider-Lastin (eds.), *Deutsche Mystik im abendländischen Zusammenhang. Neu erschlossene Texte, neue methodische Ansätze, neue theoretische Konzepte* (Tübingen: Max Niemeyer, 2000), pp. 353–408.

Hamm, Berndt, *Lazarus Spengler (1479–1534)* (Tübingen: Mohr Siebeck, 2004).

Hansmann, Lisolotte, and Lenz Kriss-Rettenbeck, *Amulett—Magie—Talisman* (Hamburg: Nikol, 1977).

Hauknes, Marius, "The Painting of Knowledge in Thirteenth-Century Rome," *Gesta* 55.1 (Spring 2016), pp. 19–47.

Hayum, Andrée, *The Isenheim Altarpiece: God's Medicine and the Painter's Vision* (Princeton: Princeton University Press, 1989).

Heckscher, William S., "*Melancholia* (1541): An Essay in the Rhetoric of Description by Joachim Camerarius," in Frank Baron (ed.), *Joachim Camerarius (1500–1574): Beiträge zur Geschichte des Humanismus im Zeitalter der Reformation / Essays On the History of Humanism during the Reformation* (Munich: Wilhelm Fink, 1978), pp. 31–120.

Henderson, John, *The Renaissance Hospital: Healing the Body and Healing the Soul* (New Haven: Yale University Press, 1999).

Herrlinger, Robert, *History of Medical Illustration: From Antiquity to 1600*, trans. Graham Fulton-Smith (New York: Editions Medicina Rara, 1970).

Hess, Daniel, and Thomas Eser (eds.), *The Early Dürer*, exhibition catalogue (Nuremberg: Germanisches National Museum; New York: Thames and Hudson, 2012).

——, and Oliver Mack, "Dürer as Painter: The Early Work up to 1505," in Daniel Hess and Thomas Eser (eds.), *The Early Dürer*, exhibition catalogue (Nuremberg: Germanisches National Museum; New York: Thames and Hudson, 2012), pp. 171–93.

Hoffman, Konrad, "Dürers 'Melencolia'," in Werner Busch, Reiner Haussherr, and Eduard Trier (eds.), *Kunst als Bedeutungsträger: Gedenkschrift für Günter Bandmann* (Berlin: Gebr. Mann, 1978), pp. 251–77.

——, "Dürer's 'Melencolia,'" *The Print Collector's Newsletter* 9.2 (May–June 1978), pp. 33–35.

Hoffmann, Rainer, *Im Zwielicht: Zu Albrecht Dürers Meisterstich* Melencolia I (Cologne: Böhlau, 2014).

Holly, Michael Ann, *Panofsky and the Foundations of Art History* (Ithaca: Cornell University Press, 1984).

——, "Interventions: The Melancholy Art," *Art Bulletin* 89.1 (March 2007), pp. 7–17.

Houtman, Dick, and Birgit Meyer (eds.), *Things: Religion and the Question of Materiality* (New York: Fordham University Press, 2012).

Hunt, E. D., *Holy Land Pilgrimage in the Later Roman Empire, AD 312–460* (Oxford: Clarendon Press of Oxford University Press, 1982).

Hutchison, Jane Campbell, *Albrecht Dürer: A Biography* (Princeton: Princeton University Press, 1990).

——, *Albrecht Dürer: A Guide to Research* (New York: Garland, 2000).

Ilatovskaya, T. A., *West European Drawing of XVI–XX Centuries: Kunsthalle Collection in Bremen—Catalogue* (Moscow: Kultura, 1992).

Jackson, Stanley W., *Melancholia and Depression: From Hippocratic Times to Modern Times* (New Haven: Yale University Press, 1986).

Jacoby, Joachim, "A Note on Dürer's So-Called Jabach Altarpiece," *Bibliothèque d'Humanisme et Renaissance* 63.1 (2001), pp. 47–62.

Jeanneret, Michel, *Perpetual Motion: Transforming Shapes in the Renaissance from Da Vinci to Montaigne*, trans. Nidra Poller (Baltimore: Johns Hopkins University Press, 2001).

Jouanna, Jacques, "At the Roots of Melancholy: Is Greek Medicine Melancholic?," in *Greek Medicine from Hippocrates to Galen: Selected Papers*, ed. Philip van der Eijk, trans. Neil Allies (Leiden: Brill, 2012), pp. 229–58.

Kahane, Henry, Renée Kahane, and Angelina Pietrangeli, "'Picatrix' and the Talismans," *Romance Philology* 19.4 (May 1966), pp. 574–93.

Kahsnitz, Rainer, *Carved Splendor: Late Gothic Altarpieces in Southern Germany, Austria, and South Tirol*, trans. Russell Stockman (Los Angeles: J. Paul Getty Museum, 2006).

——, and William D. Wixom (eds.), *Gothic and Renaissance Art in Nuremberg, 1300–1550*, exhibition catalogue, Metropolitan Museum of Art and Germanisches Nationalmuseum (Munich: Prestel, 1986).

Kauffmann, Hans, "Der sogennante Jabasche Altar und die Dichtung des Buches Hiob," *Kunstwissenschaftliche Beiträge, August Schmarsow gewidmet zum fünfzigsten Semester* (1907), pp. 153–62.

Kaufmann, Thomas DaCosta, "Hermeneutics in the History of Art: Remarks on the Reception of Dürer in the Sixteenth and Early Seventeenth Centuries," in Jeffrey Chipps Smith (ed.), *New Perspectives on the Art of Renaissance Nuremberg: Five Essays* (Austin: University of Texas Press, 1985), pp. 23–39.

Kemp, Wolfgang, "Walter Benjamin und die Kunstwissenschaft, Teil 2: Walter Benjamin und Aby Warburg," *Kritische Berichte* 3.1 (1975), pp. 5–25.

Kessler, Herbert L., "Christ the Magic Dragon," *Gesta* 48 (2009), pp. 119–34.

——, "A Sanctifying Serpent: Crucifix as Cure," in Karl F. Morrison and Rudolph M. Bell (eds.), *Studies in Medieval Empathies* (Turnhout: Brepols, 2013), pp. 161–85.

——, "Speculum," *Speculum* 86 (2011), pp. 1–41.

Kierkegaard, Søren, "At a Graveside," in *Three Discourses on Imagined Occasions*, ed. and trans. Howard V. Hong and Edna H. Hong (Princeton: Princeton University Press, 1993), pp. 71–102.

Kim, Hyun-Ah, *The Renaissance Ethics of Music* (New York: Routledge, 2015).

King, Catherine, "National Gallery 3902 and the Theme of Luke the Evangelist as Artist and Physician," *Zeitschrift für Kunstgeschichte* 48.2 (1985), pp. 249–55.

Kinsman, Robert S. (ed.), *The Darker Vision of the Renaissance: Beyond the Fields of Reason* (Berkeley: University of California, 1974).

Kirkland-Ives, Mitzi, *In the Footsteps of Christ: Hans Memling's Passion Narratives and the Devotional Imagination in the Early Modern Netherlands* (Turnhout: Brepols, 2012).

Klibansky, Raymond, Erwin Panofsky, and Fritz Saxl, *Saturn and Melancholy: Studies in the History of Natural Philosophy, Religion, and Art* (London: Nelson, 1964).

Koepplin, Dieter, and Tilman Falk, *Lukas Cranach: Gemälde, Zeichnungen, Druckgraphik*, 2 vols., exhibition catalogue (Basel: Birkhäuser, 1974).

Koerner, Joseph Leo, *The Moment of Self-Portraiture in German Renaissance Art* (Chicago: University of Chicago Press, 1993).

——, "The Fortune of Dürer's 'Nemesis,'" in Walter Haug and Burghart Wachinger (eds.), *Fortuna* (Tübingen: Max Niemeyer, 1995), pp. 239–94.

Kolve, V. A., *Chaucer and the Imagery of Narrative: The First Five Canterbury Tales* (Stanford: Stanford University Press, 1984).

Kötting, Bernhard, *Peregrinatio Religiosa: Wallfahrten in der Antike und das Pilgerwesen in der alten Kirche* (Münster: Regensbergsche, 1950).

Krohm, Hartmut, "Alter Daedalus: Zum Begriff künsterlischer Tätigkeit in Dürers 'Marienleben'," in Bodo Brinkmann, Hartmut Krohm, and Michael Roth (eds.), *Aus Dürers Welt: Festschrift für Fedja Anzelewsky* (Turnhout: Brepols, 2001), pp. 77–90.

Kühne, Hartmut, *Ostensio Reliquiarum: Untersuchungen über Entstehung, Ausbreitung, Gestalt und Funktion der Heiltumsweisungen im römische-deutschen Regnum* (Berlin: Walter de Gruyter, 2000).

Kuhrmann, Dieter, *Die Frühzeit des Holzschnitts*, exhibition catalogue (Munich: Staatliche Graphische Sammlung, 1970).

Kunzle, David, "The Art of Pulling Teeth in the Seventeenth and Nineteenth Centuries: From Public Martyrdom to Private Nightmare and Political Struggle?" in Michel Feher, Ramona Naddaff, and Nadia Tazi (eds.), *Zone 5: Fragments for a History of the Human Body* (New York: Zone Books, 1989), pp. 29–89.

Kupfer, Marcia, *The Art of Healing: Painting for the Sick and the Sinner in a Medieval Town* (University Park: Pennsylvania State University Press, 2003).

Kuriyama, Shigehisa, "Interpreting the History of Bloodletting," *Journal of the History of Medicine and Allied Sciences* 50 (1995), pp. 11–46.

Kusukawa, Sachiko, *The Transformation of Natural Philosophy: The Case of Philip Melanchthon* (Cambridge: Cambridge University Press, 1995).

Kutschbach, Doris, *Albrecht Dürer: Die Altäre* (Stuttgart: Belser, 1995).

Laín Entralgo, Pedro, *The Therapy of the Word in Classical Antiquity*, trans. L. J. Rather and John M. Sharp (New Haven: Yale University Press, 1970).

Lane, Barbara G., "'Requiem aeternam dona eis': The Beaune 'Last Judgment' and the Mass of the Dead," *Simiolus* 19.3 (1989), pp. 166–80.

Lassnig, Ewald, "Dürers 'Melencolia-I' und die Erkenntnistheorie bei Ulrich Pinder: Versuch einer Interpretation aus einer Naheliegenden Quelle," *Wiener Jahrbuch für Kunstgeschichte* 57 (2008), pp. 51–95.

Lee, Rensselaer W., "*Ut Pictura Poesis*: The Humanistic Theory of Painting," *Art Bulletin* 22.4 (December 1940), pp. 197–269.

Leonhard, Karin, "Pictura's Fertile Field: Otto Marseus van Schrieck and the Genre of *Sottobosco* Painting," *Simiolus* 34.2 (2009–2010), pp. 95–118.

——, "Painted Poison: Venomous Beasts, Herbs, Gems, and Baroque Color Theory," *Nederlands Kunsthistorisch Jaarboek* 61 (2011), pp. 128–33.

Lesses, Glenn, "Austere Friends: The Stoics and Friendship," *Apeiron* 26.1 (March 1, 1993), pp. 57–75.

Leuker, Tobias, *Dürer als ikonographischer Neuerer* (Freiburg: Rombach, 2001).

Lynch, Terence, "The Geometric Body in Dürer's Engraving *Melencolia I*," *Journal of the Warburg and Courtauld Institutes* 45 (1982), pp. 226–32.

Mandrella, David (ed.), *Dessins allemands et flamands du musée Condé à Chantilly: De Dürer à Rubens*, exhibition catalogue (Paris: Éditions de la Réunion des musées nationaux, 1999).

Massing, Jean Michel, "Dürer's Dreams," *Journal of the Warburg and Courtauld Institutes* 49 (1986), pp. 238–44.

Maué, Herman, and Sonja Brink (eds.), *Die Grafen von Schönborn: Kirchenfürsten, Sammler, Mäzene*, exhibition catalogue (Nuremberg: Germanisches Nationalmuseum, 1989).

Mayhew, Robert (ed.), *The Aristotelian Problemata Physica: Philosophical and Scientific Investigations* (Leiden: Brill, 2015).

Mayor, A. Hyatt, *Prints and People: A Social History of Printed Pictures* (Princeton: Princeton University Press, 1971).

Mayer, Anton L., "Die heilbringende Schau in Sitte und Kult," in Odo Casel (ed.), *Heilige Überlieferung: Ausschnitte aus der Geschichte des Mönchtums und des heiligen Kultes für Ildefons Herwegen* (Münster: Aschendorff, 1938), pp. 234–62.

Mazzotta, Giuseppe, *The Worlds of Petrarch* (Durham: Duke University Press, 1993).

McClure, George W., *Sorrow and Consolation in Italian Humanism* (Princeton: Princeton University Press, 1991).

McEvoy, James, "The Theory of Friendship in Erasmus and Thomas More," *American Catholic Philosophical Quarterly* 80.2 (2006), pp. 227–52.

McNeill, John T., *A History of the Cure of Souls* (New York: Harper and Brothers, 1951).

Meyer, Kathi, "St. Job as a Patron of Music," *Art Bulletin* 35.1 (March 1954), pp. 21–31.

Melion, Walter S., *The Meditative Art: Studies in the Northern Devotional Print, 1550–1625* (Philadelphia: Saint Joseph's University Press, 2009).

Mende, Matthias, *Dürer-Bibliographie* (Wiesbaden: Harrassowitz, 1971).

Merback, Mitchell B., "Nobody Dares: Freedom, Dissent, Self-Knowing and Other Possibilities in Sebald Beham's *Impossible*," *Renaissance Quarterly* 63.4 (Winter 2010), pp. 1037–1105.

———, *Pilgrimage and Pogrom: Violence, Memory, and Visual Culture at the Host-Miracle Shrines of Germany and Austria* (Chicago: University of Chicago Press, 2013).

———, "The Man of Sorrows in Northern Europe: Ritual Metaphor and Therapeutic Exchange," in Catherine R. Puglisi and William L. Barcham (eds.), *New Perspectives on the Man of Sorrows* (Kalamazoo: Medieval Institute Publications, 2013), pp. 77–116.

———, "*Pro remedio animae*: Works of Mercy as Therapeutic Genre," in Birgit Münch and Jürgen Müller (eds.), *Peiraikos' Erben: Die Genese der Genremalerei bis 1500* (Wiesbaden: Reichert, 2015), pp. 97–124.

———, "'Return to Your True Self!': Practicing Spiritual Therapy with the *Spiegel der Vernunft* in Munich," in Debra Cashion, Ashley West, and Henry Luttikhuizen (eds.), *The Primacy of the Image in Northern European Art, 1400–1700: Essays in Honor of Larry Silver* (Leiden: Brill, 2017), pp. 362–77.

——, "*Lob und Danck*: On the Social Meaning of Votive Images before the Enlightenment," in Ittai Weinryb (ed.), *Agents of Faith: Material, Place, Memory,* exhibition catalogue (New Haven: Yale University Press, 2018).

Mommsen, Theodor E., "Petrarch's Conception of the 'Dark Ages'," *Speculum* 17, no. 2 (April 1942), pp. 226–42.

Möseneder, Karl, *Paracelsus und die Bilder: Über Glauben, Magie und Astrologie im Reformationszeitalter* (Tübingen: Max Niemeyer, 2009).

Moxey, Keith, "Panofsky's Melancholia," in Moxey, *The Practice of Theory: Poststructuralism, Cultural Politics, and Art History* (Ithaca: Cornell University Press, 1994), pp. 65–78.

——, "Hieronymus Bosch and the 'World Upside Down': The Case of *The Garden of Earthly Delights*," in Norman Bryson, Michael Ann Holly, and Keith Moxey (eds.), *Visual Culture: Images and Interpretations* (Middletown, CT: Wesleyan University Press, 1994), pp. 104–40.

Müller, Christian, *Urs Graf: Die Zeichnungen im Kupferstichkabinett Basel* (Basel: Schwabe, 2001).

Müller, Jürgen, and Thomas Schauerte (eds.), *Die gottlosen Maler von Nürnberg: Konvention und Subversion in der Druckgrafik der Beham-Brüder,* exhibition catalogue (Nuremberg: Museen de Stadt Nürnberg, 2011).

Müller, Peter O., *Substantiv-Derivation in den Schriften Albrecht Dürers. Ein Beitrag zur Methodik historisch-synchroner Wortbildungsanalysen* (Berlin: Walter de Gruyter, 1993).

Murdoch, John E., *Album of Science: Antiquity and the Middle Ages* (New York: Charles Scribner's Sons, 1984).

Nichols, Ann Eljenholm, "The Bread of Heaven: Foretaste or Foresight?" in Clifford Davidson (ed.), *The Iconography of Heaven* (Kalamazoo, MI: Medieval Institute Publications, 1994), pp. 40–68.

Niehoff, Franz (ed.), *Maria allerorten: Die Muttergottes mit dem geneigten Haupt 1699–1999. Das Gnadenbild der Ursulinen zu Landshut - Altbayerische Marienfrömmigkeit im 18. Jahrhundert,* exhibition catalogue (Landshut: Museen der Stadt Landshut, 1999).

Notarp, Gerlinde Lütke, *Von Heiterkeit, Zorn, Schwermut und Lethargie: Studien zur Ikonographie der vier Temperamente in der niederländischen Serien- und Genregraphik des 16. und 17. Jahrhunderts* (Münster: Waxmann, 1998).

Nussbaum, Martha C., *The Therapy of Desire: Theory and Practice in Hellenistic Ethics* (Princeton: Princeton University Press, 1994).

Olariu, Dominic, "Thomas Aquinas' Definition of the *imago Dei* and the Development of Lifelike Portraiture," *Bulletin du centre d'études médiévales Auxerre* 17.2 (2013).

Orlandini, Alessandro, *Foundlings and Pilgrims: Frescoes in the Sala del Pellegrinaio of the Hospital of Santa Maria della Scala in Siena* (Siena: Nuova Immagine, 2002).

Osten, Gert von der, "Job and Christ: The Development of a Devotional Image," *Journal of the Warburg and Courtauld Institutes* 16.1–2 (January–June 1953), pp. 153–58.

Ousterhout, Robert (ed.), *The Blessings of Pilgrimage* (Urbana: University of Illinois Press, 1990).

Pangle, Lorraine Smith, *Aristotle and the Philosophy of Friendship* (Cambridge: Cambridge University Press, 2003).

Panofsky, Erwin, "*Imago Pietatis*: Ein Beitrag zur Typengeschichte des 'Schmerzensmanns' und der 'Maria Mediatrix'," in *Festschrift für Max J. Friedländer zum 60 Geburtstage* (Leipzig: Seemann, 1927), pp. 261–308.

——, *Albrecht Dürer*, 2 vols. (Princeton: Princeton University Press, 1943).

——, "Erasmus and the Visual Arts," *Journal of the Warburg and Courtauld Institutes* 32 (1969), pp. 200–227.

——, *Hercules am Scheidewege, und andere antike Bildstoffe in der neueren Kunst*, new edition (Berlin: Gebr. Mann, 1997).

——, and Fritz Saxl, *Dürers Melencolia I: Eine quellen- und typengeschichtliche Untersuchung* (Leipzig and Berlin: B. G. Teubner, 1923).

Parshall, Peter, "Camerarius on Dürer—Humanist Biography as Art Criticism," in Frank Baron (ed.), *Joachim Camerarius (1500–1574): Beiträge zur Geschichte des Humanismus im Zeitalter der Reformation / Essays On the History of Humanism during the Reformation* (Munich: Wilhelm Fink, 1978), pp. 11–29.

——, "Albrecht Dürer and the Axis of Meaning," *Bulletin of the Allen Memorial Art Museum* 50.2 (1997), pp. 5–31.

——, "Albrecht Dürer's *Gedenckbuch* and the Rain of Crosses," *Word and Image* 22.3 (2006), pp. 202–10.

——, "Graphic Knowledge: Albrecht Dürer and the Imagination," *Art Bulletin* 95.3 (September 2013), pp. 393–410.

——, and Rainer Schoch, *Origins of European Printmaking: Fifteenth-Century Woodcuts and Their Public*, exhibition catalogue, National Gallery of Art, Washington (New Haven: Yale University Press, 2005).

Passmore, John, *The Perfectibility of Man* (New York: Charles Scribner's Sons, 1970).

Pawlik, Anna, *Das Bildwerk als Reliquiar? Funktionen früher Großplastik im 9. bis 11. Jahrhundert* (Petersberg: Michael Imhoff, 2013).

Pericolo, Lorenzo, and Elisabeth Oy-Marra (eds.), *Perfection: The Essence of Art and Architecture in Early Modern Europe* (Turnhout: Brepols, 2018).

Pfeiffer, Gerhard, "Albrecht Dürer und Lazarus Spengler," in Dieter Albrecht, Andreas Kraus, and Kurt Reindel (eds.), *Festschrift für Max Spindler, zum 75. Geburtstag* (Munich: C. H. Beck'sche Verlagshandlung, 1969), pp. 379–400.

Pickering, F. P., *Literature and Art in the Middle Ages* (Coral Gables: University of Miami Press, 1970).

Pingree, David, "A New Look at *Melencolia I*," *Journal of the Warburg and Courtauld Institutes* 43 (1980), pp. 257–58.

Pirsig, Wolfgang, "'Dürers Mutter'—aus ärztlicher Sicht," in Michael Roth (ed.), *Dürers Mutter: Schönheit, Alter und Tod im Bild der Renaissance* (Berlin: Staatliche Museen zu Berlin / Nicolaische Verlagsbuchhandlung, 2006), pp. 17–22.

Podro, Michael, *The Critical Historians of Art* (New Haven: Yale University Press, 1982).

Porter, Roy (ed.), *Medicine in the Enlightenment* (Amsterdam: Rodopi, 1994).

Posset, Franz, *Renaissance Monks: Monastic Humanism in Six Biographical Sketches* (Leiden: Brill, 2005).

Powell, Amy Knight, *Depositions: Scenes from the Late Medieval Church and Modern Museum* (New York: Zone Books, 2012).

Prange, Peter, *Deutsche Zeichnungen, 1450–1800: Die Sammlungen der Hamburger Kunsthalle, Kupferstichkabinett. Bestandkatalog*, eds. Hubertus Gaßner and Andreas Stolzenburg, 2 vols. (Cologne: Böhlau, 2007).

Pröll, Franz Xaver (ed.), *Willibald Pirckheimer, 1470-1970: Eine Dokumentation in der Stadtbibliothek Nürnberg*, exhibition catalogue (Nuremberg: Stadtbibliothek, 1970).

Preimesberger, Rudolf, "Albrecht Dürers Jabachaltar—'Trommler und Pfeifer,'" in Ekkehard Mai (ed.), *Die Zukunft der Alten Meister: Perspektiven und Konzepte für das Kunstmuseum von heute* (Cologne: Böhlau, 2001), pp. 155–85.

Prins, Jacomien, "A Philosophic Music Therapy for Melancholy in Marsilio Ficino's 'Timmaeus Commentary,'" in Andrea Sieber and Antje Wittstock (eds.), *Melancholie— zwischen Attitüde und Diskurs: Konzepte in Mittelalter und Früher Neuzeit* (Göttingen: V&R Unipress, 2009), pp. 119–43.

Prosperetti, Leopoldine van Hogendorp, *Landscape and Philosophy in the Art of Jan Brueghel the Elder (1568-1625)* (Burlington, VT: Ashgate, 2009).

——, "Viola Animae: The Art of Jan Brueghel the Elder and the the Tradition of Devout Naturalism," *Italian Quaterly* 46.179–182 (Winter–Fall 2009), pp. 107–21.

Puff, Helmut, "Memento Mori, Memento Mei: Albrecht Dürer and the Art of Dying," in Lynne Tatlock (ed.), *Enduring Loss in Early Modern Germany: Cross Disciplinary Perspectives* (Leiden: Brill, 2010), pp. 103–32.

Remond, Jaya, "Perfection," in Daniel Hess and Thomas Eser (eds.), *The Early Dürer*, exhibition catalogue (Nuremberg: Germanisches National Museum; New York: Thames and Hudson, 2012), pp. 521–22.

Reuterswärd, Patrik, "Sinn und Nebensinn bei Dürer: Randbemerkungen zur 'Melencolia I,'" in Robert Mühler and Johann Fischl (eds.), *Gestalt und Wirklichkeit. Festgabe für Ferdinand Weinhandl* (Berlin: Duncker and Humblot, 1967), pp. 411–36.

Rheins, Jason G., "Homo numerans, venerans, or imitans? Human and Animal Cognition in Problemata 30.6," in Robert Mayhew (ed.), *The Aristotelian Problemata Physica: Philosophical and Scientific Investigations* (Leiden: Brill, 2015), pp. 381–412.

Richter, Gerhard, *Thought-Images: Frankfurt School Writers' Reflections from Damaged Life* (Stanford: Stanford University Press, 2007).

Richter, Leonhard G., *Dürer-Code: Albrecht Dürers entschlüsselte Meisterstiche* (Dettelbach: J. H. Röll, 2014).

Rittgers, Ronald K., *The Reformation of Suffering: Pastoral Theology and Lay Piety in Late Medieval and Early Modern Germany* (Oxford: Oxford University Press, 2012).

——,"Christianization through Consolation: Urban Rhegius' Soul Medicine for the Healthy and the Sick in These Dangerous Times (1529)," in Anna Marie Johnson and John A. Maxfield (eds.), *Reformation as Christianization: Essays on Scott Hendrix's Christianization Thesis* (Tübingen: Mohr Siebeck, 2012), pp. 321–48.

Robison, Andrew et al., *Albrecht Dürer: Master Drawings, Watercolors, and Prints from the Albertina*, exhibition catalogue (Washington, D.C.: National Gallery of Art / Munich: Delmonico Books, Prestel, 2013).

Roth, Michael (ed.), *Dürers Mutter: Schönheit, Alter und Tod im Bild der Renaissance* (Berlin: Staatliche Museen zu Berlin / Nicolaische Verlagsbuchhandlung, 2006).

Rousselle, Aline, *Porneia: On Desire and the Body in Antiquity*, trans. Felicia Pheasant (Oxford: Basil Blackwell, 1988).

Röver-Kann, Anne, with Manu von Miller, *Dürer-Zeit: Die Geschichte der Dürer-Sammlung in der Kunsthalle Bremen*, exhibition catalogue (Munich: Hirmer, 2012).

Rowlands, John, *The Age of Dürer and Holbein. German Drawings 1400–1550*, exhibition catalogue (Cambridge: Cambridge University Press, 1988).

——, with Giulia Bartrum, *Drawings by German Artists and Artists from German-Speaking Regions of Europe: The Fifteenth Century and the Sixteenth Century by Artists Born before 1530*, 2 vols. (London: British Museum, 1993).

Rubin, Miri, *Corpus Christi: The Eucharist in Late Medieval Culture* (Cambridge: Cambridge University Press, 1991).

Rudy, Kathryn M., "A Guide to Mental Pilgrimage: Paris, Bibliothéque de l'Arsenal ms. 212," *Zeitschrift für Kunstgeschichte* 63.4 (2000), pp. 494–515.

Sandar, Hjalmar G., "Beiträge zur Biographie Hugos van der Goes und zur Chronologie seiner Werke," *Repertorium für Kunstwissenschaft* 35 (1912), pp. 519–45.

Schade, Werner, *Cranach: A Family of Master Painters*, trans. Helen Sebba (New York: G. P. Putnam's Sons, 1980).

Schauerte, Thomas Ulrich, *Die Ehrenpforte für Kaiser Maximilian I: Dürer und Altdorfer im Dienst des Herrschers* (Munich: Deutscher Kunstverlag, 2001).

——, *Albrecht Dürer: Das große Glück. Kunst im Zeichen des geistigen Aufbruchs* (Bramsche: Kulturgeschichtliches Museum Osnabruck, 2003).

——, "Von der 'Philosophia' zur 'Melencolia I': Anmerkungen zu Dürers Philosophie-Holzschnitt für Konrad Celtis," in Franz Fuchs (ed.), *Konrad Celtis und Nürnberg: Akten des interdisziplinären Symposions vom 8. und 9. November 2002 im Caritas-Pirckheimer-Haus in Nürnberg* (Wiesbaden: Harrassowitz, 2004), pp. 117–39.

——, "*Peripeteia*: Konrad Celtis, the Nuremberg School of Poets, and Dürer's 'Ercules,'" trans. Randall Herz, in Daniel Hess and Thomas Eser, (eds.), *The Early Dürer*, exhibition catalogue (Nuremberg: Germanisches National Museum; New York: Thames and Hudson, 2012), pp. 208–20.

——, Jürgen Müller, and Bertram Kaschek (eds.), *Von der Freiheit der Bilder: Spott, Kritik und Subversion in der Kunst der Dürerzeit* (Petersberg: Michael Imhoff, 2013).

Scheidig, Walther, *Die Holzschnitte des Petrarca-Meister zu Petrarcas Werk "Von der Artzney bayder Gluck des guten und widerwärtigen"—Augsburg 1532* (Berlin: Henschelverlag, 1955).

Scheil, Elfreide, "Albrecht Dürer's *Melencholia I* und die Gerechtigkeit," *Zeitschrift für Kunstgeschichte* 70.2 (2007), pp. 201–14.

Schleif, Corine, "Albrecht Dürer between Agnes Frey and Willibald Pirckheimer," in Larry Silver and Jeffrey Chipps Smith (eds.), *The Essential Dürer* (Philadelphia: University of Pennsylvania Press, 2010), pp. 185–205.

Schleiner, Winfried, *Melancholy, Genius and Utopia in the Renaissance* (Wiesbaden: Otto Harrassowitz, 1991).

Scherbaum, Anna, *Albrecht Dürers Marienleben: Form, Gehalt, Funktion und sozialhistorischer Ort* (Wiesbaden: Harrassowitz, 2004).

Schilling, Edmund, and Kurt Schwarzweller (eds.), *Katalog der Deutschen Zeichnungen: Alte Meister*, 3 vols. (Munich: Prestel, 1973).

Schmidt, Jeremy, *Melancholy and the Care of the Soul: Religion, Moral Philosophy and Madness in Early Modern England* (Aldershot: Ashgate, 2007).

Schmitz, Hermann, *Die Glasgemälde des Königlichen Kunstgewerbe-museums zu Berlin*, 2 vols. (Berlin: Julius Bard, 1913).

Schmitz, H. Günter, "Das Melancholieproblem in Wissenschaft und Kunst der frühen Neuzeit," *Sudhoffs Archiv* 60.2 (1976), pp. 135–62.

Schneider, Friedrich, "Albrecht Dürers Tafelgemälde 'Barmherzigkeit' 1523, ehemals im Dom zu Mainz," *Mainzer Zeitschrift* 2 (1907), pp. 75–87.

Schoch, Rainer, *100 Meister-Zeichnungen aus der Graphischen Sammlung der Universität Erlangen-Nürnberg*, exhibition catalogue (Nuremberg: Germanisches Nationalmuseum, 2008).

——, Matthias Mende, and Anna Scherbaum, *Albrecht Dürer. Das druckgraphische Werk*, 3 vols. (Munich: Prestel, 2001–2004).

Schröder, Eberhard, *Dürer: Kunst und Geometrie. Dürers künstlerisches Schaffen aus der Sicht seiner Underweysung* (Basel: Birkhäuser, 1980).

Schrütrumpf, Eckart, "Black Bile as the Cause of Human Accomplishments and Behaviors in *Pr.* 30.1: Is the Concept Aristotelian?," in Robert Mayhew (ed.), *The Aristotelian Problemata Physica: Philosophical and Scientific Investigations* (Leiden: Brill, 2015), pp. 357–80.

Schuster, Peter-Klaus, "Das Bild der Bilder: Zur Wirkungsgeschichte von Dürers Melancholiekupferstich," *Idea: Jahrbuch der Hamburger Kunsthalle* 1 (1982), pp. 72–134.

——, *Melencolia I: Dürers Denkbild*, 2 vols. (Berlin: Gebr. Mann, 1991).

———, and Jörg Völlnagel, "Dürer and Rufus: *Melencolia I* in the Medical Tradition," in *Rufus of Ephesus, On Melancholy*, ed. Peter E. Pormann (Tübingen: Mohr Siebeck, 2008), pp. 197–219.

Schütz, Karl, *Albrecht Dürer im Kunsthistorischen Museum* (Vienna: Kunsthistorisches Museum Wien/Milan: Electra, 1994).

Sears, Elizabeth, *The Ages of Man: Medieval Interpretations of the Life Cycle* (Princeton: Princeton University Press, 1986).

Seiger, Johann Anselm, *Medizinische Theologie: Christus Medicus und Theologia Medicinalis bei Martin Luther und im Luthertum der Barockzeit. Mit Edition dreier Quellentexte* (Leiden: Brill, 2005).

Seitz, Hanns M., "'Do der gelb fleck ist . . .': Dürers Malaria, eine Fehldiagnos," *Wiener klinische Wochenschrift* 122, supplement 3 (October 2010), pp. 10–13.

Shank, Michael H., "The Faces of Saturn: Images and Texts from Augustus through Dürer and Galileo," in Marvin Bolt and Stephen Case (eds.), *Engaging the Heavens: Inspiration of Astronomical Phenomena V* (San Francisco: Astronomical Society of the Pacific, 2012), pp. 105–28.

Shin, Junhyoung Michael, *Et in picturam et in sanctitatem: Operating Albrecht Dürer's Marienleben* (Berlin: Verlag für Wissenschaft und Forschung, 2003).

Silver, Larry, *Marketing Maximilian: The Visual Ideology of a Holy Roman Emperor* (Princeton: Princeton University Press, 2008).

Simon, Elliott M., *The Myth of Sisyphus: Renaissance Theories of Human Perfectibility* (Madison, NJ: Fairleigh Dickinson University Press, 2007).

Simon, Erika, "Das Werk: Die Rezeption der Antike," in *Albrecht Dürer 1471–1971*, exhibition catalogue (Nuremberg: Prestel, 1971), pp. 263–64.

Slenczka, Ruth, *Lehrhafte Bildtafeln in spätmittelalterlichen Kirchen* (Cologne: Böhlau, 1998).

Smith, Jeffrey Chipps, *Nuremberg: A Renaissance City, 1500–1618*, exhibition catalogue (Austin: University of Texas Press, 1983).

———, "Dürer's Losses and the Dilemmas of Being," in Lynne Tatlock (ed.), *Enduring Loss in Early Modern Germany: Cross Disciplinary Perspectives* (Leiden: Brill, 2010), pp. 71–101.

Smith, Pamela H., *The Body of the Artisan: Art and Experience in the Scientific Revolution* (Chicago: University of Chicago Press, 2004).

Smith, Robert, "Dürer, Sexuality, Reformation," in Bernard Smith (ed.), *Culture and History: Essays Presented to Jack Lindsay* (Sydney: Hale and Iremonger, 1984), pp. 304–34.

Sohm, Philip L., "Dürer's *Melencolia I*: The Limits of Knowledge," *Studies in the History of Art* 9 (1980), pp. 13–32.

Spencer, John R., "Ut Rhetorica Pictura: A Study in Quattrocento Theory of Painting," *Journal of the Warburg and Courtauld Institutes* 20, no. 1–2 (1957), pp. 26–44.

Spier, Jeffrey, "Medieval Byzantine Magical Amulets and Their Tradition," *Journal of the Warburg and Courtauld Institutes* 56 (1993), pp. 25–62.

Spitz, Lewis W., *The Religious Renaissance of the German Humanists* (Cambridge, MA: Harvard University Press, 1963).

Stack, Joan, "Albrecht Dürer's Curls: Melchior Lorck's 1550 Engraved Portrait and Its Relationship to Dürer's Self-Fashioned Public Image," *MUSE* 42 (2009), pp. 43–75.

Starobinski, Jean, *Geschichte der Melancholiebehandlung von den Anfängen bis 1900* (Basel: J. R. Geigy, 1960).

Stechow, Wolfgang, "Alberti Dureri Praecepta," *Studies in the History of Art* 4 (1971–72), pp. 81–92.

Stiegemann, Christoph (ed.), *Caritas: Nächstenliebe von den frühen Christen bis zur Gegenwart*, exhibition catalogue, Erzbischöflichen Diözesansmuseum Paderborn (Petersberg: Michael Imhoff, 2015).

Stolberg, Michael, "Lucas Cranachs 'Melencolia'-Darstellungen und die zeitgenössische Medizin," in Stefan Oehmig (ed.), *Medizin und Sozialwesen in Mitteldeutschland zur Reformationszeit* (Leipzig: Evangelische Verlagsanstalt, 2007), pp. 249–71.

Stonberg, Jacquelyn Tuerk, "An Early Byzantine Inscribed Amulet and its Narratives," *Byzantine and Modern Greek Studies* (1999), pp. 25–42.

Strauss, Walter, *The Complete Engravings, Etchings and Drypoints of Albrecht Dürer*, 6 vols. (New York: Abaris, 1974).

——, *The Complete Drawings of Albrecht Dürer*, 6 vols. (New York: Abaris, 1974).

Strieder, Peter, *Tafelmalerei in Nürnberg 1350–1550* (Konigstein im Taunus: Langweische / Hans Köster, 1993).

Sullivan, Margeret A., "*Alter Apelles:* Dürer's 1500 *Self-Portrait*," *Renaissance Quarterly* 68.4 (Winter 2016), pp. 1161–91.

Summers, David, *Vision, Reflection, and Desire in Western Painting* (Chapel Hill: University of North Carolina Press, 2007).

Tal, Guy, "An 'Enlightened' View of Witches: Melancholy and Delusionary Experience in Goya's *Spell*," *Zeitschrift für Kunstgeschichte* 75.1 (2012), pp. 33–50.

Talbot, Charles (ed.), *Dürer in America: His Graphic Work*, exhibition catalogue (New York: MacMillan, 1971).

Terrien, Samuel, *The Iconography of Job through the Centuries: Artists as Biblical Interpreters* (University Park: Pennsylvania State University Press, 1996).

Thausing, Moritz, *Dürer: Geschichte seines Lebens und seiner Kunst* (Leipzig: E. A. Seemann, 1876).

Thompson, C. J. S., *The Mystery and Art of the Apothecary* (London: John Lane, Bodley Head, 1929).

Timken-Zinkann, R. F., "Medical Aspects of the Art and Life of Albrecht Dürer (1471–1528)," in *Proceedings of the XXIII International Congress of the History of Medicine, London 2–9 September 1972*, vol. 2 (London: Wellcome Institute for the History of Medicine, 1974), pp. 870–75.

Toccacieli, Luigi, *Melencolia I di Albrecht Dürer: Un modo di leggere un'opera d'arte incisoria* (Milan: Silvana Editoriale, 2008).

Ullmann, Ernst, *Albrecht Dürer-Selbstbildnisse und autobiographische Schriften als Zeugnisse der Entwicklung seiner Persönlichkeit* (Berlin: Academie, 1994).

Unverfehrt, Gerd (ed.), *Dürers Dinge: Einblattgraphik und Buchillustrationen Albrecht Dürers aus dem Besitz der Georg-August-Universität Göttingen*, exhibition catalogue (Göttingen: Kunstsammlung der Universität Göttingen, 1997).

Vekerdy, Lilla, "Paracelsus's *Great Wound Surgery*," in Elizabeth Lane Furdell (ed.), *Textual Healing: Essays On Medieval and Early Modern Medicine* (Leiden: Brill, 2005), pp. 77–99.

Verdon, Timothy, "Masaccio's Trinity: Theological, Social, and Civic Meanings," in Diane Cole Ahl (ed.), *The Cambridge Companion to Masaccio* (Cambridge: Cambridge University Press, 2002), pp. 158–76.

Vigarello, Georges, "The Upward Training of the Body from the Age of Chivalry to Courtly Civility," in Michel Feher, Ramona Naddaff, and Nadia Tazi (eds.), *Zone 4: Fragments for a History of the Human Body* (New York: Zone Books, 1989), pp. 149–99.

Vikan, Gary, "Art, Medicine, and Magic in Early Byzantium," *Dumbarton Oaks Papers* 38 (1984), pp. 65–86.

Voigtländer, Emmy, "Ein Selbstbildnis aus Dürers Spätzeit," *Repertorium für Kunstwissenschaft* 44 (1924), pp. 282–87.

Walker, D. P., *Spiritual and Demonic Magic from Ficino to Campanella* (orig. 1958; University Park: Pennsylvania State University Press, 2000).

Warburg, Aby, "Heidnisch-antike Weissagung in Wort und Bild zu Luthers Zeiten," *Sitzungsberichte der Heidelberger Akademie der Wissenschaften, Philosophisch-Historische Klasse*, 26 (orig. 1919; Heidelberg, 1920).

——, "Pagan-Antique Prophecy in Words and Images in the Age of Luther," in Warburg, *The Renewal of Pagan Antiquity: Contributions to the Cultural History of the European Renaissance*, trans. David Britt (Los Angeles: Getty Research Institute for the History of Art and the Humanities, 1999), pp. 597–697.

——, "Sandro Botticelli's *Birth of Venus* and *Spring*: An Examination of Concepts of Antiquity in the Italian Early Renaissance," in Warburg, *The Renewal of Pagan Antiquity: Contributions to the Cultural History of the European Renaissance*, trans. David Britt (Los Angeles: Getty Research Institute for the History of Art and the Humanities, 1999), pp. 89–156.

Weber, Paul, *Beiträge zur Dürers Weltanschauung: Eine Studie über die drei Stiche Ritter Tod und Teufel, Melancholie und Hieronymus im Gehäus,* Studien zur Deutschen Kunstgeschichte, 23 (Strassburg: Heitz & Mündel, 1900).

Weitzmann, Kurt (ed.), *Age of Spirituality: Late Antique and Early Christian Art, Third to Seventh Century*, exhibition catalogue (New York: Metropolitan Museum of Art, 1979).

Wendehorst, Alfred, "Nuremberg, the Imperial City: From its Beginnings to the End of its Glory," in Rainer Kahsnitz and William D. Wixom, (eds.), *Gothic and Renaissance Art in Nuremberg, 1300–1550*, exhibition catalogue (Munich: Prestel, 1986), pp. 11–26.

Wenzel, Siegfried, *The Sin of Sloth: Acedia in Medieval Thought and Literature* (Chapel Hill: University of North Carolina Press, 1967).

Wiesflecker, Hermann, *Kaiser Maximilian I: Das Reich, Österreich und Europa an der Wende der Neuzeit*, 5 vols. (Vienna: Verlag für Geschichte und Politik, 1971–85).

Winkler, Friedrich, *Die Zeichnungen Albrecht Dürers*, 4 vols. (Berlin: Deutscher Verein für Kunstwissenschaft, 1936–39).

———, *Albrecht Dürer: Leben und Werk* (Berlin: Gebr. Mann, 1957).

Wirth, Jean, *L'image à la fin du Moyen Âge* (Paris: Cerf, 2011).

Witt, Ronald G., *In the Footsteps of the Ancients: The Origins of Humanism from Lovato to Bruni* (Leiden: Brill, 2000).

Wolf, Norbert, *Albrecht Dürer, 1471–1528: The Genius of the German Renaissance* (Cologne: Taschen, 2010).

Wölfflin, Heinrich, *The Art of Albrecht Dürer*, trans. Alastair Grieve and Heide Grieve (London: Phaidon, 1971).

Woods-Marsden, Joanna, *Renaissance Self-Portraiture: The Visual Construction of Identity and the Social Status of the Artist* (New Haven: Yale University Press, 1998).

Yates, Frances A., *The Occult Philosophy in the Elizabethan Age* (London: Routledge and Kegan Paul, 1979).

———, "Chapman and Dürer on Inspired Melancholy," *University of Rochester Library Bulletin* 34 (1981), pp. 25–44.

Zak, Gur, *Petrarch's Humanism and the Care of the Self* (New York and Cambridge: Cambridge University Press, 2010).

Zehnder, F. G. (ed.), *Stefan Lochner Meister zu Köln: Herkunft — Werke — Wirkung*, exhibition catalogue (Cologne: Wallraf-Richartz-Museum, 1993).

Zika, Charles, *Exorcising Our Demons: Magic, Witchcraft and Visual Culture in Early Modern Europe* (Leiden: Brill, 2003).

———, "Wild Riders, Popular Folklore and Moral Disorder," in Zika, *The Appearance of Witchcraft: Print and Visual Culture in Sixteenth-Century Europe* (London: Routledge, 2007), pp. 99–124.

Zöllner, Frank, "The 'Motions of the Mind' in Renaissance Portraits: The Spiritual Dimension of Portraiture," *Zeitschrift für Kunstgeschichte* 68.1 (2005), pp. 23–40.

Index

Works by Dürer are listed under their titles. Page numbers in italics represent illustrations.

Timanthes of Cythnus, 235–38.

Toccacieli, Luigi, *55, 56, 62, 63.*

Tovar, Antonio, 302 n.14.

Traut, Wolf, *255.*

Treasury of Merits, 91.

Trinity, 110, 224. See also *Adoration of the Holy Trinity; Holy Trinity* (woodcut).

Tristia (spiritual sadness), 14.

Trithemius, Johannes, 261.

Trostblatt, 44–45, 159, 183–85, 238–39, 260. *See also* Consolation.

Tschertte, Johann, 233.

Two Musicians (Dürer), 214, *215, 217,* 220–21; self-depiction in, 214, *217,* 223.

ULSEN, DIRK VAN (THEODORICUS ULSENIUS), *12,* 218, 271 n.39.

Universal healing, 252.

VASARI, GIORGIO, 10, 267 n.2

Venatorius, Thomas, 194.

Venice, 232.

Veronica, sudarium of, 87, *88.*

Verticality, 67–69; vertical and horizontal pathways, 69–70, 223–24.

Vexierbilder, 101.

Vienna: Maximilian's court in, 39, *155,* 256, 260; Schottenstift Monastery, 166; Turkish siege of, 11.

Vier Bücher von menschlicher Proportionen (Four books on human proportions), 15, 54.

Virchow, Rudolf, 302 n.15.

Virgil, 153.

Virgin and Child Seated by a Wall (Dürer), 56–57, *58.*

Vischer, Peter the Younger, 303 n.1.

Vision of St. Eustace (Dürer), 323 n.11.

Visual devotion, 87–91, 114.

Vitruvius, 225; *De architectura,* 54, 315 n.38.

Votive objects, 91, 216, 222. *See also* Devotional images.

WARBURG, ABY, 46, 133, 156, 274 n.16; on Alberti, 203; "Francesco Sassetti's Last Injunctions to His Sons," 207–209; idea of "humanist's consoling image," 44, 45, 159, 183, 299 n.93; on cosmology and magic, 43, 152, 275 nn.24,28; understanding of the magic square in narrative terms, 158–59.

Warburg Institute (Hamburg), 43, 276 n.32.

Water, 80, 284 n.9.

Weiditz, Hans (Petrarch Master), *Von Verstand* woodcut from German edition of Petrarch, 63–66, *65.*

Weixlgärtner, Arpad, 273 n.16.

Weyden, Rogier van der, *Last Judgment Altarpiece,* 249.

Weyer, Johann, 293 n.25.

Wind, 203–204, 207, 209; Boreas, 153, *155,* 203; Four Winds, 203–204, 252.

Winkler, Friedrich, 239, 306 n.29, 319 n.82.

Witchcraft, 133, 293 n.25; *Witches' Sabbath* by Hans Baldung Grien, *137.*

Witch Riding Backward (Dürer), 203.

Wölfflin, Heinrich: on the ambiguity of the ladder, *55,* 69, 280 n.11; on the "chaos of objects" in *Melencolia,* 35; on *Melencolia* and *St. Jerome,* 270 n.32; on "speculative" thought, 48–49, 51.

YATES, DAME FRANCES, 43, 44, 130–31, 260.

ZAK, GUR, 18, 270 n.27.

Zika, Charles, 133.

Zwölfbrüderhaus (House of the Twelve Brethren), 248–49, 252.

Zone Books series design by Bruce Mau
Typesetting by Meighan Gale
Image placement and production by Julie Fry
Printed and bound by Maple Press